Studies in Big Data

Volume 88

Series Editor

Janusz Kacprzyk, Polish Academy of Sciences, Warsaw, Poland

The series "Studies in Big Data" (SBD) publishes new developments and advances in the various areas of Big Data- quickly and with a high quality. The intent is to cover the theory, research, development, and applications of Big Data, as embedded in the fields of engineering, computer science, physics, economics and life sciences. The books of the series refer to the analysis and understanding of large, complex, and/or distributed data sets generated from recent digital sources coming from sensors or other physical instruments as well as simulations, crowd sourcing, social networks or other internet transactions, such as emails or video click streams and other. The series contains monographs, lecture notes and edited volumes in Big Data spanning the areas of computational intelligence including neural networks, evolutionary computation, soft computing, fuzzy systems, as well as artificial intelligence, data mining, modern statistics and Operations research, as well as self-organizing systems. Of particular value to both the contributors and the readership are the short publication timeframe and the world-wide distribution, which enable both wide and rapid dissemination of research output.

The books of this series are reviewed in a single blind peer review process.

Indexed by zbMATH.

All books published in the series are submitted for consideration in Web of Science.

More information about this series at http://www.springer.com/series/11970

K. G. Srinivasa · Siddesh G. M. · S. R. Mani Sekhar
Editors

Artificial Intelligence for Information Management: A Healthcare Perspective

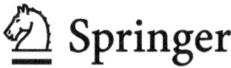 Springer

Editors
K. G. Srinivasa
Department of CSE
National Institute of Technical Teachers
Training and Research
Chandigarh, India

Siddesh G. M.
Department of ISE
Ramaiah Institute of Technology (MSRIT)
Bangalore, India

S. R. Mani Sekhar
Department of ISE
Ramaiah Institute of Technology (MSRIT)
Bangalore, India

ISSN 2197-6503   ISSN 2197-6511   (electronic)
Studies in Big Data
ISBN 978-981-16-0414-0   ISBN 978-981-16-0415-7   (eBook)
https://doi.org/10.1007/978-981-16-0415-7

This Springer imprint is published by the registered company Springer Nature Singapore Pte Ltd.
The registered company address is: 152 Beach Road, #21-01/04 Gateway East, Singapore 189721,
Singapore

Preface

Artificial Intelligence (AI) defines various procedures that allow the system to perform tasks more efficiently and effectively. With the advance in digitalization of data acquirement, AI techniques play a vital role in human healthcare and wellbeing organizations.

As the dataset is increasing day by day Machine Learning (ML) and Artificial Intelligence can generate productive results by incorporating different task at once and refining the previous results. These techniques can be used in collecting, storing, analysis, of different healthcare data, which differ in inpatient history to the diagnosis methods. Subsequently, it provides intelligent approaches to finding out the possible solutions in health care. Some of the areas where AI tools can be used include early finding & treatment of cardiology, stroke, diabetes, cancer, etc.

The book is divided into four parts and fifteen chapters. Part I discusses the introduction to AI and ML in Healthcare. Subsequently, Part II highlights the different analytics techniques used in healthcare. After that, Part III provides the various security, privacy & visualization methods used in healthcare. Finally, Part IV exemplifies the different applications in health data analytics. This book also provides a platform for the most recent research on using AI and ML-based solutions for healthcare problems.

Part I: Introduction to Artificial Intelligence and Machine Learning in Healthcare

Chapter "Introduction to Healthcare Information Management and Machine Learning" presents an overview to the Machine learning techniques and a brief overview of Information Management in healthcare. The chapter gives the outline of some chosen machine learning calculations, for example, direct relapse, straight discriminant examination, bolster vector machine, innocent Bayes classifier, neural systems, and choice trees.

Chapter "Introduction to Artificial Intelligence" explores the files of Artificial Intelligence and its types. The chapter also brief about the various classification techniques. They also discussed the challenges and application of AI.

Chapter "Healthcare Data Analytics Using Artificial Intelligence" highlights the relationship between AI and healthcare, healthcare data collection and storage system, medical data pre-processing, AI algorithms for healthcare, AI methodology for medical and medicinal diagnosis, selection and extraction of features using AI, disease diagnosis with AI, medical image processing with AI and patient care and treatment with AI.

Chapter "Data Collection and Processing in Health Care" tells the process of Data collection and processing in healthcare. Later the author discussed the importance of data collection and its challenges. Finally, the chapter gives the overview of various concepts used for data collection and process.

Part II: Healthcare Analytics

Chapter "Sensor Data Analytics for Health Care" discuss how the sensor data analysis works in healthcare industry. They also illustrated how the increasing popularity of smart systems have paved the way for it to be integrated into every part of people's lives. Later, various sensor technologies have been explored in this chapter with two case studies to emphasize on the importance of combining the forces of healthcare with sensor technology and data analysis.

Chapter "Social Media Analytics for Health Care" presents the importance of social media in healthcare. Later, it focuses on the different SMA approaches used in healthcare, followed by certain recent case studies of SMA in healthcare. The research areas that can be ex-plored for SMA in healthcare is also discussed along with certain drawbacks.

Chapter "Multi-modal Data-Driven Analytics for Health Care" emphasize the importance of multi modal system where instead of relying on a particular data source or a particular field of data analytics; one can combine multiple sources and apply multi domain techniques to extract information to even greater extent. The high quality information retrieved from the analysis can be further used to determine and diag-nose more symptoms and hence help in providing accurate solutions.

Part III: Security, Privacy and Visualization

Chapter "Security and Privacy Issues in Health Care" illustrate the challenges, threats and concerns with respect to healthcare data and the solutions to the problems are looked at. Here we try and understand how these issues are handled by the various technology industries by looking at the several case studies in this area of healthcare and how the integrity of the data is maintained.

Chapter "Healthcare Data Visualization" presents an attempt to summarize healthcare data through exploratory data analysis and Process mining control-flow discovery techniques. How they helps in identifying the discrepancies between planned and actual healthcare processes. Later the chapter present Process Mining based control flow visualizations on real-time event log detailed in healthcare information systems.

Chapter "Data Science Tools and Techniques for Healthcare Applications" discuss the different data science-oriented tools and methods for healthcare analytics. A case study on the usage of different tools and techniques is also presented at the end of the chapter that provides the complete life-cycle of the analytics phase for healthcare applications.

Part IV: Applications in Health Data Analytics

Chapter "Management of Dementia Through Self-help and Assistive Technologies" highlights a scenario of the mentioned self-help that could be achieved by the patients and their caregivers themselves. They have showed how assistive technologies can support the patients and their family members to counter the societal restrictions of dementia while involving assistive instruments and tools such as mobile, smart device, and smart sensors. Further, the chapter present various benefits and limitation related to assistive technologies.

Chapter "Classification and Prediction of Leukemia Using Gene Expression Profile" tells how the proposed system, is going to classify Leukemia into Acute Lymphocytic Leukemia (ALL) and Acute Myeloid Leukemia (AML) and also going to predict who is at cancer risk by monitoring gene expressions. The main motivation is to help the society to reduce the cost of treatment for cancer as many people cannot afford the cost of chemotherapy

Chapter "Estimation of Basic Reproduction Number and Herd Immunity for COVID-19 in India" shows how the estimation of basic reproduction number and herd immunity has become an important question which might support policy makers to take decisions for improvement of current scenario of COVID-19. The chapter shows how the auto regressive integrated moving average (ARIMA) tool has been used to estimate confirm cases, discharge, deaths and case fatality rate due to COVID-19 in India.

Chapter "Artificial Intelligence in Medicine: Diabetes as a Model" discuss how AI is used for monitoring of diabete patient health data. Later the author has discussed the scope and need for AI in clinical care. Later the chapter presents the various application in Non- communicable Diseases, diabetes etc.

Chapter "Smart Healthcare: Using IoT and Machine Learning-Based Analytics" discuss a portion of the healthcare challenges and information analysis development. They also illustrated the process of screen the health states of an individual, support from sensors and IoT gadgets.

The editors are very thankful to all the members of Springer (India) Private Limited, for the given opportunity to edit this book.

Chandigarh, India   Dr. K. G. Srinivasa
Bangalore, India   Dr. Siddesh G. M.
Bangalore, India   Dr. S. R. Mani Sekhar

Contents

Editors and Contributors

About the Editors

Dr. K. G. Srinivasa received his Ph.D. in Computer Science and Engineering from Bangalore University in 2007. He is the recipient of All India Council for Technical Education – Career Award for Young Teachers, Indian Society of Technical Education – ISGITS National Award for Best Research Work Done by Young Teachers, Institution of Engineers (India) – IEI Young Engineer Award in Computer Engineering, Rajarambapu Patil National Award for Promising Engineering Teacher Award from ISTE – 2012, IMS Singapore – Visiting Scientist Fellowship Award. He has published more than 100 research papers in International Conferences and Journals. He has visited many Universities abroad as a visiting researcher – He has visited University of Oklahoma, USA, Iowa State University, USA, Hong Kong University, Korean University, National University of Singapore, University of British Columbia, Canada are his few prominent visits. He has authored three text books namely File Structures using C++ by TMH, Soft Computing for Data Mining Applications by LNAI Series – Springer and Guide to High Performance Computing by Springer. He has edited research monographs in the area of Cyber Physical Systems and Energy Aware Computing with CRC Press and IGI Global respectively. He has been awarded BOYSCAST Fellowship by DST, for conducting collaborative. Research with Clouds Laboratory in University of Melbourne in the area of Cloud Computing. He is the principal Investigator for many funded projects from AICTE, UGC, DRDO, and DST. He is the senior member of IEEE and ACM. His research areas include Data Mining, Machine Learning and Cloud Computing. His recent research areas include Innovative Teaching Practices in Engineering Education, pedagogy; outcomes based education, and teaching philosophy.

Dr. Siddesh G. M. is currently working as Associate professor in Department of Information Science & Engineering, M S Ramaiah Institute of Technology, Bangalore. He has published a good number of research papers in reputed International Conferences and Journals. He is a member of ISTE, IETE etc., He has authored books on Network Data Analytics, Statistical Programming in R, Internet of Things with Springer, Oxford University Press and Cengage publishers respectively. He has edited research monographs in the area of Cyber Physical Systems, Fog Computing and Energy Aware Computing, Bioinformatics with CRC Press, IGI Global and Springer publishers respectively. His research interests includes Internet of Things, Distributed Computing and Data Analytics.

Dr. S. R. Mani Sekhar is currently an Assistant Professor at the Department of Information Science & Engineering, Ramaiah Institute of Technology, Bangalore. He is a member of ISTE. He has published a good number of research papers and book chapters. He has authored a book title "Programming with R", Cengage publisher. He has also edited a book title "Statistical Modelling and Machine Learning Principles for Bioinformatics Techniques, Tools, and Applications", Springer. He is also an associate editor for "International Journal of End-User Computing and Development". His research interests include bioinformatics, data science, data analytics, and software engineering.

Contributors

K. Aditya Shastry Department of Information Science & Engineering, Nitte Meenakshi Institute of Technology, Yelahanka, Bangalore, Karnataka, India

Mumtaz Irteqa Ahmed Ramaiah Institute of Technology, Bengaluru, India

R. Aravind Shreyas Ramaiah Institute of Technology, Bengaluru, India

Dheeraj Bhat Ramaiah Institute of Technology, Bengaluru, India

Divya Ramaiah Institute of Technology, Bengaluru, India

Amit Doegar National Institute of Technical Teachers Training and Research, Chandigarh, India

Vivek Dosaya Department of Information Science and Engineering, Ramaiah Institute of Technology, Bangalore, India

V. Gaurav Ramaiah Institute of Technology, Bengaluru, India

Gouri Gavimath Department of Information Science and Engineering, Ramaiah Institute of Technology, Bangalore, India

Moumita Ghosh Department of Biotechnology and Medical Engineering, National Institute of Technology Rourkela, Rourkela, Odisha, India

R. Hanumantharaju Department of Computer Science and Engineering, M S Ramaiah Institute of Technology (Affiliated to VTU), Bangalore, India

Srinidhi Hiriyannaiah Ramaiah Institute of Technology, Bengaluru, India

Anita Kanavalli Department of Computer Science and Engineering, M S Ramaiah Institute of Technology (Affiliated to VTU), Bangalore, India

S. Krutika Ramaiah Institute of Technology, Bengaluru, India

Manoj Kumar Department of Information Science & Engineering, Nitte Meenakshi Institute of Technology, Yelahanka, Bangalore, Karnataka, India

Gumpeny Lakshmi Assistant Professor, Department of General Medicine, Gayatri Vidya Parishad Institute of Healthcare & Medical Technology, Visakhapatnam, India

Poulami Majumder Department of Biotechnology, Maulana Abul Kalam Azad University of Technology, Kolkata, West Bengal, India

M. V. Manoj Kumar Department of Information Science and Engineering, Nitte Meenakshi Institute of Technology, Bengaluru, India

Sunilkumar Manvi School of C & IT, REVA University, Bangalore, India

Kushagra Mishra Member of Technical Staff a t Nutanix, San Jose, USA

Minal Moharir RV College of Engineering®, Bengaluru, Karnataka, India

B. Naga Sri Ram Department of CSE, Koneru Lakshmaiah Education Foundation, Guntur, Andhra Pradesh, India

G. Navya Krishna Department of CSE, Koneru Lakshmaiah Education Foundation, Guntur, Andhra Pradesh, India

L. M. Patnaik National Institute of Advanced Studies, Bengaluru, India

K. R. Pavan RV College of Engineering®, Bengaluru, Karnataka, India

D. Pradeep Kumar Department of Computer Science and Engineering, M S Ramaiah Institute of Technology (Affiliated to VTU), Bangalore, India

B. S. Prashanth Department of Information Science and Engineering, Nitte Meenakshi Institute of Technology, Bengaluru, India

Anant Raj Ramaiah Institute of Technology, Bengaluru, India

Pothuraju Rajarajeswari Department of CSE, Koneru Lakshmaiah Education Foundation, Guntur, Andhra Pradesh, India

Partha Pratim Ray Department of Computer Applications, Sikkim University, Gangtok, Sikkim, India

G. Sai Pooja Department of CSE, Koneru Lakshmaiah Education Foundation, Guntur, Andhra Pradesh, India

Kolli Saivenu Ramaiah Institute of Technology, Bengaluru, India

B. L. Sandeep Department of Information Science and Engineering, Ramaiah Institute of Technology, Bangalore, India

H. A. Sanjay Department of Information Science and Engineering, Nitte Meenakshi Institute of Technology, Yelahanka, Bangalore, Karnataka, India

S. Seema Department of Computer Science and Engineering, M S Ramaiah Institute of Technology (Affiliated to VTU), Bangalore, India

S. R. Mani Sekhar Department of Information Science and Engineering, Ramaiah Institute of Technology, Bangalore, India

Aditya Shastry Department of Information Science and Engineering, Nitte Meenakshi Institute of Technology, Bengaluru, India

Siddesh G. M. Department of Information Science and Engineering, Ramaiah Institute of Technology, Bangalore, India

Nabeel Siddiqui Duke University, Durham, NC, USA

Tilak Singh Department of Information Science & Engineering, Ramaiah Institute of Technology, Bangalore, India

H. R. Sneha Department of Information Science and Engineering, Nitte Meenakshi Institute of Technology, Bengaluru, India

B. J. Sowmya Department of Computer Science and Engineering, M S Ramaiah Institute of Technology (Affiliated to VTU), Bangalore, India

Gumpeny R. Sridhar Endocrine and Diabetes Centre, Visakhapatnam, India

Nikitha Srikanth RV College of Engineering®, Bengaluru, Karnataka, India

K. G. Srinivasa National Institute of Technical Teachers Training & Research, Chandigarh, India

Pramod Sunagar Department of Computer Science and Engineering, M S Ramaiah Institute of Technology (Affiliated to VTU), Bangalore, India

A. Thirugnanam Department of Biotechnology and Medical Engineering, National Institute of Technology Rourkela, Rourkela, Odisha, India

V. Yamini Radha Department of CSE, Koneru Lakshmaiah Education Foundation, Guntur, Andhra Pradesh, India

Introduction to Artificial Intelligence and Machine Learning in Healthcare

Introduction to Healthcare Information Management and Machine Learning

S. R. Mani Sekhar, Siddesh G. M., Sunilkumar Manvi, and Vivek Dosaya

Abstract Health information management deals with the collection, storing, analysis, and management of health data. It consists of various fields such as computer science, information science, information management, medicinal, business and data analytics. Machine Learning (ML) in healthcare evolving as an emerging field for healthcare industry. They help in analyzing the health data more effectively and timely. ML is one of the vital regions in the field of software engineering. It gives a streamlined answer for this present reality issues by utilizing past learning or past experience information. There are distinctive kinds of machine learning calculations present in software engineering. This chapter gives the outline of some chosen machine learning methods, for direct relapse, straight discriminant examination, bolster vector machine, innocent Bayes classifier, neural systems, and choice trees. Every one of these techniques is described in detail, which thus helps the reader to create our own answers for the given issues.

Keywords Health care · Machine learning · Healthcare information management · Classifier

1 Introduction

In current trends, healthcare data is increasing day by day in digital form. These data are related to the patient's information, lab reports, doctor prescription, demographic data, etc. This information can help the research in understanding current population health issues, subsequently, can help in the prediction of upcoming health issues [1, 2]. This information can make billing and administration processes more efficient.

S. R. M. Sekhar (✉) · S. G. M. · V. Dosaya
Department of Information Science and Engineering, Ramaiah Institute of Technology, Bangalore, India

S. Manvi
School of C & IT, REVA University, Bangalore, India

© The Author(s), under exclusive license to Springer Nature Singapore Pte Ltd. 2021   3
K. G. Srinivasa et al. (eds.), *Artificial Intelligence for Information Management: A Healthcare Perspective*, Studies in Big Data 88,
https://doi.org/10.1007/978-981-16-0415-7_1

As digital medical data is increasing rapidly, the organization and management of these data is a challenging task. The organization should have the necessary application and tool to maintain the privacy, security and effectiveness of the patient's data. This helps in achieving the future goals of high-quality care, effective management of data, and in avoiding needless expenses.

Due to the increase in digital records, informatics can help in filling the gap between physical clinical records and digital technology. The tools can help the physician to maintain and to organize the patient's records. In turn, this recorded information can help the physician and administrative staff to focus on critical information.

2 Health Information Management

Health information management [3] deals with the collection, storing, analysis and management of health data. It consists of various fields such as computer science, information science, information management, medicinal, business, and data analytics. These fields help in the improvement of the system quality by providing timely, quality care. In the hospital, the staff uses an electronic device to record the patient information in place of paperwork. These devices help inpatient information gathering and for patient data analysis.

Health information management should make regular up to date changes with the latest issues related to the privacy, security, information governance, interoperability, data analytics fields.

- Privacy and Security: To prevent and secure electronic health data from hackers.
- Information governance: To incorporate new policies, panels, structures for proper management of the organization's data.
- Interoperability: Effective communication of data between organizations and stakeholders.
- Data analytics: Analysis of raw data for real-time decision-making.

3 Machine Learning in Health Care

Machine Learning (ML) is the branch of artificial intelligence [4], it helps machines learn from experiences and improves without being coded by humans. Its aims at designing algorithms that can effectively use data to learn. Here, learning involves taking data from different sources, observing data, drawing out patterns from it, and take better decisions in the future taking those patterns in mind. The primary aim is to enable machines to learn automatically without any intervention from humans.

In today's world there is data everywhere, no matter where you are or what you do, data will be generated. Up until 2005, mankind had created 130 exabytes of data (1 exabyte = 1 billion gigabytes). In 2010 the data generated reached 1,200 exabytes, by 2015 it grew to 7,900 exabytes and it is estimated that by 2020 it will grow to 40,900 exabytes. The growth in data generated is exponential and it will continue to grow.

ML in healthcare evolving as an emerging field for healthcare industry. They help in analyzing the health data more effectively and timely. Some of the application of health care using machine learning is.

- Identification of illness
- Prediction of new drug
- Analysis of medical image
- Smart health System
- Crowdsourced Information Gathering.

4 What is Predictive Analytics in Health Care?

Predictive analytics includes a diverse range of statistical methodology such as information mining, predictive modelling, and ML that read through and try to understand current and historical factual information to predict the future.

In today's business, predictive healthcare analytical models use outlines initiate in historical information to identify risks and opportunity to use to our own benefit. Models recognize relations among several issues to allow qualitative assessment of risk related with a specific set of conditions, instructing decision-making for individual candidate communications.

Predictive methodology is a field of statistics that extracts information from raw data and use it to predict trends and rhythmic behaviour patterns. It provides a predictive score for each entity such as medical patient, product, vehicles, and machines to determine processes that affect a large number of entities. For example, we have a model for analysis of patient illness, identification of drug, analysis of medical report and smart hospital record system, etc.

4.1 Forms of Healthcare Data Analytics

As we know the amount of healthcare data generated every second is enormous, but all this data is unstructured data. We need to structure this data in such a way that it makes sense. Data analysts use their experience and skill set to structure data as well as draw of significant information out of this data. This is the field where forms are data analytics come into picture. Data-driven insights play a big role in providing businesses the ability to come up with new initiatives to benefit themselves.

There are four major types of data analytics used today:

- *Descriptive Analytics*: As the name suggests, descriptive analytics takes up raw data and converts it in such a way that humans can easily understand it. Each event which occurred in past is described in detail. This is helpful in deriving a pattern from past events so that the future strategies are more efficient and implementable.

- *Diagnostic Analytics*: It helps a data analyst to acquire more information of an issue so that the source of that issue can be identified. Both descriptive and diagnostic analytics plays major role in today's modern businesses to improve.
- *Predictive Analytics*: It provides foresight to businesses. It is basically using current events to determine the future trends or estimating the precise timings of it happening. It uses predictive analytical models. For example, we can use a patients diet, exercise, medical record information to predict if the patient will have any health complications in future or not, or we can solve the customer churn problem for banks by using customers information, such as balance, number of credit cards, age, and smoking habits.
- *Prescriptive Analytics*: Predictive analytics aims at finding the best course of action for a given situation. It provides a step by step procedure to overcome a situation or minimizing its effects by choosing an alternate path.

5 How Does Predictive Analytics Work in Health Care?

Predictive analytics uses predictive modelling. It usually includes a machine learning algorithm in its approach to estimate future trends in health care. These models are trained on data already available and can be tested for new values, predicting the results beneficial for a business.

There are two types of predictive models. They are as follow:

- Regression Models
- Classification Models.

5.1 Regression Models [5]

Regression models are used to predict a real value the following formula is used for Simple Linear Regression,

$$Y = B0 + B1 * X \tag{1}$$

Equation 1 represents an equation of a line in a two-dimensional space. Here, 'Y' is the dependent variable which tells how it depends on 'X', whereas 'X' is an independent variable, a variable that causes the dependent variable to change. Similarly 'B1' is the coefficient for the 'X', it tells how a unit change in 'X − 1' changes 'Y'. While 'B0' is the constant term, which tells the base value of 'Y'. It basically fitting a line that best fits the data.

It uses ordinary least squares method to plot the best fitting line. According to it the sum of square of differences of the 'Y' values in the data set and the corresponding 'Y' values on line should be minimum. The line which gives the minimum sum is the best fitting line.

5.1.1 Multiple Linear Regression (Preacher, K. J., Curran, P. J., & Bauer, D. J. 2006)

Multiple linear regression is a statistical measure that usages various descriptive variables to find the result of a response variable, given by the Eq. 2

$$W = A0 + A1 * F1 + A2 * F2 + \cdots + An * Fn \tag{2}$$

Here 'W' is our dependent variable and $F1, F2, \ldots, Fn$ are our independent variable.

Dummy Variable: In measurements and econometrics, especially in case of relapse investigation, a fake variable (otherwise known as a pointer variable, structure variable, one-hot encoding, Boolean marker) is one which takes the binary values of 0 or 1 to demonstrate the nonappearance or closeness of some unmitigated condition that might be required to shift the result.

Dummy Variable Trap: Let us consider an attribute called city name, which includes either London or Delhi. Let this categorical column will be split into two columns of binary values ie either 0 or 1 (corresponding to London(D1) or Delhi(D2)). Here we see that always $1 - D1$ is equal to D2 if we know that the value of D1 is 0 then obviously the value of D2 will be 1 and vice versa.

Because of this condition the model cannot distinguish between the effects of D1 $- 1$ and D2. And this condition is called as the dummy variable trap. And therefore it won't work properly. Hence we cannot have both D1 and D2 in our model, we will have to exclude one of them, if you have 4 then remove 1 and have only 3 in your model, if you have 100 then include only 99.

The p-value: In factual speculative testing, the p-esteem or likelihood esteem or asymptotic centrality is the likelihood for a given measurable model that, when the invalid theory is valid, the measurable summary (such as the example mean distinction between two looked at gatherings) would be more prominent than or equivalent to the genuine watched outcomes.

How to Build Models?

We know that in multiple linear regression with a large number of independent variables. There is a famous saying that the more the garbage in the more the garbage out, i.e., if you throw in a lot of stuff in a model, it won't be a good model, you need to select which independent variables will be going in your model. This is logical as not all the attributes are important to make an efficient model as there will always be certain attributes which will be garbage.

We will talk about five ways of building model. These are the following:

i.   *All In:*

     This means throwing in all the independent variables you have. As discussed earlier we know this is very inefficient but at times you might not have a choice. This happens when you have a prior knowledge that all the variables go in or when you are just forced to do it by your executive.

ii. *Backward Elimination*: This is also called the step by step method.

     - Step 1: Choose a significance level to stay in your model and this has to be done before you start. For example (S = 0.5).
     - Step 2: Fit the model with all possible independent attributes. This is just like the ALL IN method.
     - Step 3: In this step, you start getting rid of the unnecessary attributes. Select the attributes with the highest p-value. If P > S then go to Step 4, otherwise go to finish.
     - Step 4: Remove the variable with P > S.
     - Step 5: Start fitting the model without the removed attribute.

     After the Step 5 go to Step 3 and continue this until you reach a point where the highest P-values of your model are less that the significance level.

iii. *Forward Elimination*: Process of forward elimination is discussed below:

     - Step 1: Choose a significance level to enter your model. For example, S = 0.05
     - Step 2: Fit all the simple linear regression models Y ~ Xn and then choose the model in which the P-value is the lowest.
     - Step 3: Keep this variable and add fit all possible models with the one extra attribute added to the one/ones you already have
     - Step 4: Choose the attribute with the lowest P-value. If P < S, then goto Step 3, otherwise go to Step 3.
     - Step 5: Keep the previous model
       Since this is computationally very intensive we barely ever use this method.

iv. *Bidertional Elimination*: This merges both forward and backward elimination.

     - Step 1: Choose a significance level to enter and stay in the model. For example SENTER = 0.05, SSTAY = 0.05
     - Step 2: Perform the step coming immediately in forward elimination, that is the variable with P < S enters the model
     - Step 3: Perform all the step of backward elimination that is that the older variables must have P < S to stay Repeat Step 2 and 3 till the conditions are satisfied
     - Step 4: Now no new variables will enter and none of the old variables will leave

v.   All Possible Models
Here we make all possible regression models, i.e., $2^n - 1$ number of total combinations. Then select the one with the best conditions. This method is barely used for its immensely computationally intensive approach. We will use backward elimination for its robust nature and less computationally intensive processing and implementation.

Support Vector Regression (SVR): (Cortes & Vapnik, 1995): It is straightforward direct relapse in a higher dimensional space. SVR can be thought of as though every datum point in the preparation set is speaking to its own measurement. At the point when your portion is assessed between a test point and a point in the preparation set, the esteem acquired, therefore, gives us the organize of your test point in that specific measurement. When we assess the test point for every one of the focuses in the preparation set, k, we get a vector. After you understand that vector you can utilize it to play out a straight relapse.

Random Forest Regression: [6, 7] The overall approach for random forest regression was first introduced by Ho in 1995. Ho designed a woodlands of trees part with one-sided hyperplanes can choose up accuracy as they progress without facing overtraining, as lengthy as the backwoods are haphazardly limited to be touchy to just chosen highlight measurements. An resulting work sideways the corresponding lines inferred that other part strategies, as long as they are randomly bound to be unfeeling to some component measurements, carry on comparatively. Note that this perception of a progressively perplexing classifier (a bigger timberland) getting increasingly precise about monotoni-cally is in sharp difference to the basic conviction that the multifaceted nature of a classifier can just develop to a specific dimension of exactness before being harmed by over-fitting. The clarification of the backwoods plan's fortification from overtraining can be initiated in Kleinberg's hypothesis.

It is one of the gathering (which means gathering) strategies. These models chip away at the standard of Wisdom of the group. To put it plainly, it is smarter to consider supposition of a 1000 unique individuals with very little information than consider the conclusion of just a single expert (provided the 1000 individuals have precision superior to arbitrary speculating, i.e., over half). Doesn't bode well? I will clarify it.

Consider a marginally one-sided coin which has a likelihood of arriving on heads 51% of the time. In the event that this coin is hurled a 1000 unique occasions, the likelihood that there will be more number of heads than tails is 75%. This likelihood crosses 99% if the coin is hurled multiple times. You can crunch the numbers yourself.

Presently consider if these coins are models, and each model's exactness is simply higher (51%) than unadulterated speculating (half). What's more, on the off chance that you think about 1000 such models, the likelihood that they will all in all give the right outcome is 75%. What's more, on the off chance that there are 10,000 such models, they will by and large give an exactness of more noteworthy than 99% (provided they are autonomously constructed, which isn't actually the reasonable case, yet this guideline works great).

This is actually what random forest regression models do, they fabricate many (sometimes even thousands) singular (trees can be relapses and orders) that are constructed utilizing some division of the information. And afterward they anticipate the yield by joining the yields of these trees, by casting a ballot or normal or anything reasonable.

5.2 Classification Models

5.2.1 K-Nearest Neighbours (K-NN) [8]

Let's imagine that we have a scenario where we have two categories already present in our data and also we've identified two categories, one is carrier one on the left which is red card two is green on the right. And for simplicity's sake we're just going to take into consideration two variables or two columns in our data set so all of this grouping is happening based on these two columns $x - 1$ and $x - 2$. And now let's say we add a new data point into our data set.

The question is should it fall into the red category or should fall into the green category.

How do we decide that. So how do we classify this new data point to a cluster of points. As a red data point or a green data point and that's where the nearest neighbours algorithm will come to assist us. At the end of performing this algorithm we'll be able to identify whether it's a red or green point.

So how does the K-nearest neighbour algorithm work. How did it do that. We're going to build a step by step rule guides to the K and then. And as you'll see this is a very simple algorithm. All right so the first step is to choose a number k of neighbours that you're going to have in your algorithm so you go to you have to identify whether K is equal to 1 2 2 3 5 or some other number. And one of the most common default values for k is 5, to take the K-nearest neighbours of the new data point according to their Euclidean distance.

Now here you can if you don't have to use Euclidean distance you can use other distances such as a Manhattan distance or any other distances that you might be considering. But in most cases Euclidean distance is so we're to stick to those. So once you've taken the nearest neighbours among these K neighbours you need to count the number of data points in each category.

So how many data points fell into one category to the other carrier and so on if you might even have more than two categories in your data set. So you just need to calculate how many fall into each category and then you need to assign the new data point to the category where you counted the most neighbours. As simple as that, that's why it's called K-nearest neighbours. And then your model is ready as it is it's a very simple algorithm and moral which is going to do a manual exercise right now to really solidify this knowledge. So let's move onto that.

So here we've got the new data point that has been added to our scatterplot as we saw previously. How do we find the nearest neighbours of this new data point. Well, let's have a look at the Euclidean distance that we're going to use so quickly and distance is a very basic type of distance that we define in geometry it's the one we use in geometry. And basically if you have two points over here one and two then the distance between the two points is measured according to this formula.

So x − 2 minus X the difference between the x-coordinates and then squared plus the difference between the y-coordinates squared and then you take a square root out of all that. And that is basically if you look at it this way it's a right-angled triangle as suiting you to in. Cathedral's and you squaring it you take in other theatres and it's growing it's taking you adding them up you're taking a square root and that gives you the length of the high poisoner's. That's how Euclidean distance work. Again you could use any type of distance but this is the geometrical distance and this is what we're going to stick to.

So basically o n ascatterplot a two-dimensional kind of polygon just draw the lines and see what is closer. So here on your data point how are going to identify which other closest five neighbours. we just look at them and we see the distances here so we can see that's the closest one that's probably the second closest ONE-THIRD closest fourth closest fifth closest So let's outline those.

So now all we have to do is step three among these neighbours then count the number of data points in each category is in category 1 in the red when we have 3 neighbours in category 2 we have two neighbours. So therefore Step 4 is assigned the new data point to the category where you counted the most neighbours. That means we need to assign it to the read category as simple as that. Now we have classified this new point and your model will be ready.

5.2.2   Support Vector Machine (SVM) [9]

SVM is where at first created during the 1960s then they were refined again during the 1990s and just at this point they're winding up prevalent in machine learning since they are showing that they can be very powerful in light of the fact that they are to some degree distinctive to other machine learning calculations. What's more, we'll discover how they're unique towards the finish of the story. Be that as it may, for the present we should see how support vector machines really work.

Here we have a common focuses on a two-dimensional space for the good of simplicity. We have only two sections x − 1 and x − 2. Also, we are very brave some as of now have concurred so we've effectively arranged them however at this point how do we determine a line that is going to isolate them. So how would we really isolate these focuses. Since that is a detachment or then again as it were that choice limit will be imperative for us going ahead when we begin including new focuses with the goal that's that is the purpose of our order. That is the motivation behind receptiveness since we need to make a limit between these two with the goal that when we later on include new indicates that we need to arrange that haven't been characterized yet we will know where they will fall either in the more noteworthy green territory or in the red region. So how might we separate these focuses we see here. Well one route is to draw a line like that in our two-dimensional space and after that express anything to one side will be green anything to one side will be red and if another point falls some place on this space we will know immediately if it's red or green since we'll know where it falls. Anyway there's another way we can draw a level line that way or we can draw a slanting line like that. We can really draw another corner to corner line or we can draw another askew. So there are loads of various lines that we can make that will accomplish a similar outcome they'll isolate our focuses to two classes.

And yet they all, later on, will have distinctive results so when we include new focuses contingent upon where that point will fall it'll either be classed as a major aspect of the Green Zone and part the Reds or we need to locate the ideal line and that is the thing that fields are about. They're tied in with finding the best line or the best choice limit which will enable us to isolate our space into classes. So how about we discover how the SVM really scans for this light. Well the line is sought through the most extreme edge so here you can see a line and this is the line.

Furthermore, SVM would draw. Thus fundamentally the line isolates these two Klaas' of focuses. Also, in the meantime it has the most extreme edge which implies this separation so this line is drawn equidistant starting here and this brings up we'll discover precisely why these focuses in a second. And afterward the separation between the line and every single one of these focuses that is equidistant. Furthermore, that is edges so, the aggregate of these two separations must be boosted all together for this line to be the aftereffect of the SVM.

What's more, these two points are really called the help vectors for what reason they're called vectors was around an hour and a second. In any case, so fundamentally these two points are supporting this entire calculation. So regardless of whether you dispose of the remainder of the focuses that thing will change the calculation will be actually the equivalent. So these different focuses they don't add to the consequence of the calculation just these two are contributing and along these lines they called the supporting vectors you can call them supporting focuses yet truly they are vectors. This is the reason on the grounds that in a multi-dimensional space when you have something beyond two factors you can have three-five 10 or 100 factors.

Each point is very longer a point since you can't picture it on a two-dimensional plane or indeed, even a three-dimensional space and consequently every one of those focuses that we see here is considered, i e., vector in a multi-dimensional space so the more broad term for focuses that we see here are vectors and this is something that is considered in arithmetic in college or secondary school science also, fundamentally. So as a rule they are on the whole vectors just in this specific model and we have two measurements at that point we can call them focuses yet as a general rule there are pictures and that is for what reason they're called help vectors. So thus these two explicit vectors are the ones supporting sort of supporting this choice limit or then again along these lines we're fabricating this calculation that is for what reason they're essential and that is the reason this entire calculation is known as the help vector machines. So now what else do we have here. Well we have the line in the centre which is known as the most extreme edge hyperplane or the greatest edge classifier.

The two-dimensional space it's much the same as a classifier is only the line. Be that as it may, very a multi-dimensional space it's a hyperplane. What's more, I realize it's an extremely confounding term yet that is what is known as a most extreme edge hyperbola. So those the majority of the ones that we saw were additionally hyperplane yet there weren't the most extreme edge mixture edges and you can watch that yourself so you can draw an alternate hyperplane here and simply look at the negligible. It'll generally be less in light of the fact that this is the one with the greatest edge. And after that, you have the green and the red dabbed lines. So the green one is known as the positive hyperplane and the red was known as the negative hyperplane. It doesn't generally make a difference in which request you name them simply the fact of the matter is that one of them is certain also, negative or fundamentally anything to the directly of the positive is delegated the green classification or on the other hand the positive classification anything to one side to group as a negative classification or the red class for our situation.

With the goal that's the means by which the supervision machine calculation works obviously there's some confused arithmetic behind it yet the substance of its natural piece is actually this that we're working with a directly divisible informational collection where we can really it's given to us as a matter of course that we can put a line through an outline which will isolate the two classifications and afterward we're simply looking for the one with the greatest edge. So reasonably when you consider it's really an entirely straightforward calculation when you consider it thusly.

In the event that I was going into the arithmetic and the inquiry is what's so unique about SVM is for what reason are they so prominent and for what reason are they diverse to other machine learning calculations and that is actually what we're going to discuss at the present time. So envision you're attempting to show a machine how to recognize apples and oranges how to group a natural product into either an apple an orange. So you're telling a machine that. Good I'm going to give you some test information so view these apples. These are apples and oranges. Dissect them. See them see what parameters they have and afterward next time they're going to give you. I'm going to give you a natural product which will be either an apple or an orange and you're going to need to group it and reveal to me whether it's an apple or an orange. Right. With the goal that's sort of a standard machine learning issue.

Presently for our situation here you can see suppose on the correct we have oranges on the left we have apples. So what predominately machine Algren's would do is they would take a gander at the most Apple the apples and the most orange the orange so they would take a gander at the most stock standard regular kind of apples and the most stock standard regular kind of oranges and now case would be Apple some more there in that in the very heart of the apple Clauss far from the oranges. What's more, for the oranges would be someplace over yonder. So additionally in the very heart of the orange Clauss far from the Apple so they were attempted.

A machine would endeavour to gain from the apples that resemble apples so it would realize what an apple is. What's more, it likewise endeavoured to gain from oranges so it would recognize what an orange really is and that is the means by which most of the machine learning calculations work and afterward dependent on that it is ready to think of a few expectations and arranging four new information components and factors that you would get it on account of support vector machine. It's somewhat unique. Rather than taking a gander at the most stocks standard apples and stocks and oranges what this help victualling machines do is they really take a gander at the apples that are particularly similar to an orange so here you can see an apple which isn't your standard Apple is orange and shading right. So it's anything but difficult to mix this apple of an orange and they would take a gander at oranges which are not stock standard oranges which are more similar to apples than everything else so you can arrange the Lemon here. So those of us in the picture simply out of the oranges the SVM would pick the one that will be that looks the most like an apple for this situation. We have a green orange. It's not typical to have a green orange when you consider orange you consider orange.

The help vectors you can see that they're in reality very near the limit so they're near the apple or the red one would be near the green ones and the orange or the green imprint here would be exceptionally near the red ones and in this manner the help vector machine in that sense you can consider it resembles an increasingly extraordinary sort of calculation an insubordinate kind of calculation a dangerous sort of calculation since it takes a gander at an exceptionally extraordinary case which is very near the limit and it utilizes that to build its investigation. Also, that in itself makes the help vector machine calculations extremely extraordinary altogether different from the vast majority of the other machine learning calculations.

5.2.3   *Decision Tree Classifier* [7]

It represents arrangement and relapse trees and this term is an umbrella term for two kinds of trees which are what we see calcifications trees and relapse trees. Presently the thing that matters is that arrangement trees enable you to order your information so they won't give absolute factors, for example, male or female apple or orange or diverse kinds of hues and factors of that sort. While animosity trees are intended to enable you to anticipate results which can be genuine numbers so, for example, the pay of an individual or the temperature that will be outside and things like that. So those are the two distinct sorts and we will discuss order trees in this segment of the course. So here we have a precedent with bunches of focuses on our two-dimensional scatterplot. Presently how completes a choice tree work. So it will do is cut it up into cuts in a few emphasis so we should see. So they'll be part one. They'll be part two so part one split our information at X t o rise to 60 split to part our girl $X - 1$ parallels 50 split three. In any case, our. Intriguing or 70 and split for split our information at $x - 2$. It's not appeared here it's around 20. So that is the way a choice tree works and the reason for the split. So how are these parts chosen how does the calculation realize where to choose the parts. Well essentially on the off chance that you view it now and, at that point the split is done in such an approach to boost the number classification in every one of these parts so to amplify, for example, we need most extreme read's classes here and here is the reason it's as yet the equivalent yet then the following split expands the quantity of green here and them progressively red here. It's an essential method to clarify it.

Truly there's some mind-boggling arithmetic occurring in the foundation. The split is attempting to limit entropy. As it's enlightening entropy it's an intriguing term. It would take a long stretch of time and hours for us to experience the majority of that at this moment. Thus in the event that you need to get into the more profound science behind this calculation, at that point you surely can examine that. In any case, for us it's adequate that we're simply searching for the ideal split or the calculations going to find ideal parts that will amplify the quantity of various focuses in every single one of these new pockets are really called leaves. So we have the beginning scatterplot and after that toward the end you've got these leaves and the last leaves are really called a terminal rent. With the goal that's the manner by which this will happen. Presently allows rewind a bit and we should do that entire method once more. Be that as it may, while we're playing out the parts we're going to begin developing a choice tree a genuine choice tree. How about we see. So there is our part number one. Furthermore, what it's doing is it's part our little girl at the 60 level. So now how about we build a choice tree that will make that inquiry. So is X excessively more prominent than 60 or under 60 so if is incredible and 6 it falls into one branch if it's less than 60 it will fall into the following extent.

So there we go X − 2 is under 60. No yes and no. Next is part two just parts t that is over 60 × to verbal. We're just managing information that is above X − 2, so it's at this very moment we're checking. So I'm returning at this point. Presently we are checking as part to occur at 50 for the X − 1 variable. So here we go x X − 1 is under 50 yes or no. So if and here you can see that immediately this split as of now you can disclose to us in the case of something is green or on the other hand red. So in the event that it's less so on the off chance that we're as of now over 60 and, at that point underneath 50 at that point it's green which we can see here in the event that we are over 50, at that point it's red which we can see here. With the goal that's the manner by which this grouping works and all, we should arrange off the rest.

6 Case Studies

6.1 *SVM Model to Predict Diabetes [2]*

The support vector machine (SVM) has been widely deployed in taking care of issues in biomedical fields that require some form of classification. This approach for classification is largely information driven. Hence, it is used particularly in those situations where test sizes are little and the number of parameters taken into consideration is large in number. The most common real-time application of this approach is to create a robotized order of sicknesses and to enhance techniques for identifying ailments in the healthcare sector. One of the most common medical morbidity on the rise is diabetes. The tests conducted for confirmation of this metabolic disorder involve glucose tolerance test which takes into consideration random blood sugar, fasting blood sugar, and glycosylated haemoglobin.

According to reports in the United States, diabetes influences an expected 23.6 million individuals. Among these, about 33% are unconscious that they have the illness. Another 57 million individuals are pre-diabetic. Ongoing examinations show that diabetes can be avoided by way of life changes among people with pre-diabetes. The SVM approach has been used to deal with recognizing people with either unfamiliar diabetes and recognize them from people that don't have both of these conditions. The elements used to make the SVM were compelled to clear clinical estimations that don't require a look into centre tests.

Two distinctive characterization plans were conceived. In the first technique, classification strategy I, the gathering of people with diabetes was recognized from those without diabetes, incorporating people who were pre-diabetic. The second technique consisted of classification strategy II, the gathering of people with either undiscovered diabetes or who were pre-diabetic, was recognized from those without diabetes. Around fourteen factors were chosen among various included in usual health records. These were selected on whether or not they were connected with the hazard for diabetes. These included factors such as family ancestry, age, sexual orientation, race and ethnicity, weight, stature, midsection outline, BMI, physical action, hypertension, smoking, liquor use, instruction, and family salary. The factors incorporated into the choice were those with the best discriminative execution.

The SVM calculation plays out a characterization by developing a multidimensional hyperplane that ideally separates or demarcates between two classes by augmenting the edge between two information groups. This calculation accomplishes high discriminative power by utilizing uncommon nonlinear capacities called bits. These are then used to change the space obtained as input.

The essential thought behind the SVM strategy is to build a $n - 1$ dimensional isolating hyperplane to segregate 2 modules in an n-dimensional space. An information point is seen as a n-dimensional vector. Two factors in a dataset will make a two-dimensional space; the isolating hyperplane would be a straight line (one dimensional) partitioning the space down the middle. At the point when more measurements are included, SVM looks for an ideal isolating hyperplane called the greatest edge isolating hyperplane. The separation between the hyperplane and the closest information point on each side is augmented. The best situation is that two classes are isolated by a straight hyperplane. In any case, true circumstances are not generally that straightforward. A few information focuses on an issue that the two classes may fall into a 'dark' territory that isn't anything but difficult to be isolated. SVM takes care of this issue by two methods. First, it permits a few information to focus to the wrong side of the hyperplane by presenting a client determined parameter C. This parameter indicates the exchange off among the misclassifications and augmentation of edge. Secondly, it utilizes bit capacities to enhance more measurements to the low dimensional space. Therefore, 2 classes could now be distinct in the high dimensional space.

The SVM approach will in general group elements without giving appraisals of the probabilities of class enrolment in the dataset, which is a key distinction from different strategic relapse. Two key parameters for the pieces, C and gamma, were pre-chosen to produce an ideal SVM display. Parameter C powers over-fitting of the model by determining resistance for misclassification. Parameter gamma controls the level of nonlinearity of the model. LibSVM, an unreservedly accessible SVM programming library, was utilized to produce the SVM models.

To create the information collection for model preparation, various non-cases were chosen to coordinate the quantity of cases in the preparation informational collection. As per the required information design input, estimations of chosen highlights were standardized to values from -1 to $+1$. Estimations of absolute factors, for example, race are subjectively allocated to numbers between - 1 and $+ =1$. Estimations of ceaseless factors were changed into qualities between -1 and $+1$ by partitioning them by a fitting number. An utility incorporated into the LibSVM bundle (grid.py) was utilized to locate the ideal limits for punishment parameter C and gamma under 5-crease cross-approval. Diverse functions were tried and chose for the models dependent on execution.

MLR was performed utilizing the equivalent chose hazard factors or highlights and case status as the result variable. The evaluated β coefficients were connected to the test informational collection to compute for every individual the likelihood of being a case. Test informational indexes were utilized to survey the execution of the models. Approval, utilizing the test informational indexes, kept away from the potential inclination of the execution gauge due to over-fitting of the model to preparing informational collections. For the SVM display, the information records in the test informational collections were arranged by the necessity that variable qualities be standardized to values from -1 to $+1$; the main segment of the information informational collection was set to 0.

To assess the strength of the appraisals from the SVM, tenfold cross-validation was performed in the preparation informational collection. The preparation informational index was parcelled into 10-break even with size. Every subsection was utilized as a test informational index for a module prepared on all cases and an equivalent number of non-cases arbitrarily chosen from the 9 remaining information subsets. This cross-approval process was rehashed multiple times, enabling every subdivision to serve once as the test informational collection.

In the first strategy of classification that was concerned with analysed or undiscovered diabetes versus no diabetes or pre-diabetes, eight different factors, namely, family ancestry, age, race, weight, stature, BMI, and hypertension yielded the best execution. In the second strategy, undiscovered diabetes or pre-diabetes versus no diabetes, ten factors including family ancestry, age, race and ethnicity, weight, tallness, midsection periphery, BMI, gender, and physical movement achieved best.

6.2 Naive Bayes to Claim Fraud Diagnosis (Viaene, Derrig, & Dedene, 2004; (Peng, Kou, Sabatka, Matza, Chen, Khazanchi, & Shi, 2007)

Insurance protection misrepresentation costs Americans, in any event, $80 billion every year. Roughly analyzing, the expense of extortion can't be exactly roughly 2% of the all-out yearly premium pay for the European protection industry. In Canada, it has been gauged that CAN$1.3 billion worth of general protection claims paid in Canada consistently is deceitful. Distributed work in the protection writing will, in general, affirm these requests of greatness, at any rate utilizing a wide meaning of what establishes a fake case. Delivering definite figures, notwithstanding, stays troublesome as extortion by its very nature is an incognito task and not surely knew. There is no uncertainty, be that as it may, that protection misrepresentation has advanced into a common and expensive issue. The best method to battle extortion is, obviously, to avert maltreatment of the framework. Back up plans have been enhancing their candidate screening offices, giving uncommon preparing to front-office and cases dealing with staff, building up unique examination units, escalating correspondence and participation inside the business and between the business and indictment and police specialists to battle protection misrepresentation, supporting state- or nation-level extortion agencies, and carrying out to an approach of bringing hard lawbreakers under the watchful eye of the courts. Regardless, fraudsters are prestigious for their deftness and inventiveness with regard to finding better approaches for abusing the inactivity of complex frameworks, particularly when there are huge measures of cash included. It is basic that the fake action is distinguished at the most punctual conceivable minute and that miscreants are quickly found.

Models that are of the predictive type can be used to name high-uncertainty arrangements and help agents to concentrate on suspicious records and quicken the case taking care of procedure. To accomplish the objective, this task ponders the qualities, preprocesses values, and creates order replicas utilizing a three-advance approach. The initial step is shown development. A prescient model is built in view of preparing dataset, which incorporates predefined class names for every value. The second step is demonstrating approval. This progression utilizes approval dataset to tune the model loads amid estimation and survey the arrangement precision of the model. The third step is shown utilization. The arrangement demonstrated, created, and approved in the first and second step is utilized to group future obscure information into predefined classes.

Naive Bayes classifier technique can be used for this purpose. The protection information is from Mutual of Omaha insurance agency. There are five datasets that give data about approach types, claims, makers, and customers. The traits incorporate numeric, absolute, and data types. These datasets were joined into one dataset utilizing a typical one of a kind key. An objective quality demonstrates the session of every value of the information. These records have a place with either normal or unusual class. Information arrangement evacuates unimportant factors and missing qualities, conducts connection investigation to comprehend the connection among characteristics and the objective trait, chooses qualities for order displaying, and changes to suitable structures for the three classifiers. On the off chance that all occurrences of a variable are absent, this variable has no utilization in the characterization and was evacuated. Naive Bayes (NB) process is a basic probabilistic classifier that processes the probabilities of cases having a place with each predefined class and appoints cases to the class that has the most astounding likelihood.

It is proposed for this venture for two reasons. Initially, numerous factors chosen by connection investigation are straight out and this classifier is intended to arrange downright information. Secondly, in spite of its innocent structure, the Naive Bayes classifier works well in some certifiable circumstances and beats some mind-boggling classifiers. Naive Bayes delivers a lot higher arrangement precision. For test information, the classifier accomplishes 99% order exactness for a category of records.

6.3   Real-Time Applications of Neural Networks [10]

This section explains four genuine artificial neural network applications. Neural networks has seen a blast of enthusiasm throughout the most recent couple of years and is in effect effectively connected over an uncommon scope of issue spaces in the zone. Along these lines, let us begin with their description.

Handwriting Recognition: Handwriting acknowledgment has turned out to be vital. This is on the grounds that handheld gadgets like the Palm Pilot are winding up exceptionally prominent. Consequently, we can utilize neural systems to perceive written by hand characters.

Travelling Salesman: The making a trip sales reps issue alludes to find the briefest conceivable way to travel through all urban areas in a region. We could utilize neural networks to tackle this issue.

Neural system calculation: A hereditary calculation begins with arbitrary introduction of the system to take care of the issue. This calculation picks a city in an arbitrary way each time and finds the closest city. Along these lines, this procedure proceeds with a few times. After each emphasis, the state of the system changes and system meets to a ring around every one of the urban communities. The utilized calculation limits the length of rings. Along these lines, we can evaluate the voyaging issue.

Customer churn problem: Neural networks can be used to help banks identify the reason behind their customers leaving their banks and well as tell the banks about which customer has the highest probability of leaving its bank. This uses an artificial neural network and input parameters are credit score, amount, age, gender, ethnicity, loans, etc. ANN using these parameters predict if the customer will leave the bank or will stay in it.

6.4   Real-Time Applications of Decision Trees

As graphical portrayals of intricate or basic issues and questions, choice trees have an essential job in business, in fund, in undertaking the board, and in some other territories. A choice tree is a chart portrayal of conceivable answers for a choice. It indicates diverse results from a lot of choices. The graph is a generally utilized basic leadership device for investigation and arranging. The graph begins with a container (or root), which diverges into a few arrangements. That is why, it is called choice tree. Choice trees are useful for an assortment of reasons. Not just they are straightforward outlines that help you 'see' your considerations, yet in addition since they give a system to assessing every conceivable option. What's more, choice trees enable you to deal with the conceptualizing procedure so you can think about the potential results of a given decision.

Illustration One-Basic insight: Branches are lines that interface hubs (nodes), showing the stream from inquiry to reply. Every hub regularly conveys at least two hubs stretching out from it. In the event that the leaf hub results in the answer for the choice, the line is left unfilled. To what extent should the choice trees be? A choice tree should range insofar as is expected to accomplish an appropriate arrangement. Hypothetically, when you are portraying a choice tree you should include each conceivable choice and result in the tree. This will assist you with investigation, arranging and will permit you dodge awful astonishments. Presently we are going to give increasingly basic choice tree models.

Illustration Two-Simple example: Suppose you are pondering whether to leave your place of employment or not. You need to think about some imperative focuses and questions. Here is a case of a choice tree for this situation.

Illustration Three-Project Management Decision: Envision you are an IT anticipate supervisor and you have to choose whether to begin a specific undertaking or not. You have to consider critical conceivable results and outcomes. The choice tree models, for this situation, may help yield the required result. Remember that in every choice tree, there is dependably a decision to do nothing!

Illustration Four-Financial Decision: With regard to the money territory, choice trees are an extraordinary instrument to enable you to compose your considerations and to think about various situations. Suppose you are pondering whether it's value to put resources into new or old costly machines. This is an established monetary circumstance.

Illustration Five: Money related Decision: The choice tree model can be used for speaking to the monetary results of putting resources into old or new machines. It is very clear that purchasing new machines will bring us substantially more benefit than purchasing old ones.

6.4.1 Ventures for Creating Decision Trees

- Compose the principle choice: Start the choice tree by illustrating a case (the root hub) on 1 edge of your paper. Compose the fundamental choice on the case.
- Draw the lines: Draw line driving out from the container for every conceivable arrangement or activity. Make no less than 2, however, preferred not any more over 4 lines. Keep the lines as far separated as you can to expand the tree later.
- Delineate the results of the arrangement toward the finish of each line: A tip; It is a decent practice here to draw a circle if the result is unsure and to draw a square if the result prompts another issue.
- Keep including boxes and lines: Proceed until there are no more issues, and all lines have either questionable results or clear consummation.
- Completion of the tree: The containers that speak to dubious results stay as they seem to be. A tip: An exceptionally decent practice is to allot a score or a rate shot of a result occurring. For instance, on the off chance that you know for a specific circumstance, there is half opportunity to occur, place that 50% on the fitting branch.

When you complete your choice tree, you're prepared to begin investigating the choices and issues you face.

7 Conclusion

Going through this chapter the author state that healthcare predictive modelling with machine learning is a very powerful tool in solving real-world health problems but it is not limited to health issue problems. The scope and potential are enormous and these technologies are destined to change the face of technology in no time. Before the finish of this part per user will ready to comprehend the idea of various machine learning calculations and will ready to make their own answer for the genuine world issues. We should come up with ways in which these techniques can benefit our environment and quality of life as author believe that one day these technologies will take us to put off all our current problems.

References

1. Nyce, C.: Predictive Analytics White Paper (PDF), American Institute for Chartered Property Casualty Underwriters/Insurance Institute of America (2007)
2. Yu, W., Liu, T., Valdez, R., Gwinn, M., Khoury, M.J.: Application of support vector machine modeling for prediction of common diseases: the case of diabetes and pre-diabetes. BMC medical informatics and decision making (2010)
3. Pratt, W., Unruh, K., Civan, A., Skeels, M.M.: Personal health information management. Commun. ACM **49**(1), 51–55 (2006)

4. Panch, T., Szolovits, P., Atun, R.: Artificial intelligence, machine learning and health systems. J. Glob. Health Dec;**8**(2) (2018)
5. Draper, N.R., Smith, H.: Applied Regression Analysis. Wiley (1998)
6. Rokach, L., Maimon, O.Z.: Data mining with decision trees: theory and applications. World Scientific (2008)
7. Quinlan, J. R.: Induction of decision trees PDF. Mach. Learn. (1986)
8. Altman, N.S.: An introduction to kernel and nearest-neighbor nonparametric regression. Am. Stat. **46**, 175–185 (1992)
9. Cortes, C., Vapnik, V.: Support-vector networks. Mach. Learn. **20**, 273–297 (1995)
10. Data Fair. Artificial Neural Network Applications—4 Real World Applications of ANN. https://data-flair.training/blogs/artificial-neural-network-applications/

Introduction to Artificial Intelligence

Moumita Ghosh and A. Thirugnanam

Abstract Artificial Intelligence (AI) is the branch of computer science, which makes the computers to mimic the human behavior to assist humans for better performance in the field of science and technology. Replicating human intelligence, solving knowledge-intensive tasks, building machines, which can perform tasks, that require human intelligence, creating some system which can learn by itself are the few specific goals of AI. Machine learning and deep learning are two subsets of AI which are used to solve problems using high performance algorithms and multilayer neural networks, respectively. With the help of machine learning process, structured data like genetic data, electrophysical data, and imaging data are properly investigated in medical diagnosis. AI provides advanced devices, advanced drug designing techniques, tele-treatment, physician–patient communication using Chatbots and intelligent machines used for analyzing the cause and the chances of occurrence of any disease in the field of health care.

Keywords Artificial intelligence · Machine learning · Deep learning · Drug development · Healthcare systems

1 Introduction

Artificial Intelligence (AI) is a domain of computer science which deals with the development of intelligent computer systems, which are capable to perceive, analyze, and react accordingly to the inputs [1, 2]. It is well-known fact that humans are considered as the most intelligent and smart species on earth. The features which have helped them to bag this title include the ability to think, apply logic, do reasoning, understand the complexity, and make decisions on their own. They can also do planning, innovation, and solve problems to a greater extent. Since the era of invention of fire to reaching the Mars, man has invented many things for the benefit of humans. One such

M. Ghosh · A. Thirugnanam (✉)
Department of Biotechnology and Medical Engineering, National Institute of Technology Rourkela, Rourkela 769008, Odisha, India
e-mail: thirugnanam.a@nitrkl.ac.in

invention is the computer, which plays a significant role in reducing the workload of humans and solving many complex mathematical and logical problems. However, for researchers, it can be considered that sky is not the limit for new inventions. So, they tried to create a "man-made homosapien" species, which can be related to the world of computers in the form of AI (which are *Artificial,* i.e., manmade, and *Intelligence,* i.e., has thinking power). If a system can have the basic skills like learning, reasoning, self-improvement (by learning from experience), language understanding, and solving problems, then it can be assumed that there is the existence of AI. The AI has been used and implemented in many fields especially in technological domain and is expected to provide 2.3 million jobs by 2020. It is a cutting-edge technology which has its impact in almost every field, be it business, defense, aerospace, or health care systems. It can also be denoted as the method of simulation of human intelligence designed or programmed by humans. With the help of AI, a well-equipped life is generated where the automated machines work for humans, saving their time and energy. Basically, two types of assistants are considered for humans, manual (in the form of robots), and digital (Chatbots) which can perform risky, repetitive, and troublesome tasks. The task of developing such machines is accomplished by minutely studying the human behavior and implementing the logic in the form of algorithms resulting in inventions of software, devices, robots, etc., making human race smarter.

There are many areas which contribute to artificial intelligence which includes mathematics (used for developing algorithms), biology, philosophy, psychology, neuroscience (for studying human mind and its behavior), statistics (for handling huge data), and last but not the least, computer science (to run the algorithm for implementing the concepts). The basic aim of AI is to provide more transparent, interpretable, and explainable systems which can help to establish a better-equipped system used as an intelligent agent. The concept of trusting machine as a replica of human started with the invent of turing test in which the machine is tested irrespective of the knowledge of examiner upon the instructions given considering it as human and if it passes the test, the machine is considered as intelligent. No wonder AI has affected many aspects of the society and presented a new modern era in this digital revolution.

1.1 Types of AI (Based on Capabilities)

The various types of artificial intelligence based on the capabilities can be classified as

- Weak or narrow A I
- General AI
- Strong AI.

Weak or narrow AI: it is a type of AI which can perform a predefined narrow set of instructions without exhibiting any thinking capability. It is the most widely used type of AI in this world. Some famous examples are Apples's Siri, Alexa, Alpha Go, IBM's Watson supercomputer, Sophia (the humanoid) all belong to the weak AI type [3].

General AI: it is the type of AI which can perform the tasks like what human can do. Till now it is not achieved, there are no such machines which works like human or can think as perfectly as human, but it may happen in near future.

Strong AI: it is the type of AI in which it is expected that the machine will surpass the capacity of human. It will perform better than humans, though it is tough, but it is not impossible. It may be the situation when it can be said that the machines will be the master and overtake humans. It has been considered as a great threat to the society by scientists including Stephen Hawking.

1.2 Types of AI (Based on Functionality)

Based on the functionality, artificial intelligence can be classified as per the following types:

(i)   Reactive machines
(ii)   Limited memory
(iii)   Theory of mind
(iv)   Self-awareness.

Reactive machines: these are the machines which works on the data available in the form of predefined dataset. It does not have the facility of data storage for storing the past and future data. It completely depends on the present data. IBM's chess program which defeated famous champion Garry Kasparov and the deep blue system, Google's AlphaGo are some of the examples for reactive machines [3].

Limited memory: these are the machines which can store the past experience or store the memory for limited period of time. An example for limited memory AI is the self-driving cars (it can store the information like speed, distance, speed limit required for the navigation of the car).

Theory of mind: these are types of machines, which are expected to understand the psychological and emotional aspects of human mind and work accordingly. So far such machines are a dream but scientists are working to develop such machines in near future.

Self-awareness: these machines belong to a hypothetical concept that will be considered as super-intelligent machines, which can think, act, and will be self-aware as they will have consciousness and sentiments like humans. Research is carried out to develop such machines and considered as future AI.

1.3 Domains of AI

The major domains of AI (Fig. 1) are neural network, robotics, expert systems, fuzzy logic systems, natural language processing (NLP).

Neural networks: these can be described as the representation of human neural system, i.e., neurons and dendrites in the form of layers and nodes representing data. It comprises algorithms that understand the relationships between the data while mimicking the human brain. These are widely used in AI in the form of machine learning and deep learning. Some of the typical examples are pattern recognition of face and image recognition in medical diagnosis.

Robotics: it is the domain of AI which is mostly associated with the development of intelligent machines in the form of robot which obeys human instructions. The use of robots or humanoids is a new trend and is being appreciated and adopted worldwide. Robots used in industry, medical surgery, restaurants, etc., are classified under this category.

Expert system: these are systems which make decisions with the help of data present in the knowledge base and getting guidance by an expert. These are basically computer applications developed to solve complex problems with intelligence and expertise.

Fuzzy logic system: this domain is considered as resembling the human thinking method and decision-making. It is quite similar to the way humans decide between 0 and 1, but it also deals with all the possibilities between 0 and 1. Examples of fuzzy logic systems used are in consumer electronics, automobiles, comparison of data, etc.

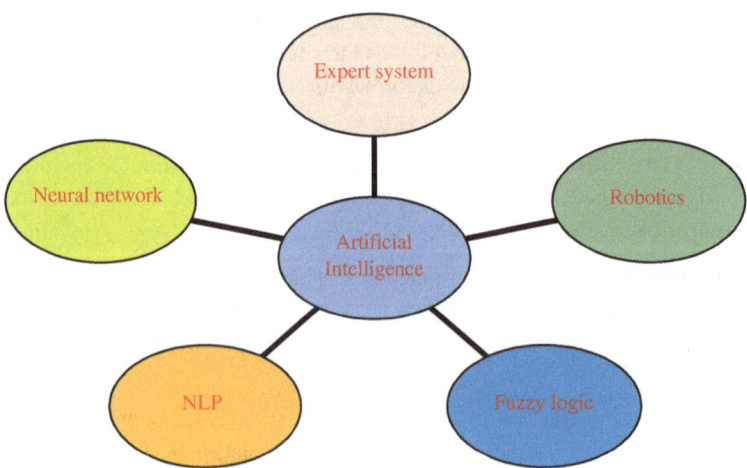

Fig. 1 Various domains of Artificial Intelligence

Natural language processing (NLP): this domain deals with bridging the gap of communication between the computer and human languages. It is basically the interaction between computer and human in a smart way. Google translator and spell check are some of the examples under NLP domain.

2   Subsets of Artificial Intelligence

Artificial intelligence has emerged as a boon for the society for the furtherance of advanced techniques to deal with the real-life problems. The major two subsets of AI are Machine Learning (ML) and Deep Learning (DL). ML is considered as the subset of AI and DL is considered as the subset of ML. The pictorial representation of the relationship between AI, ML, and DL is shown in Fig. 2.

2.1   Machine Learning

As humans can think, improve by self-improvement cycle, and learn from the past experiences, AI machines can also learn from the past experiences with the help of the concept known as Machine Learning (ML). The machine learning deals with the development of algorithms that enables the computer to learn from its data and past experiences on their own [4]. In this method, the machine analyzes the available data set which is also known as training data and with the help of the algorithms predict the possible output over the given input. More the data (information) is provided, more perfect is the performance or prediction. In other words, the relationship between the data and efficiency is that the machine can improve its efficiency by gaining

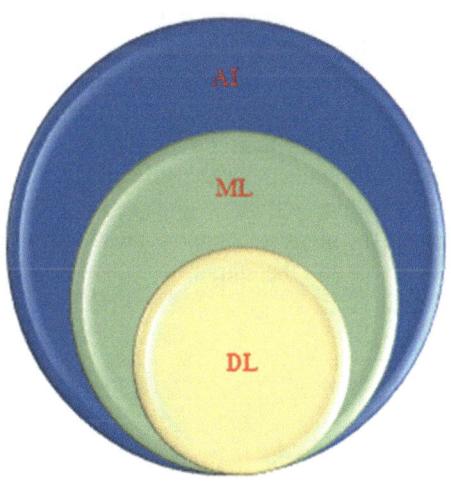

Fig. 2 Relationship between AI, ML, and DL

more and more data. It can learn from the data and improve automatically. This is very much helpful for dealing with huge data of complex problems, which are difficult for humans to deal with and they also consume more time in solving. In this process of computing the machine receives data as input and provides result using an appropriate algorithm.

Classification of Machine Learning

Based on the nature of the learning signal or response that the machine gets; machine learning can be classified into following categories:

(i)   Supervised learning
(ii)   Unsupervised learning
(iii) Reinforcement learning.

Supervised learning: according to the literal meaning, this method correlates with the method of learning of student under the supervision of a teacher. As a teacher illustrates the student with many good examples to help in grasping the concept perfectly, the machine is provided with many labeled data to help in obtaining the perfect output from the given input. The algorithms under this method are classified into two categories, i.e., regression and classification. One example of this method is spam filtering [5, 6].

Unsupervised learning: in this method the machine has to train itself without any supervisor, i.e., the data provided at the input are not labeled or classified. The algorithm has to train itself by searching the degree of similarities among the given data and figure out the appropriate output for the given problem. The algorithm helps to refine the data which can be correlated with the desired output. The algorithms are classified into clustering and association types [6, 7].

Reinforcement learning: this method is typically a feedback-based learning method. In this method the machine is given a reward for every right action taken by it and a penalty for any wrong action, so it is a self-learning method done by analyzing its past performances. The objective of the algorithm is to achieve maximum reward points. Examples for reinforcement learning is a robotic dog learning by its own mistakes and performances, computer playing video games by their own.

The machine learning algorithm is widely being used in multiple fields such as medical diagnosis, image processing, web search engines, photo tagging applications, finance and marketing sector, fraud detection, weather forecasting, and many more. The main advantage is the repetitive process and self-learning methods that it applies to find the output.

2.2   Challenges and limitation of ML

The basic challenge and limitation for ML are that it requires huge amount of data. Without quality data, ML algorithm cannot provide accurate results for further analysis. The prediction can be considered best if the analysis is done over a large amount of data. Another point is that the data need to be heterogeneous as well. With wide range of inputs or datasets, the efficiency of the algorithm will be enhanced with appropriate output. It is similar to that of a new entrant in an organization making mistakes as junior and eventually improves by self-learning and provides output with required accuracy and efficiency.

2.3   Deep Learning

Deep Learning (DL) is considered as the subdomain of ML and thereby the subset of AI. In ML, the system is provided with given input data sets and subjected to self-learning from the past experiences and give predictions as output. Deep learning can be denoted as the next level of machine learning where the system is similar to human nervous system and mimic the working of the neurons. In ML the system is mostly put either in supervised or unsupervised learning method with multilayers of algorithms undergoing such learning methods. As the number of layers increases, it is called as deep learning or Deep Neural Network (DNN) [8]. The initial layer is denoted as the input layer, the last layer is called the output layer and the intermediate layers are termed as the hidden layer, where all the layers are interconnected [9]. The amount of the depth of the network in terms of layers decides how efficient the algorithm can do the dense representation of any data (for example, in an image, the edge, boundaries, etc., are the required data needed for representation). This method has the capability of working upon unstructured data and provides efficient results. This includes intake of large amount of data known as bigdata and assures better performance with respect to the complex data [10]. It helps in enhanced feature extraction, pattern recognition of complex dataset and high-level data extraction. The main advantage is that it can learn without any predefined data and does not require explicit programming by the programmers. The process of deep learning begins with the understanding the problem given, identifying the data, selecting the proper algorithm followed by training and testing the model.

2.3.1   Types of Neural Networks

Basically neural networks can be classified into two categories, namely,

I.   **Shallow neural network** (in which there is only one single hidden layer between the input and output layer) as shown in Fig. 3a [11].

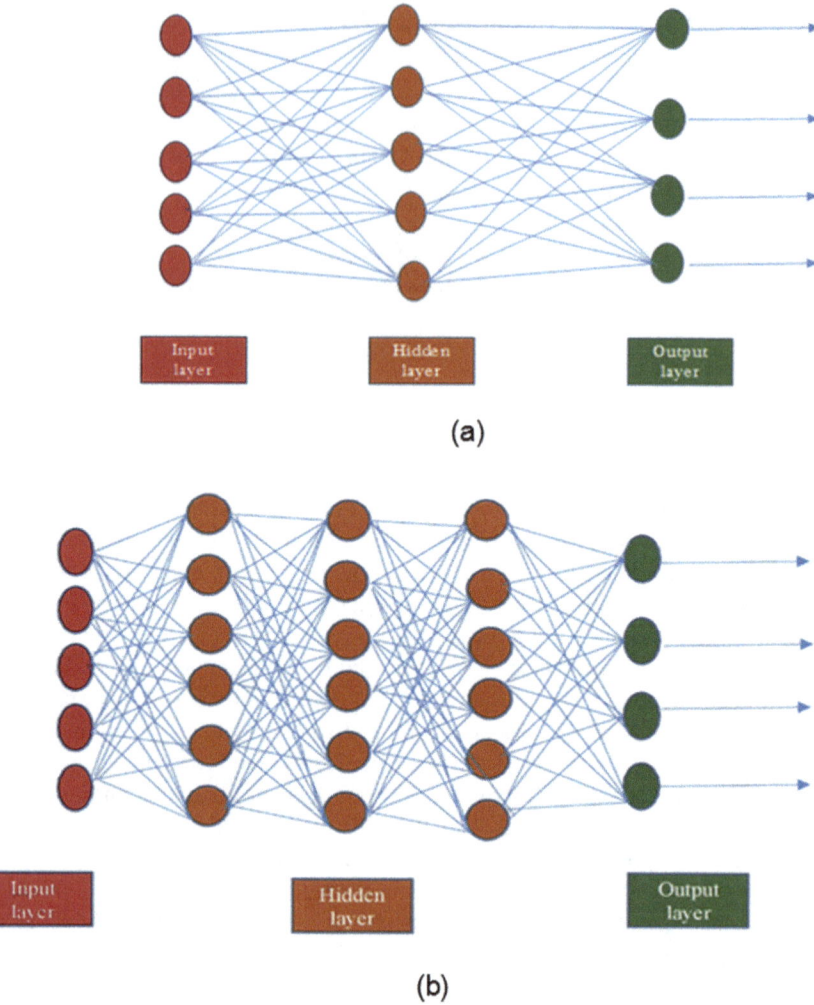

Fig. 3 Schematic diagram of **a** simple and **b** deep learning neural network

II.   **Deep neural network** (in which there are multiple hidden layers between the
      input and output layer and it is the most widely used network) as shown in
      Fig. 3b.

   The deep neural networks are further broadly classified into three categories:

(a)   *Feed-forward neural networks*: it is the single way data transmission type of
      network in which the data moves towards the output layer through the input
      layer. It does not contain any recurrent movement of information.
(b)   *Recurrent neural networks*: in Recurrent Neural Networks (RNN), there is a
      recurrent flow of data from the output to the input to generate the memory for

the system, learn from the data and produce results. Some of the major applications of the RNN are the Chatbots, fraud detection algorithms in monetary transaction, providing caption for images, and many more [11].

(c) **_Convolutional neural networks_**: the Convolutional Neural Networks (CNN) are the most widely used neural networks which have multi-layered neural network. The CNN is considered to be the most efficient form of neural network which is basically used for feature extraction of images and pattern recognition. It has a wide range of application in the field of medical diagnosis and has helped in medical image analysis. Deep CNN has its great usage in radiology and pathology as well. For instance, it can help in esophageal endoscopy for detecting esophageal cancer [12]. The schematic diagram (Fig. 4) describes how the image recognized by the network [13, 14]. The CNN network is widely used method and algorithm in the application of deep learning and is basically used for image identification and classification. The algorithms are developed in a manner to deal with the pixel data. The basic CNN network consists of two parts, i.e., feature extractor and classifier. The feature extractor contains the convolutional and pooling layers whose purpose is to extract the minute features from the image in terms of pixel data. The convolutional layer deals with the feature extraction of the image and preserving the relevant data about the pixels. It reveals the information like edge, boundaries of a image. The pooling layers reduce the dimensionality of an image while retaining the important information. As CNN is a multilayer neuron network, the role classifier part of the network is to classify the information obtained from convolution and pooling layers. This role is played by the fully connective layer whose motive is to connect each node of a layer with other nodes. As a result, whatever image

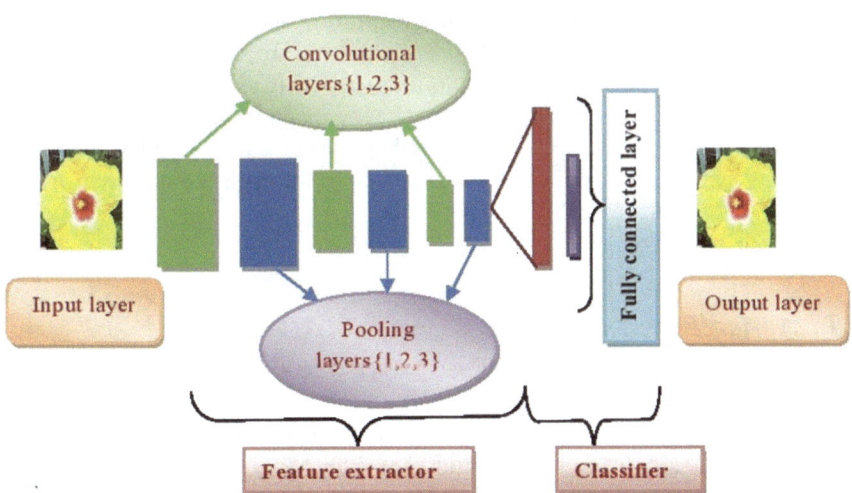

Fig. 4 Schematic diagram depicting the image recognition of the input image using CNN

is placed in the input layer is produced in the output layer if passed through a simple image detection CNN network.

The biggest challenge and limitation of DL is to acquire large amount of data and label it accurately to help the machine while learning the data. Another challenge that could arise is the degree of interpretability which should be high and accurate.

3 Applications of Artificial Intelligence in Modern World

Artificial intelligence has been evolved as one of the most important technology in this world, with its impact on almost every field of human endeavor. It was all started in the year 1950s, after its invention by John McCarthy (the father of AI). With time, it has played a significant role in helping the human generation to become more advanced and equipped than ever before. It can be mentioned that it has spread the broad spectrum of its application from "the soil to the space". The 24×7 Internet facility, the invention of cloud technology, the concept of big data, sensors, and other technological advancements have turned up as a boon for the development of AI. Although AI has not yet replaced humans completely, it has assisted humans to a great extend in solving and handling the problems which are difficult and risky. In the form of intelligent machines, it has played the role of representative of human beings. Today, AI has found wide applications in agriculture, business, education, entertainment industry, medical, defense, and space technology where it has crucial and admirable effects. It has a great impact in the health sector which has helped to bridge the gap between technology and medicine, in diagnosing the patients. It requires data accuracy and security and the trust of the patients on the system. It has also many amazing applications of robotics in the form of robots performing surgery or assisting in diagnosis. Basically, AI deals with large amount of data to obtain the required results, and accordingly the algorithms are designed to reduce the chances of error and provide accurate results. As already mentioned, the spectrum of its application has spread from soil to space as a booming technology for the betterment and development of human life. Following are few of the application areas of AI and data based on some case studies.

3.1 Agriculture

The agriculture is the backbone of any country and hence improving this sector with the help of technology is essential. Considering the world scenario, the agriculture sector shall be capable of producing almost 50% more food than being produced now. The implementation of AI and its technologies has significantly played its role in improving the situation of agriculture industry. Going with the phases of farming, AI is used in the analysis of soil and its monitoring, advancement in crop sowing phase, moving forward in the pest/weed control methods and lastly to the crop harvesting and supply of produce to the right place and at justifiable rate [15, 16]. With the advent of AI, sensor technology and Internet this industry has benefitted to a large extent. In soil analysis and monitoring, AI can help us to know about the soil and seed relationship. In this regard, it tells which seed should be opted for specific type of soil. It predicts in reducing the use of harmful chemical fertilizers used to enhance the plant growth and monitors the irrigation method thereby saving water. According to a study done in Alfalfa, California, the use of Geographic Information System (GIS), in the irrigation method has helped to enhance the crop output by 35% and reduction in the amount of water used for irrigation. AI-based apps, basically with the help of sensors, pictures, and infrared rays help to determine the quality and properties of soil. Hence it helps in improving the agriculture process assuring better yield and profit for the concerned farmers.

Moving to the next application is the sowing process enhancement by the use of AI sowing app. According to a study in 2016, pilot project with 175 farmers was initiated by ICRISAT (The International Crop Research Institute for the Semi-Arid Tropics) with partnership of Microsoft in Kurnool district of Andhra Pradesh, India whose objective was to increase the level of output (about 30%) with decrease in the investment done prior to the farming. It was equipped with the alert messages provided to the farmers regarding the most suitable dates for cropping, land preparation, and usage of fertilizer using this app which works and gives required results by taking the images uploaded by the farmers from the user end. In another study, the development of machine learning technology along with integrated computer vision applications by Blue River Technologies aimed to optimize the herbicide and pest control. This technology helps to distinguish between the affected and normal parts of the plant. The "see and spray" project of Arkansas, USA, using this technology, got reduction in the required amount of expenses for weedicides per acre of land. In a different study done on the crop harvesting, it was found that the time taken by AI-based robots in tomato farms in Japan, is lesser than the time taken by the human.

3.2 Business, Banking, and Finance

This industry or sector is very important and delicate to protect the data and records of millions of customers. The prime factor is the trust, data transparency, and security of the customers. But unfortunately, till date, AI is unable to stop any fraud cases. However, with the help of AI many fraud detection methods and technologies are now offered to make the system more robust. Similarly, the business and retail market are also getting benefited by improvised methods of customer handling and providing faster and safer services. The world of e-commerce is highly affected by its high-level of customer interaction.

In the finance and banking sector, AI has come up with many technological aids either in form of apps or methods to prevent from frauds, enhance better customer data storage/retrieval, and many more. A study by a bank helped online fraud detection solution provider, i.e., Teradata which helps to manage the false positive cases and detection of real frauds. Another study revealed that the payment fraud over anomaly of data is nicely dealt by a client bank using the software Feedzai, using which the bank got a hike of 78% of new customers. DataVisor software helped a bank in USA to detect the fraud in loan and repayments and get profit by 30% with a high accuracy of 90%. Similarly, in business sector, AI has helped many IT firms like Deloitte, IBM, Infosys to bloom in the market as a better technological service provider. Elsevier undergone a digital transformation from being a publisher to a tech with the help of big data and machine learning.

3.3 Education

This is the sector of any nation which transforms the nation after all students are the future of the nation. Considering India only where it is assumed that almost more than half of the population is of age lesser than 25, therefore, it is much more crucial to protect the data shared by the students and provide the best form of education. In this pandemic year, it is not unknown how technology has equipped the education sector to continue the process of education be it in schools, colleges, or research. Apps like Zoom, Microsoft Teams have made it possible or easy to impart knowledge online and from distance. AI has helped the students worldwide to get access to the huge amount of data in the forms of syllabus, curriculum, textbooks, research articles and papers, and e-learning to a greater extent [17].

According to Content Technologies Inc., which is an AI research and development company, smart, and customized educational content can be created and developed which help the students to get access of the customized study materials. It basically uses the concept of deep learning. In a hackathon (organized by NITI Ayog), ReadEx was featured which helped to generate real-time questions using natural language processing and also provided content recommendations and flashcard creation. In a recent study, the Andhra Pradesh government (India) was aided by a predictive analysis done with the assistance of Microsoft using some Azure machine learning process to find the dropouts of students in an academic institution. It successfully detected 19,500 students record who are more likely to dropout in Visakhapatnam district for the year (2018–2019) so that precautionary counseling sessions could be arranged to counsel the students. Not only the students, teachers also got benefitted from these technologies as it optimized searches in Wikipedia or e-learning courses from various organizations. A case study depicts the use of Pearson's Write-To-Learn app for the betterment of writing skills. This app provides tips, hints, and personalized feedbacks to improve the writing skills of the learner be it student or any teacher. In another study, AI has put the fact of how Wikipedia handled the situation of decreased level of content writers by 40% and the problem of controlling abusive comments by the users. It uses AI and associate technology to deal with it and now its AI who writes for Wikipedia which has really changed the world.

3.4 Entertainment and Gaming

This industry does not need much introduction and effect of AI in this. The highly efficient digitally strong technologies have provided awesome movies and work pieces which includes high power editing, imaging, and sound effects. It has transformed the media industry. Starting from the camera effects to the action effects everything has been improved. Probably the superpowers having a huge fan following are nothing using technology. The famous Netflix uses AI and big data to manage the search and provides the better content recommendation and many more ways to help users for better access of data. Gaming industry also uses AI to improve the quality of the game and secure the data provided by the users. It has made the online game in social media possible with multiple participants. Ludoking, PUBG, and many other games have touched and captured the hearts of millions of teenagers.

3.5 Health Care

Artificial intelligence has its maximum effect in this sector and has totally transformed the way of treatment and diagnosis. The goal of having a very effective healthcare system of a nation can now be achieved in many way by difficult task accomplishments with the help of technology and AI. The three basic steps of treatment which are detection, diagnosis and analysis, and treatment are now improvised and enhanced with the advent of artificial intelligence in this sector. The main two factors which are of major concerned are the patient's data privacy and security. Any technology which is introduced mainly focus on these two factors. This includes development of different apps including data collection apps, digital Chatbots for consultation on primary basis, image detection, and analysis using specific algorithms. Since the broad discussion has been done later in this chapter here the focus is on the role of AI in COVID-19 pandemic in India and worldwide.

Role of AI in Handling COVID-19 Pandemic

The role of AI in medical field is tremendous as the planet witnessed a pandemic due to Corona outbreak, which has affected the entire human population with huge number of death cases. In this scenario, AI has come with its technologies to help the people from getting infected with the virus. It cannot assure to avoid death but can assure prevention and precaution by the following ways:

(i) *It has served as high-level data mining tool*: with the help of AI, researchers can get help to fight the disease. Information like the nature of the virus, the symptoms, crucial data from other research papers, and records of past incidents are available by data mining methodologies.

(ii) *As a predictor*: the Corona outbreak was reported in Wuhan, China. The fact that it turned into a pandemic and all such related information were predicted with help of AI and ML. It is being identified that BlueDot and Metabiota uses AI and ML to predict the pandemic outbreak.

(iii) **Quick diagnosis**: it is true that AI alone cannot treat patients but has assisted a lot for the quick diagnosis in terms of image analysis of the lungs (CT scan) of suspected and positive cases.

(iv) **Tracking the patients**: it is the most prevalent job that is being done to keep the record of the active, recovered, and death cases. Microsoft developed a Corona online tracker to track the status of the virus and its possible predictions based on the present data. Similarly, the Indian government also developed its own website to track Corona infected persons. The very famous *Aarogya Setu* App developed by the Ministry of Telecommunication and Information Technology, Government of India, helped to guide citizens in tracking the nearby affected patients and to take necessary preventive measures. AI has helped to fight back the pandemic from this deadly virus.

3.6 Smart Cities and Transportation

This is the area in which the application of AI has its specific and unique role. Smart city is a term, which has become a point of measure of urbanization of a nation. A smart city can be described as the city with technologies to make the life of people much easier and advanced. Similarly, smart transportation signifies the way of handling the transportation and controlling the traffic and accidents which is really a matter of concern due to large number of deaths on highways and roads [18]. As people in smart cities are more likely to use smart technologies, it is obvious that the data security will become a major concern. Be it smart homes, parks, robotic equipped restaurants, or the home delivery of food, it is all because of AI. They also play a crucial role in crowd management and cybersecurity in smart cities.

Considering smart mobility and transportation, AI has given autonomous vehicles the power to detect the chances of accidents and protect the person. It may be the automated airbags or the water splashes to the alarming sounds if the driver gets to sleep while driving. The broader applications of intelligent transportation systems are the use of CCTV cameras installed in the highways to keep track and record of all the activities. Google map needs no extra explanation how it is helping in tracking the one who is traveling and tracing the places one needs to travel. It also helps in suggesting different routes to control the congestion. Based on a study it was found that almost more than 500 train accidents occurred from 2012 to 2017 in India, out of which 53% was due to the derailment. So, the Ministry of Railways, India used AI technology to help in detecting the problems in the track and avoided many such accidents. These technologies are being used and will be used further for the betterment of the nation and the world.

3.7   Space Exploration

In the present scenario it has become almost impossible to imagine the world without technology and the effects of AI in space exploration. The world is aware of the space mission of Chandrayan-2 and the mission to Mars of ISRO which is not possible without the help of AI and its application. Starting from the satellite communication to the rovers moving around the Mars surface many activities needs to be performed by its own or without any instruction from the space station. Be it NASA or ISRO or any other space organization, no one can deny the use of AI in space exploration and how it has enhanced the quality of space exploration. The satellites sending the images from space are decoded and extraction of useful information from the images is done with the help of machine and deep learning. As per a study in 2015, it has been known that the space mission of SpaceX Falcon 9 was accomplished with the help of machine learning which helped it for successful landing at the Cape Canaveral Air Force Station. Application of deep learning has assured the automatic landing of many aircrafts, accurate data collection and transmission without minimum chances of human error.

From another study it was reported that SKICAT (Sky Image Cataloging and Analysis Tool) performed beyond the expectations of human and was able to classify many images having lower resolution during the span of second Palomer Sky Survey. With the help of AI, NASA and Google discovered two obscure planets in 2017 [Kepler-90i and Kepler-90 g]. From these studies, it can be assumed how strongly AI and its subset-based technologies have changed the world in the space exploration and definitely, many more to come with the strengths of AI technology in creating a world of intelligent machines.

4   Artificial Intelligence for Advanced Medical Diagnosis

Medical field is the area where the AI has put its most important impact which has changed the way of medical diagnosis. It has made the diagnosis process much more effective, efficient, faster, and much more reliable. It never aims to replace the doctors but to help them in making their service easier. It basically acts as an assistant to the physician. The role of AI in medical diagnosis is classified into two types, i.e., virtual and physical. Virtual branch deals with clinical data management and the physical branch mostly deals with the use of robots [19]. It has many applications such as assisting in diagnosis, in surgery, with the help of specifically designed robots and equipment helping in guiding the patients about the particular disease. It also helps to aware them and restricts them from getting affected with the help of Tele-treatment technologies. It is also used in signal and image processing along with some crucial predictions regarding the organs. It has also assisted the physicians in maintaining their daily schedule by acting as a reminder to them. It also helps the patients in keeping track with the doctor regarding their pre- and post-surgery conditions. The medical data and records maintenance, the payment facility, and many more applications are used in the healthcare system. Since healthcare system is one of the most important sectors for any nation, it really needs to be improved a lot to facilitate the people and enhance quality treatment in this sector. All this has been possible due to the introduction of AI, cloud technology (for data storage and fast retrieval), the concept of big data, and the use of mobile computing in the healthcare system. Eventually the combination of AI, Robotics, Internet of Things (IoT), and Internet of Medical Things (IoMT) is the new era of healthcare solution system and an important milestone in the process of fourth industrial revolution. Following image (Fig. 5) depicts the most important use cases of AI and robotics as a whole in the healthcare system [20].

As per the data from a case study a project named as the project DeepDream which was developed by Google in 2015 helped to create images of given input and also imagine all possible features that the image should have. This method includes the training of the neural network-based software with millions of images as an input and then asked to produce images from the selected. Based on some case studies on the combating technologies for the most common deadly disease which is cancer a software was introduced by the IBM, namely, Watson for oncology, including both ML and NLP technologies, in 2016. It helped the patients to get to know about the correct

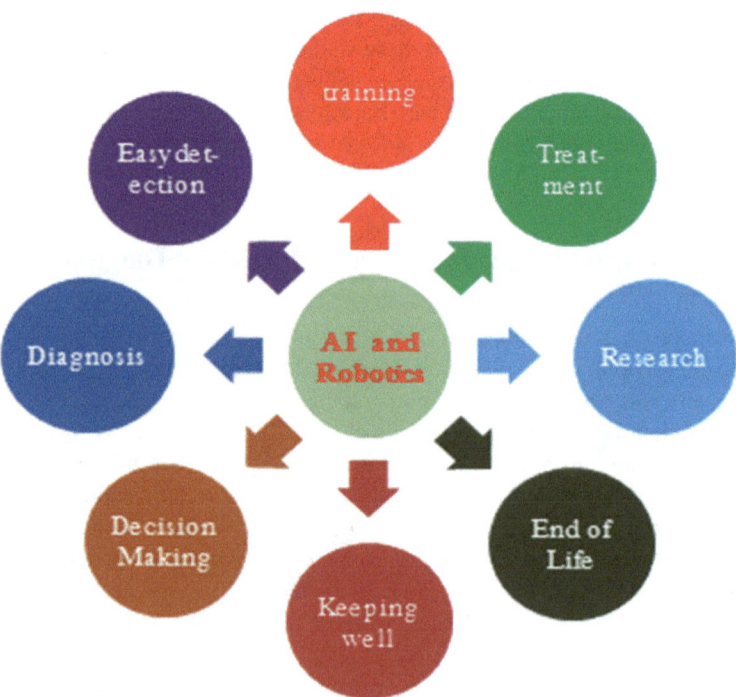

Fig. 5 Use cases of AI for healthcare system

mode of treatment required for them based on their symptoms and health conditions. A similar project for fastening the cancer therapy process is the AI developed by NITI Ayog organization of Indian government which is named as Digital Pathology which contained the images of annotated and curated pathology images. Another ongoing project is the Biobank for cancer patients which helped to bridge the gap between the imaging done by radiologists and by the machine and find out some very minute details. One more case study talks about the e-healthcare and consultation service provided by the UK-based AI Babylon in 2018. In a case study, it explains how the nurse robot Molly which helps the physician in organizing the patients' symptoms and follow up the treatment process. An app developed by National Institutes of Health named as AI AiCure to manage the patient's prescriptions and manage the health condition of patient.

The basic things on which any AI developer put focus are the data generation, data management, and disease detection and management. There are many examples of medical imaging being improved by the implementation of deep learning algorithms be it in detecting the correct disease at the right time or throughout the diagnosis process like eye diseases such as diabetic retinopathy, diabetes detection, risk prediction and control, and also the heart disease monitoring systems [21, 22]. There are also many cases where the drug discovery is done with the help of AI, machine learning, and deep learning technologies and help to find the best solution for a disease. There is no limit to its application under proper implementation and ideologies. But there are few challenges that AI must face in the field of medicine and health care such as the data accuracy, security, integrity, and the interpretability. These factors are very much important for any technology to be trusted and used by the general public. Another factors includes the rate of availability of the services to the people in need at correct time which aims at the digitizing the nation totally because it is known that the rural areas lack the facilities and also the doctors move to town and cities for their improvement. So, the rural remains the same in most of the cases, thereby the prime job is to provide the service where it is much needed. Still, with all these challenges AI has been working with much accuracy in health care and not only diagnosis or treatment it has gone beyond that and provided with some advanced level of medical applications which are being discussed later in this chapter.

4.1 Database Management

In healthcare system, the application of AI, ML, DL, cloud computing, and IoMT has created excellent technologies for the development and services to the healthcare system. Currently, the whole world is going digitized at a higher rate and is in the grip of technology assisted services. With the help of technologies, such as cloud storage and devices based on mobile computing methods, the digital universe is existing and working efficiently. It provides lots of data to store, keep track of and retrieve at a higher speed. Based on a report by the International Data Corporation (IDC), the data size of this digitized universe will be almost 40,000 Exabytes (EB) by the end of 2020. Similarly, by the use of AI and relevant technologies in healthcare system, it is generating large amounts of data in the form of EHR (Electronic Health Record), EMR (Electronic Medical Record), PHR (Personal Health Record), MPM (Medical Practice Management software), and other digital records related to the patients and physicians. The biggest challenge is to manage, maintain the privacy and security norms of all these data. In such cases, an advanced level of algorithms by AI and ML are required to handle big data efficiently ensuring no loss of security and integrity of the data. For instance, the AI and ML approaches have been used to find useful information from the "data lakes" which are large data sets of information extracted from Electronic health records [23]. This huge amount of data is stored in the data warehouse and then analysis is done to produce the effective and feasible outcomes. One of the important features of the healthcare big data is that it is unstructured and heterogeneous type which again becomes more challenging in terms of proper management.

In this scenario ML, DL, and NLP works as a boon to this sector which helps to solve many problems related to database management. Whether it is the data extraction from various medical images (CT, MRI, X-ray, ECG, EMG, PET, and EEG) or to manage the medical records; is very easy with use of advanced level of algorithms [24]. But it must accept the challenges for the proper management of database and accomplish the task of managing the healthcare big data. Some of the basic challenges are data storage, accuracy, availability, data cleaning, data integrity, data sharing, and security. With proper data management and data analysis, AI helps to manage the analytics of the huge data and provides better access to patients and doctors.

4.2 Advanced Medical Devices

In medical and healthcare services, AI and its related technology has spelled its magic in the development of medical devices used for treatment. Talking about the devices, it is only the machinery and equipment that come into our mind which mostly includes surgical equipment, image capturing, and analyzing devices. But to a large extent, software is the most essential medium used in the device to analyze, interpret, and solve health-related problems in diagnosis and treatment of diseases. The classification of medical devices is primarily based on three basic categories (Fig. 6) and all the recent developments are classified based on these major classifications.

In 2016, Medtronic a leading medical device company, in collaboration with IBM Watson developed the SugarIQ App including the AI technology. This app helps the diabetic patient to monitor the sugar levels along with the proper guidance for food habits and all the information regarding healthy eating habits. In 2017, the Medtronic again introduced a device asserting automatic insulin control and stabilization in the body throughout the day. The device named as MiniMed 670G system was launched with the approval of Food and Drug Administration (FDA). In 2017, computerized

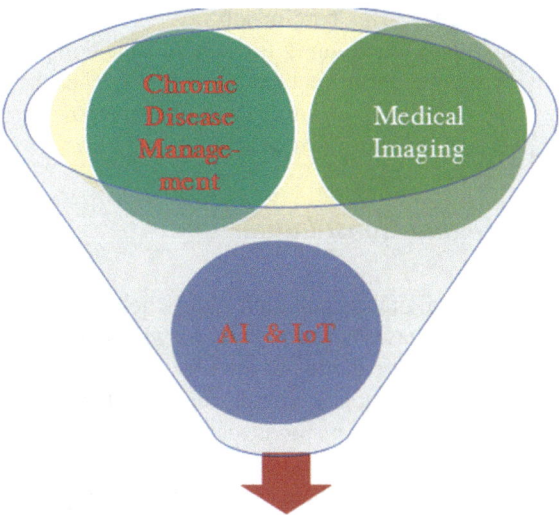

Fig. 6 Image depicting three main categories of medical devices development

New trends of medical devices

CT scans was introduced by the GE health care in collaboration with NVIDIA. It enhanced the medical imaging process and ensures the capture of minute details of affected body parts which is not possible to get by physically looking at the scan data.

The invention of IoT and AI has given many devices in form of various mobile apps to monitor the body required to maintain good health. Patient monitoring system is also a device or system for monitoring the patients' detailed activity and helps to control the deterioration of the body by giving feedback and suggestions. One such development is IntelliVue Guardian Solution, which was done by Philips Healthcares which uses the concept of artificial intelligent and makes appropriate predictions for effective and early managing of health status of a patient.

4.3   Drug Design

Artificial intelligence has already marked its significance in drug discovery and now drug design is also becoming a chief application of AI in drug development process. The basic drug development process includes various steps such as the drug target identification and validation, new drugs design, repurposing of drugs, improvement in research and development, asserting biomedicine conformation, and finally the clinical trials on patients [25]. AI has also successfully helped in the drug discovery method by determining the correct drug molecule and the information about the reaction of proteins in the body before going for design. For drug design, AI is used to determine the proper candidate molecules from the reduced graph of the drug to be designed. This type of job was performed by the company Tessella. AI can also help in differentiating the non-suitable compounds for the drug design which are not suitable for the patient body. It also takes the help of computer-aided design techniques to design the drugs for specific requirements [26].

4.4   Digital Consultation

AI provides digital consultation to the whole world in the form of healthcare chatbots. These are AI-based software solution which provides customized service in form of messages to the patients or the users without making them realize that they are talking to any person or any device [27]. These basically make use of the natural language processing methods and help the healthcare industry to provide digitized service. They also provide consultation regarding food habits, exercise, and other tips to stay healthy. It helps to take necessary preventive measures by the users in order to protect themselves from getting affected with any disease and keep track of their health. Many services companies like Sensely, Your.MD, Babylon HealthTap+ , Pact., Woebot, and others provide a platform for digital consultation to the patients with the help of AI and related technologies like ML, NLP, and DL.

4.5   Genome Editing

This is totally a different aspect of AI application in which the focus is on the features of genetic composition of a person. They try to get the relationship between the occurrence of the disease and the changes it made to the genes. Using the AI and ML techniques, scientists are now able to know the genomic data using gene editing and sequencing techniques. Gene editing can be described as the technique involved in DNA mutations with some alterations in the target sequence such as insertion, deletion, and substitutions [28]. It is known that the gene sequence consists of base pairs made up of (A, T, C, G); general DNA sequencing took much time but after the invent of a technology called as high throughput sequencing (HTS) which helps to perform the DNA sequencing in less than a day. The alterations done in that sequence is termed as gene editing. Many AI platforms have been developed to enhance the HTS for a better representation of genome such as DeepVariant. Overall, AI has efficiently aided the healthcare system and expected to do more in near future related to genome editing and more advancements including the genetic screening tools for the infants.

5 Conclusion

Artificial intelligence and its related technology like machine learning, deep learning, natural language processing has invaded the world undergoing fourth phase of industrial revolution in a very strong manner. It has put its incredible and efficient impacts on almost every sector, from agriculture to education and even to the space technology. It has greatly assisted the healthcare system for making it more efficient in providing the services to the patients and being affordable and feasible for use. The use of machine learning in health care has really modified the scenario in the healthcare system and still there is more scope for research and development. The various application of deep learning and machine learning has helped in better disease detection and diagnosis process. Furthermore, the use of deep learning in image analysis and data extraction from medical images has helped in detecting some deadly diseases. It has also its impact in radiology and the use of robots in medical diagnosis process has its own significance. Artificial intelligence has also spread its spectrum to advance level of medical application and many more research results are leading to a new venture of application in health sciences. It has greatly changed the daily activities by digitalizing the universe and getting benefits from the predictive analysis. The common advantages of AI include reducing the workload of humans and making it easier for them to get much lesser error-prone results for any given set of problems. But considering the assumption of AI creating new employment opportunities it also predicts the risk of increase in unemployment. Furthermore, the cost of implementation and the complexity of the used algorithms if can be reduced will be of much use in health care systems. In conclusion, it can be said that AI is the new way of living with and making it the assistance of human.

References

1. Spector, L.: Evolution of artificial intelligence. Artif. Intell. **170**(18), 1251–1253 (2006)
2. Kamble, R., Shah, D.: Applications of artificial intelligence in human life. Int. J. Res. **6**(6), 178–188 (2018)
3. Singh, H.: Artificial intelligence revolution and India's AI development: challenges and scope. Int. J. Sci. Res. **3**(3), 417–421 (2017)
4. Simeone, O.: A brief introduction to machine learning for engineers. Found. Trends Signal Process. **12**(3–4), 200–431 (2018)
5. Wang, X., Lin, X., Dang, X.: Supervised learning in spiking neural networks: a review of algorithms and evaluations. Neural Netw. **125**, 258–280 (2020)
6. Jiang, F., Jiang, Y., Zhi, H., Dong, Y., Li, Hao:, Ma, Sufeng: , Wang, Yongjun:, Dong, Q., Shen, H., Wang, Y.: Artificial intelligence in healthcare: Past, present and future. Stroke Vasc. Neurol. 2(4), 230 - 243 (2017).
7. Simeone, O.: A very brief introduction to machine learning with applications to communication systems. IEEE Trans. Cogn. Commun. Netw. **4**(4), 648–664 (2018)
8. Herzog, S., Tetzlaff, C., Wörgötter, F.: Evolving artificial neural networks with feedback. Neural Netw. **123**, 153–162 (2020)
9. Reggia, J.A.: Neural computation in medicine. Artif. Intell. Med. **5**(2), 143–157 (1993)

10. Lobo, J.L., Del Ser, J., Bifet, A., Kasabov, N.: Spiking Neural Networks and online learning: an overview and perspectives. Neural Netw. **121**, 88–100 (2020)
11. Schmidhuber, J.: Deep Learning in neural networks: an overview. Neural Netw. **61**, 85–117 (2015)
12. Kiryu, S., Akai, H., Yasaka, K.: Deep learning application in the oesophageal endoscopy. J. Med. Artif. Intell. **2**, 22–22 (2019)
13. Yamashita, R., Nishio, M., Do, R.K.G., Togashi, K.: Convolutional neural networks: an overview and application in radiology. Insights Imaging **9**(4), 611–629 (2018)
14. Tian, C., Xu, Y., Zuo, W.: Image denoising using deep CNN with batch renormalization. Neural Netw. **121**, 461–473 (2020)
15. Barbedo, J.G.A: Detecting and Classifying Pests in Crops Using Proximal Images and Machine Learning: A Review. Artif.Intell. 1(2), 312 - 328 (2020).
16. Talaviya, T., Shah, D., Patel, N., Yagnik, H., Shah, M.: Artificial Intelligence in Agriculture Implementation of artificial intelligence in agriculture for optimisation of irrigation and application of pesticides and herbicides. Artif. Intell. Agric. **4**, 58–73 (2020)
17. Hernández-Blanco, A., Herrera-Flores, B., Tomás, D., Navarro-Colorado, B.: A Systematic Review of Deep Learning Approaches to Educational Data Mining. Complexity, 2019, (2019).
18. Dickmanns, E.D.: Vehicles capable of dynamic vision. IJCAI Int. Jt. Conf. Artif. Intell. **2**, 1577–1592 (1997)
19. Hamet, P., Tremblay, J.: Artificial intelligence in medicine. Metabolism **69**, S36–S40 (2017)
20. Mani Sekhar, S.R., Siddesh, G.M., Tiwari, A., Anand, A.: Bioinspired Techniques for Data Security in IoT. In: Alam M., Shakil K., K. S. (eds) Internet of Things (IoT):Concept and Applications(2020). pp. 167 - 187, Springer, Cham (2020).
21. Xu, Q., Wang, L., Sansgiry, S.S.: A systematic literature review of predicting diabetic retinopathy, nephropathy and neuropathy in patients with type 1 diabetes using machine learning. J. Med. Artif. Intell. **3**, 1–13 (2020)
22. Riihimaa, P.: Impact of machine learning and feature selection on type 2 diabetes risk prediction. J. Med. Artif. Intell. **3**, 1–6 (2020)
23. Shah, F., Kendall, P., Khozin, N., Goosen, S., Hu, R., Laramie, J., Ringel, J., Schork, M.: Artificial intelligence and machine learning in clinical development: a translational perspective. npj Digit. Med. **2**, 69 (2019)
24. Abbod, M.F., Linkens, D.A., Mahfouf, M., Dounias, G.: Survey on the use of smart and adaptive engineering systems in medicine. Artif. Intell. Med. **26**(3), 179–209 (2002)
25. Mak, K.K., Pichika, M.R.: Artificial intelligence in drug development: present status and future prospects. Drug Discov. Today. **24**(3), 773–780 (2019)
26. Tang, C., Ji, J., Tang, Y., Gao, S., Tang, Z., Todo, Y.: A novel machine learning technique for computer-aided diagnosis. Eng. Appl. Artif. Intell. **92**(February), 103627 (2020)
27. Colace, F., De Santo, M., Lombardi, M., Pascale, F., Pietrosanto, A., Lemma, S.: Chatbot for e-learning: a case of study. Int. J. Mech. Eng. Robot. Res. **7**(5), 528–533 (2018)
28. Manghwar, H., Lindsey, K., Zhang, X., Jin, S.: CRISPR/Cas system: recent advances and future prospects for genome editing. Trends Plant Sci. **24**(12), 1102–1125 (2019)

Healthcare Data Analytics Using Artificial Intelligence

Siddesh G. M., S. Krutika, K. G. Srinivasa, and Nabeel Siddiqui

Abstract Artificial Intelligence (AI) is alleged as the greatest transformative technology of the twenty-first century. AI can be defined as the science and engineering of creating intelligent machines, specifically intelligent computer programs. The application of AI in different domains indicates the widespread involvement of this technology. One such application is in healthcare. Healthcare is one of the aspects which regulate health. Healthcare can be referred to as the systematized facility of medical care to the people and societies. Recently, the role of AI in healthcare is defined as "Augmented Intelligence" by the American Medical Association, declaring that AI is going to be designed and used to improve human intelligence rather than substituting it. AI in healthcare predominantly speaks about hospitals and doctors accessing enormous datasets of possibly lifesaving information. The application of AI algorithms in the field of medicine and healthcare would assist doctors to establish improved approaches and treatment strategies for patients. AI is used in all three traditional medical tasks: diagnosis, prediction, and therapy. This chapter discusses the relationship between AI and healthcare, healthcare data collection and storage system, medical data pre-processing, AI algorithms for healthcare, AI methodology for medical and medicinal diagnosis, selection and extraction of features using AI, disease diagnosis with AI, medical image processing with AI, and patient care and treatment with AI.

Keywords Artificial intelligence · Healthcare · Augmented intelligence · Medical diagnosis · Disease diagnosis · Treatment

S. G. M. (✉) · S. Krutika
Ramaiah Institute of Technology, Bengaluru, India
e-mail: siddeshgm@gmail.com

K. G. Srinivasa
National Institute of Technical Teachers Training Institute, Chandigarh, India

N. Siddiqui
Duke University, Durham, NC 27708, USA

© The Author(s), under exclusive license to Springer Nature Singapore Pte Ltd. 2021   45
K. G. Srinivasa et al. (eds.), *Artificial Intelligence for Information*
Management: A Healthcare Perspective, Studies in Big Data 88,
https://doi.org/10.1007/978-981-16-0415-7_3

1   Introduction

1.1   Artificial Intelligence

Artificial Intelligence (AI) is alleged as the greatest transformative technology of the twenty-first century. According to John McCarthy, the father of Artificial Intelligence, "Artificial Intelligence (AI) can be defined as the science and engineering of creating intelligent machines, specifically intelligent computer programs." Generally, the determination of AI can be well defined as the capability of a program or system to carry out all categories of works as we individuals do in our day today's life. For example, gaining knowledge from a specific source of data, Face Recognition, Problem-Solving, and Speech Recognition [1]. AI can also be referred to as the simulation of human intelligence in machines that are programmed to think like humans and mimic their actions [2].

AI can also be well defined as the study of "intelligent agents" which means that any device or agent that can observe and comprehend its surroundings and therefore take suitable actions to exploit its probabilities of accomplishing its objectives [3].

AI can be broadly categorized into two types: Type 1 and Type 2.

Type 1

- **Narrow or Weak Artificial Intelligence**:

This type of AI primarily emphasizes on one particular kind of problem which means that it functions within a limited background and is a simulation of human intelligence. It may be beneficial in saving the time of humans which includes a smaller amount of intelligence.

Examples include Google Search, IBM's Watson, Image Recognition Software, Self-Driving Cars, Alexa, Siri and other personal assistants, and Home Automation where it largely emphasizes precise complications associated with the house [1, 4].

- **Artificial General Intelligence or Strong Artificial Intelligence**:

This type of AI may be referred to as a system that executes similar tasks as that of humans which means that it is a machine with general intelligence as well as much similar to a human being, it can relate that intelligence to resolve any kind of problem.

An example of this kind of intelligence can be seen in the movies like the Data from Star Trek: The Next Generation or the Robots from Westworld.

Type 2:

- **Reactive Artificial Intelligence**:

The most basic kinds of AI machines are purely reactive. This type of AI machine generally does all that they see in the environment and takes the decisions based upon the actions they see. They don't have the capability to form memories or to use previous experiences to make decisions.

The best example for this type of AI is the "IBM's Deep Blue, Chess-Playing Supercomputer", which defeated the international grandmaster chess champion Garry Kasparov in 1990's [5].

- **Limited Memory Artificial Intelligence**:

This type of AI system makes use of previous observations or actions to execute the task but these observations don't have the capability to permanently exist on the memory.

The best example for this type of AI is the "Self-Driving Cars or the Automation Cars" where they observe other cars' speed and direction, decide when and at which moment the break must be applied, decide which lane must be chosen.

- **Theory of Mind**:

In the succeeding more innovative class, machines should form representations about the world and, on the other hand, they must also form representations about the other agents or entities in the world. This is known as the "Theory of Mind" which means the understanding that individuals, living being and objects in the world may have opinions and emotions which influence their own conduct. This type of AI system must be capable in detecting the sentiments, expectations, opinions, and beliefs of other people and should be intelligent to interact accordingly.

- **Self-Awareness**:

This type of AI system will be excellent, intelligent, and self-aware and will be capable of doing all kinds of work that humans do, meaning these will be the exact replica of the humans. These will be the systems built which will be able to form representations about themselves.

1.2 Healthcare

Healthcare is one of the aspects which regulate health [6]. Healthcare can be referred to as the systematized facility of medical care to the people and societies [7]. Healthcare can be defined as the maintenance or improvement of health by means of anticipation, cure of disease or recovery, diagnosis, illness, injury, treatment, and other physical and mental damages in people. Healthcare comprises of hospital care, medication, outpatients' official visit to medicinal providers, and nursing homecare. Health specialists provide healthcare in the associated health fields. Physicians and physician's associates are a part of these health specialists. Audiology, Dentistry, Medicine, Nursing, Occupational Therapy, Optometry, Pharmacy, Psychology, Physical Therapy, Athletic Training, and additional health specialists are all part of healthcare. It comprises of the work done in Primary Care, Secondary Care, and Tertiary care, in addition to community health. As the world's population is growing progressively, the significance of health is well thoughtout to be one of the topmost urgencies in this current society [8].

Healthcare systems are indeed the recognized organizations that satisfy the health requirements of the target communities. The best-functioning healthcare system according to the World Health Organization (WHO) requires a support mechanism, a very well-trained and adequately paid staff, reliable knowledge on which to base verdicts and strategies, and excellently-maintained healthcare facilities to offer quality medicine and innovations. An effective healthcare system may lead to a substantial portion of the county's economy, growth, and industrialization [9].

Health Information Technology (HIT) is the application of information technology that includes both computer software and hardware which manages the storage, retrieval, exchange, and usage of healthcare information, data, and knowledge for interaction and decision making. The HIT components are as follows:

- **Electronic Health Record (EHR)**: An EHR includes the detailed medical background of a patient and can contain records from several providers.
- **Electronic Medical Record (EMR)**: An EMR includes standardized medical and clinical data collected in one's providers' office.
- **Personal Health Record (PHR)**: A PHR is the medical background of a patient which is confidentially maintained, for personal usage.
- **Medical Practice Management (MPM) Software**: It's built to simplify the everyday activities of managing medical facilities.
- **Health Information Exchange (HIE)**: It enables patients and healthcare professionals to access the vital medical information of a patient appropriately and to share it securely electronically.

1.3 Relationship Between Artificial Intelligence and Healthcare

The current generation is witnessing a radical change in technology with the rise of AI. The application of AI in different domains indicates the widespread involvement of this technology. One such application is in healthcare. Humans and machines individually have their strengths and weaknesses and also they can accompaniment to each other in providing and enhancing healthcare. AI is questionably the best-stimulating automation industry and is emerging recently in healthcare. Recently, the role of AI in healthcare is defined as "Augmented Intelligence" by the American Medical Association, declaring that AI is going to be designed and used to improve human intelligence rather than substituting it. The American Medical Associations opinion highlights the partnership between man and machine, which has significant suggestions for the use of AI in healthcare [10].

AI in healthcare predominantly speaks about hospitals and doctors accessing enormous datasets of possibly lifesaving information. This includes approaches to treatment as well as their outcomes, rates of existence and speed of care met across millions of patients, geographic circumstances, numerous health situations, and occasionally interrelated health conditions. Modern computational technology could identify and analyze small and large data patterns and also predict them using machine learning to classify possible health outcomes [11].

The application of AI algorithms in the field of medicine and healthcare would assist doctors to establish improved approaches and treatment strategies for patients. As well as provide doctors all the required data to make the best appropriate indication. The AI applications are being developed which are aimed at several diverse aspects of the field of medicine by most of the technology companies worldwide. In this field, the most obvious application of AI is management of the information, in which gathering, storing, standardizing or normalizing, and tracking information paths are the first step in modernizing the medical system today [12].

AI offers itself to healthcare conveyance quite well. Indeed, in recent years, there has been an exponential growth in the utilization of AI in clinical situations. As modern medication is facing an important challenge of applying, exploring, and securing organized and unstructured data to treat the diseases, AI systems with their data mining and pattern recognition abilities prove to be useful. Medical AI is chiefly worried about the advancement of AI systems that help with detection, diagnosis, management, and treatment of diseases. Medical AI application utilizes representative disease models and analyzes their connection to signs and symptoms of patients. For instance, diagnostic AI applications collect and integrate clinical data, and compare information to assist with diagnosis and treatment with pre-defined categories like diseases. Medical AI applications are not only utilized to help the diagnosis of diseases but are also used in the development of drugs, patient monitoring, and treatment protocols development [13].

AI is used in all three traditional medical tasks: diagnosis, prediction, and therapy, but it is primarily used in medical diagnosis.

Figure 1 illustrates the medical diagnostic–therapeutic cycle. In general, the cycle

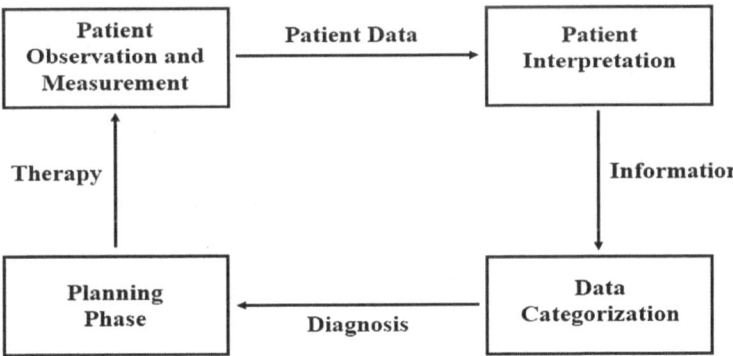

Fig. 1 Medical diagnostic–therapeutic cycle

of medical diagnosis includes patient assessment and evaluation, patient data collection, data analysis utilizing clinical expert knowledge and experience, and then the physician's formulation of the diagnosis and a treatment plan. If the medical diagnostic cycle is contrasted with the idea of an intelligent agent system, the practitioner will become the intelligent agent, the input will be the patient data and the diagnosis will become the corresponding outcome. There are many approaches by which AI systems may reproduce this diagnostic process and help practitioners with a medical diagnosis.

2   Healthcare Data Collection and Storage System

Data collection is the process of collecting and assessing targeted variable information, which further guides one in responding to the appropriate answer and evaluating the results. Data can be gathered from two data sources that are categorized as primary and secondary data sources.

- Primary Data: Data collected for the first time. Examples include Observation, Survey, Interview, and Focus groups.
- Secondary Data: Data which is already collected and analyzed by someone else. Examples include Articles on research, the Internet, and library.

In the healthcare industry, an enormous amount of data which is generated rapidly lacks information. There are many techniques through which data can be gathered for research and management of healthcare. As healthcare data are diverse in nature it is possible to collect data using both primary and secondary sources. Hospitals continue to always have data collection and reporting information systems, staffs are trained to collect data on admissions and registration, as well as an organizational culture acquainted with the quality enhancement tools, they are fairly well equipped to obtain demographic data from patients. Healthcare includes a diverse range of private and public data collection systems, like health reviews, organizational registration, and accounting records and medical information utilized by multiple organizations, like CHCs, doctors, health plans, and hospitals [14].

Collecting data from as well as on behalf of patients is a crucial part of healthcare, especially when it is essential to analyze that data to deliver the best and greatest appropriate treatment. Through the development of digitalized disease registries, the Internet has now become an immense source of information for healthcare organizations which would handle more data quickly and deliver accurate and reliable results to speed up the treatment. Providers small and large must have a strategy in place not just for the collection but also for the processing of the collected data [15].

2.1 Patient-Generated Health Data

Since technology continues to grow and expand, there are resources available which enable patients to gather and send data to their doctors and medical personnel. As the use and availability of electronic health record repositories increases, patients may use intelligent technology to share data in real time via a secure and safe platform on their phones, computer, and tablets, and also remote monitoring devices. Patient-generated health data (PGHD) may include the medical history of a person, current symptoms, biometric information, lifestyle details, and much more. This data is then sent electronically to help with diagnosis and treatment by medical professionals. Using PGHD can be beneficial in keeping providers updated regarding the progress and condition of a patient between in-person visits and allowing for ongoing health information collection. Such data can also help providers to identify and manage chronic medical needs [15].

2.2 Health Information System (HIS)

Health Information System (HIS) relates to a framework for managing data related to health care. It includes systems that collect, store, maintains and transfers a patient''s Electronic Medical Record (EMR), hospital administrative management, or decision-making systems which provides healthcare policies. Everybody in healthcare can use HIS including patients, clinicians, and public health officials. They gather data and organize it in a format which may be used to make decisions about healthcare [16]. The different types of HIS are as follows.

- **Electronic Health Record (EHR) and Electronic Medical Record (EMR) Data Systems:**

An EHR and EMR are essentially a digital representation of a patient's medical record, or chart, containing both structured and unstructured data. At a practical stage, clinical details are incorporated into systems by healthcare professionals. An EHR may comprise the medical background of a patient, health reviews, symptoms, medications, clinical findings, immunization records, image reports, test reports, and more. Several EMRs run reports mostly on information contained among them based on various areas, like diagnoses, treatments, or dates of rendered services.

However, information could be difficult to extract and manual processing is needed for certain kinds of data, such as radiological images or faxed laboratory results. Also, as each provider or health system manages its own personalized EHR system from hundreds of potential base items, individuals might have been associated with several EHR records, each formatted somewhat differently, causing issues in the quality of data. When attempting to obtain a complete image of an individual who has multiple records across systems, that can be problematic [16, 17].

- **Master Patient Index (MPI)**:

MPI links databases to separate records of the patient. For each patient, the index does have a record registered at a healthcare institution and indexes several other records for that patient. MPIs are being used to minimize redundant records of the patient and incorrect details of the patient that results in refusals of claims.

- **Patient Portals**:

Patient portals enable patients to get their personal health data, like appointment details, medicines, and laboratory outcomes over an Internet connection. A few patient portals provide for regular contact with their doctors, requests for prescription refills, and the chance for scheduling the appointments.

- **Remote Patient Monitoring or Telehealth**:

It enables medical sensors to transmit data about patients to healthcare specialists. For patients with chronic diseases, it regularly tracks blood glucose levels and blood pressure. The information is utilized to identify medical conditions which need treatment, which can become part of a broader study of health in the population.

- **Claims Processing System**:

Usually, standardized data are data developed for determinations of qualifications and billing purposes. Every healthcare payer, including private insurers, Medicaid, and medicare collect claims and other details which are described earlier. Although claim data provides a lot of knowledge about the health status of the person, it doesn't comprise the complete medical record, with the exception of the unstructured, free text and accurate demographic information. In addition, claim data is confidential to the payer and as a person can alter several times through the course of a lifespan, healthcare policies pose difficulties in knowing the full medical history of a patient.

- **Practice Management System**:

Irrespective of the existence or absence of an EHR system, healthcare facilities can also have a practice management storing and organizing patient demographic data, monitoring the services they get, and displaying insurance claims data. These systems also provide details on the cost of the services rendered and the amounts of profit obtained. HIPAA needs structured data and processing regulations when these systems exchange details electronically with payer systems.

- **Pharmacy data Systems**:

Usually, pharmacies collect the data on drugs, prescriptions, prescribers, patients, and billing that is exchanged with payers and healthcare delivery systems.

- **Public Health Departments**:

Departments of Public Health gather several kinds of details as mentioned so far, and can make it accessible in a number of different ways. Surveillance systems, registries of diseases, and reports of results are also available by request. Several health departments handle dashboards or publicly available portals with open data.

- **State Healthcare Databases**:

Majority of the states possess some kind of comprehensive system for gathering data regarding healthcare services. Certain states can collect data directly from hospitals or appoint agencies to develop reporting systems for different kinds of groups. Certain states possess databases, named All-Payer Claims Databases (APCDs), which store dental, medical and pharmaceutical claims from various public and private insurers. State specifications detail is for limited members only.

- **E-Prescribing**:

Sometimes, if the handwriting is not easily readable, a paper prescription may easily be missed and even misinterpreted. E-prescribing substitutes paperwork by enabling the doctors to directly communicate via a database to the pharmacy. Rather than turning up to pick off a prescription with the doctor''s written sheet of paper, the pharmacy could easily pull the details from the database on their computer [18].

- **Electronic Dental Records**:

The Electronic Dental Record (EDR) is basically a dental chart which is accessible in an electronic database, as per the Health Resources and Services Administration. An EDR's concept is exactly similar to an EHR because it is intended to assist the dental health specialist regarding the details required to document electronically, rather than utilizing paperwork. The electronic approach includes almost the same charting as before, like clinical reports, dental diseases, diagnosis, treatments, X-ray records, and much more. It actually makes it easier to collect all the details by integrating and arranging them together.

- **Personal Health Record**:

A personal health record is described as a record which is held by the particular patient, instead of the providers, as per the Alliance for Health Reform. It enables a patient keeping track of details from doctor's appointments, and it can also assist them to monitor their blood pressure, food consumption, and exercise schedules on their own time to help them gain a greater comprehension of their overall health.

- **Secure Messaging**:

Secure messaging is the communication system which enables patients and providers to use a standardized database to transfer medical and personal data. It essentially involves the same way as email but is subject to greater security and privacy. This makes it easier for the provider and the patient to interact on a daily basis, without thinking if they could fit it into each other's schedule.

3 Medical Data Pre-processing

The most significant and necessary steps in the acquisition of fine and final data which can be chosen as right and ideal for more tasks in data mining are Data Collection and Data Pre-processing. The data gathered by healthcare organizations can be structured or unstructured and include a broad range of data such as hospital information, physician information, patient and medical records, etc. Medical data includes text, numbers, pictures, and videos. The integration and transformation of these large and diverse data into one format require effective pre-processing tools [14].

Data mining has become much more prevalent in the healthcare industry due to the exponential progress of medical data. Data mining is perhaps the most suitable practice intended for evaluating and identifying valuable medical information. Data pre-processing plays a key role in the healthcare sector. The method of data collection is loosely regulated, culminating in missing values, data inconsistency, noisy data, etc. Such data types could generate uncertain outcomes in the analytical process. Therefore, the data must be in a processed format to produce the correct result. Therefore, the data representation and data quality are first and foremost before the analysis is performed.

Data pre-processing involves data cleaning, normalization, transformation, feature selection, and extraction, etc. The final training set is the outcome of data pre-processing. Raw data is extremely subject to noise, unpredictability, and missing values. Data pre-processing is the perfect option for improving data quality and is one of the most important phases in the process of data mining which is concerned with preparing and transforming the original dataset.

The medical data are frequently incomplete, inconsistent, or inadequate in many mistakes. The raw medical data is sometimes insufficient for even taking the correct decisions. Although the pre-processing methods produce accurate results. Nowadays, healthcare organizations produce a wide range of structured, unstructured, and semi-structured data formats. The medical data obtained from different sources of data such as hospitals, clinics, doctor's notes, patient records, and the Internet. Large and diverse data obtained from different sources can be integrated utilizing ETL tools or standard pre-processing techniques such as Excel, SQL databases, etc. Then, transforming them into a single standard format is done by several existing pre-processing tools and techniques.

The healthcare knowledge data is crucial to the victory of medical decision and treatment. Medical data pre-processing techniques also follow the normal data preprocessing techniques like data cleaning, integration, transformation and reduction. Handling of medical data is indeed a very complex challenge because it contains real-time data.

Data Pre-processing methods are classified into four categories:

- Data Cleaning—Handling missing values, data inconsistency and noisy data in the cardiac diseases database and database of other diseases.
- Data Integration—Combining data from multiple sources like physicians or doctors notes, laboratory records, etc.
- Data Transformation—Multiple data formats consolidated into a single standardized format.
- Data Reduction—Transformation of volumes of data into a minimal number of summarized reports.

3.1 Data Cleaning

Many data mining techniques depend on the dataset, which is obviously complete or noise free. Although, real-world data is very distant from being clean and complete. It's indeed prevalent to use methods in data pre-processing either to remove the noisy data or to impute i.e., to fill in the incomplete data. Medical data comprise numerous incomplete details, such as lacking many fields to be filled in by patients due to emergency situations, data collected can be noisy in some cases.

3.1.1 Missing Values Imputation

It is a quite complicated task to fill the missing values in the medical records. Managing the missing values incorrectly can quickly lead to the extraction of poor information and even to misconclusions. Missing values has been documented to induce lack of efficiency in the process of knowledge extraction. Incorrect substitution of value particularly in the medical field results in incorrect decision and treatment.

3.1.2 Noise Treatment

Two important methods are frequently used in the data pre-processing studies for treating of noise in data mining. Firstly, by using data cleaning methodologies it corrects the noisy values. It is believed that even minimal noise correction is effective however it is a challenging process and typically restricted to specific amount of noise. The second would be to utilize noise filters that recognize and delete the noisy instances in the training data, which do not require modification of the data mining methods.

3.2   Data Integration

Integration of the medical data which is stored in EMR, HER and PHR is a challenging issue. The issue of heterogeneity in the database relates equally to medical data representing individual patients and to biological data that describe our genome. Databases, in particular, are extremely heterogeneous in terms of the data models they use, the data schemas they define, the query languages they support and the terminologies they recognize. Various database systems are trying to combine the various databases by offering uniform conceptual schemas which fix representative heterogeneities and by offering querying capabilities which aggregate and integrate distributed data. Throughout this field, research has employed a wide range of databases and data mining techniques like modeling of semantic data, definition of ontology, translation of queries, optimization of queries and mapping of terms.

3.3   Data Transformation

It is a method of converting data from source format into the appropriate destination format. Medical data gathered from different sources in various formats, like database file, Excel sheet and XML document. The initial stage of data transformation is data mapping. Data mapping establishes the relation amongst the data elements of two applications, and provides guidelines on how the data is converted from the source application prior to actually being loaded into the target application. Data mapping generates the crucial metadata needed before conversion of the actual data. Several methods of transformation are introduced to transform source format into target format. They are:

- Smoothing: Removes the noise from the data.
- Aggregation: Summarization, construction of the data cube.
- Generalization: The concept of climbing hierarchy.
- Normalization: Scaled to fall within a specified limited range.
- Attribute or Feature construction.

Not all existing techniques of transformation are suitable for medical data. Data is important in making treatment decision and analysis.

3.4   Dimensionality Reduction

Data mining techniques experience the curse of dimensionality problem once datasets become huge in amount of samples or amount of predictor variables. This is a significant issue because it will obstruct the process of several data mining techniques as computational cost increases. This step can highlight the utmost important dimensionality reduction techniques according to the partition developed in Feature Selection (FS) and approaches based on space transformation. Reduction of medical data is a little challenging because each example plays a significant role in several other analysis. The data analysis allows for hospital management, fraud detection, patient care and diagnosis, etc.

3.4.1 Feature Selection

This is the method of recognizing and eliminating unnecessary information as much as possible. The aim is to get a subset of features from the actual issue which still describes it properly. This subset is widely used in training a learner, through the advanced research reporting additional benefits. Feature Selection will eliminate inappropriate and unnecessary features that can lead to unintended similarities in learning algorithms, decreasing their capacity to generalize. In the data collection phase, Feature Selection could be used to save time costs, detecting, sampling and staffs used to collect data.

3.4.2 Space Transformation

Feature Selection isn't the solitary method to deal with curse of dimensionality by decreasing the amount of magnitudes. Rather than choosing the best favorable characteristics, the techniques of spatial transformation produce up an entire new c collection of features by bringing together the original ones. Such a collection may be rendered by following various requirements. The first methods, are based on linear approaches as Factor Analysis and Principal Component Analysis (PCA).

3.4.3 Instance Reduction

Using Instance Reduction techniques is a common method to reduce the effect of the extremely large data sets. They decrease the dimension of the collected data without reducing the standard of the information which could be extracted. It is a complimentary task concerning Feature Selection. This decreases the amount of data by either eliminating the examples or creating fresh ones.

3.4.4 Instance Selection

At present the selection of instances is perceived as essential. The key challenge, is to find appropriate examples from an extremely large number of examples and later arrange them as inputs of data mining. Therefore, selection of instance is made up of a sequence of methods which should be ready to select a subset of data which may substitute the actual dataset and thus satisfy the objective of a data mining application by removing noisy and unnecessary examples from the real training data. Through contrast, methods of instance generation could produce and substitute the existing data with new artificial data, in addition to selecting data. This method enables it to cover areas within the problem domain, which do not have illustrative instances in real data, or to condense huge volumes of examples in few instances. Methods of generation of instance are also known as methods of generation of prototype, since the artificial instances generated tend to represent an area or a subset of the actual instances.

4   AI Algorithms for Healthcare

Currently, AI has transformed and id trying to transform several industries and one among them is the healthcare sector. Recently the use of machine learning and deep learning in medicine is increasing rapidly. Deep learning itself is a subsection of Machine Learning, where Machine Learning is a subsection of AI. It uses layered architecture to interpret the data in an algorithmic manner. Machine learning is a special form of computer programming in such a way that it uses an algorithm to use statistical operations against inputs to turn them into outputs without much human intervention. Even though machine learning techniques are becoming progressively better in their function, they still have to be regulated and guided to some extent. While a deep learning model can determine by itself whether or not a prediction is true through neural networks [19].

In machine learning, an algorithm requires a human with engineering and domain knowledge and experience to transform data into understandable representations for the learning algorithm to detect patterns for it. But deep learning needs less data pre-processing techniques and is capable of developing its own representations from raw data for pattern detection. The healthcare industry has thus far been suspicious about deep learning methods and recommended traditional machine learning because it can be explained. However, we can see a rise in the use of deep learning in recent years, particularly in various visual-based tasks.

Currently, there has been an enormous volume of data flowing into the healthcare system but most of the data is unreadable meaning the data is not labelled correctly and feature selection is subjective. It i s important to completely analyze and evaluate such kind of data. The deep learning network can recognize such kind of data because of its architecture. The algorithm is indeed responsible of filtering and processing data tasks which programmers would have to handle when other machine learning algorithms were to be used. While the data flows through its layers, deep learning techniques learn the features indirectly and eventually the useful data points become identifiable which means that a model becomes increasingly accurate as it processes the most data through learning from the past results [20].

Machine learning models and deep learning models learn in two different ways:

- Supervised Learning: Physicians teach an algorithm, i.e., they label and choose a set of diagnosis based on the specific clinical symptoms.
- Unsupervised Learning: Detecting data patterns without predictions, i.e., at the early phase of drug development where an algorithm is expected to make its own assumptions.

The commonly used AI algorithms in healthcare are.

4.1   Artificial Neural Networks

ANN's are a group of deep learning techniques motivated by the nervous system. More specifically, they have been motivated by a neuron organization in animal brains. They consist if units called artificial neurons which receive, process and send a signal from the previous layer to the next layer. These networks can learn from the examples by analyzing and without any direct human intervention. ANN has a lot of other uses, from pathologists using it for diagnosis to biochemical analysis. Convolutional Neural Networks (CNN) and Recurrent Neural Networks (RNN) are the two different types of neural networks that are generally used in the field of medicine [21].

4.1.1   Convolutional Neural Networks (CNN)

Imaging is indeed a significant part of medical science because it can enable a doctor to be aware of a disease long before the symptoms appear. Because of this, there are numerous screening methods like Colonoscopy, Mammograms and Pap smears. In this segment, CNN has proven crucial as the algorithm is well appropriate for binary classification and multi-class classification problem. CNN is a feed-forward neural network, a deep learning algorithm which integrates an input image, assigns weights and biases to different features of the input image, and after doing so, it is capable of distinguishing images from one another. With sufficient training, it can "learn" features and filters that need to be programmed manually in primitive AI methods. CNN can only absorb the input of fixed size and thus produce the output of fixed size.

4.1.2   Recurrent Neural Networks (RNN)

Recurrent Neural Networks are often more complicated and can absorb arbitrary inputs, producing arbitrary output data sizes while requiring even more input data than that of the CNN. Recurrent Neural Networks has proven to be important when it is used in the analysis of medical time series data for pattern recognition.

4.2   Discriminant Analysis

Discriminant Analysis is indeed a machine learning technique used to determine the appropriateness of classification of objects, as well as to assign one object to single or multiple classes. Discriminant analysis has been applied in the healthcare sector from early diagnosis of diabetic peripheral neuropathy to refining the diagnostic features of images of the blood vessels. It can also be used for detecting symptoms of mental health disorientation and for management of electronic health record systems.

4.3   K-Nearest Neighbor

It is a nonparametric ML technique, a simple classifier in which the input data sample classification is based on the class of their nearest neighbor. This is mainly used in the classification of heart disease.

4.4   Linear Regression

It is a linear statistical and machine learning technique for modeling and determining the similarity between the independent and dependent variables. Currently, linear regression is being used for predicting disease based on the risk factors.

4.5   Logistic Regression

It is a machine learning technique which makes use of regression method to determine the condition of a categorical dependent variables by using predictor variables. This is used to classify and predict the probability of an event, such as a risk assessment of disease, a function which helps doctors in making medical decisions which are critical. Also it assists medical institutions identify more vulnerable patients and curate behavioral treatment strategies to improve their daily health behaviors.

4.6   Naive Bayes

This is one of the utmost effective classification algorithms in machine learning. It is based on Bayes theorem with the assumption that the observed features are strongly independent. Because the probability distribution is high, an optimal result can be obtained by the Bayes classifier. This algorithm is commonly used for classification of medical data and for prediction of diseases.

4.7 Random Forest

It is a ML technique which constructs multiple Decision trees to perform classification and regression at the training time. It solves the problem of overfitting of decision trees. This technique is commonly used for prediction of disease risk based on the patient's past medical records and also in the analyses of Electrocardiogram (ECG) and Magnetic Resonance Imaging (MRI).

4.8 Support Vector Machine

SVM's are perhaps the most popular machine learning algorithm used by the health-care industry. SVM's use the supervised learning model for classification, regression and detection of outliers. In recent times, this algorithm has been used to predict the sensitivity of heart patients to medications, and has enabled millions to prevent severe effects, such as hospital re-admission and even death. Support Vector Machine is also used for classification of proteins, categorization of text and segregation of images. SVM's are widely used in clinical or medical research to identify imaging biomarkers, to diagnose cancer or neurological diseases and generally to classify the data from imbalanced datasets or missing value datasets.

5 AI Methodology for Medical and Medicinal Diagnosis

In recent years AI has become a particularly major topic in medicine and healthcare. The application of AI in medicine seems to have a sense of tremendous potential. Computers are now becoming smarter; in response to a specific set of conditions, they can now predict, identify and even provide suggested actions. Artificial medical intelligence provides a chance for improved treatment for people, with greater quality and precision. Applying AI to medical diagnosis has many advantages for the healthcare sector to develop. AI-based software can tell if a patient is suffering from a certain disease well before obvious symptoms appear.

- **Digital Imaging**

By using intelligent machines which are equipped with digital imaging tools, the performance of laboratory testing with AI is significantly greater. AI-based diagnostics though the AI-based medical diagnostic devices offer a shorter turnaround time than conventional microscopic testing when it comes to diagnosis [22].

- **Cloud-based Platform for Interaction**

Pathologists can send data and images to various specialists across the globe though the AI-based medical diagnosis which significantly improves research, diagnosis and collaborative diagnosis, without any need to physically migrate the sample from one location to another. In pathology, the automated technologies of AI, including AI for medical research, considerably reduce the manual errors which are often seen in physical inspections.

- **Automated Diagnosis**

Digital pathology's automated design is driven by AI that enables a pathologist to increase their efficiency by a substantial margin by reducing manual processes and tedious parts of pathology report generation. Machine learning enables more precise and timely diagnosis.

- **AI Lab Testing**

AI laboratory testing translates into intelligent algorithms capable of recognizing general and specific patterns which can then provide logical and accurate predictions for patient diseases. Medical diagnosis based on AI utilizes automated testing tools to provide a shorter response time than conventional microscopic tests.

- **Image Analysis**

AI-based medical diagnosis tends to cause an immediate transition, in which pathologists in the digital world no longer deal with glass, however with pixels that would be sent for highly specialized analysis to any part of the globe. Using image analysis techniques, AI in medical testing enables for automatic detection produced via the software's research foundation and documented data.

- **Predictive Analytics**

AI systems exploit the technology of predictive analytics to assist physicians in detecting susceptibility to the disease before it starts. That promotes a culture of preventive care rather than remedial treatment. Patients who have been susceptible to a certain disease are flagged by intelligent machine learning and hence grab the attention of a physician who will then guide on long-term care.

AI plays a significant role in medical diagnosis in pathologists by accurately identifying uncommon objects in blood, other body fluids, urine, and also in tissues. In medical diagnostic solutions, anomalies in body fluids and tissue could be detected automatically using AI.

5.1   AI Applications in Medical Diagnostics

Most of today's modern diagnostic and therapeutic applications in machine learning generally fall under the following groups [23]:

- **Chatbots**: Organizations use AI-chatbots capable of speech recognition to recognize patterns in patient's symptoms in order to establish a possible diagnosis, mitigate illness, and suggest suitable remedial actions.
- **Oncology**: Deep Learning is used by researchers to train techniques for the identification of cancer cells at a stage equivalent to that of qualified physicists.
- **Pathology**: It is the medical discipline involved with disease diagnosis dependent on the laboratory examination of body fluids like blood, urine and tissues. Machine vision and other ML techniques will increase efforts typically left only to microscopic pathologists.
- **Rare Diseases**: Machine learning is combined with facial recognition software to help clinicians diagnose rare diseases. In order to identify phenotypes that associate with rare genetic disorders, patient images are studied utilizing facial recognition and deep learning.

Below are some of the examples which currently use AI in medicine:

- **Decision-Support Systems**: DXplain originates through a series of potential diagnoses that could be relevant to the identified symptoms provided a set of symptoms [24, 25].
- **Laboratories Data Management Systems**: Germ watcher is developed to identify, monitor, as well as examine the infections in the patients who are hospitalized. This aims to minimize the cases of hospital-acquired infections by tracking the laboratory environment of a hospital, defining the community of microbiology it identifies, and reporting the findings to the National Center for Disease Control and Prevention in the US.
- **Minimizing Human Errors**: Babylon is an online platform where patients throughout UK may schedule regular examinations, appointments, as well as contact a specialist online, find symptoms, seek guidance, track their wellbeing and request testing kits.
- **Robotic Surgical Systems**: The hand movements of the doctor are converted into the robotic arms of the machine inside the da Vinci robotic surgical system. Accurate and consistent movements and magnified vision enable the doctor to conduct operations with very small cuts, and see the very pinnacle of AI in medicine inside the body in 3D.
- **Therapy**: Medication for anxiety and depression can now be accessed by signing in to AI Therapy, an online platform which provides patients with instructions about how to recognize the roots of their anxiety and depression, and a list of services tailored to meet their needs.

While both the healthcare sector and AI continue to develop and have a lot of difficult problems to be solved, AI is already the case in medical diagnosis. Below is a list of the most successful approaches using AI for solving medical problems [26]:

- **IBM's Watson for Health**: It encourages hospitals, government agencies, researchers and patients by delivering workflow-enhancing tools, improving decision-making processes, defending against fraud, and facilitating a cost-effective approach to scientific research.
- **Google Health**: It supports patients in evaluating their wellness routine and gives details on their medical problems, closest hospitals, and medication alert.
- **AI-Rad Companion Chest CT**: This is a Siemens Healthiness AI-powered healthcare solution which reads the chest CT images, performs automated measurements and prepares the medical report with useful clinical images and quantitative measurements.
- **AI-Pathway Companion**: I t i s yet another solution developed by Siemens Health-iness to improve treatment strategies by collecting all of the patient data and enabling diagnosis and therapeutic decisions along disease-specific pathways.

Industry experts are anticipating that not only current methods for using AI in medical diagnosis will be strengthened, but new methods of converging with medicine will also arise. For example, AI is expected to speed up the process of drug development. Drug development is a highly costly process. Machine Learning can help to make most of the research methods associated with the drug production most effective. It does have the ability to take off years of research and to invest hundreds of millions [27] (Fig. 2).

AI has already been widely used in all 4 major phases of drug development.

i.   **Identify Targets for Intervention**:

The very first phase of development of drugs requires knowing both of a diseases biological origins as well as its resistance mechanisms. Then the suitable goals and objectives for curing the disease (usually proteins) needs to be identified. The increasing development of high-throughput methods, like deeper screening and short hairpin RNA screening (shRNA), have greatly enhanced the amount of data required to recognize viable targeted routes. Furthermore, integration of a large amount and

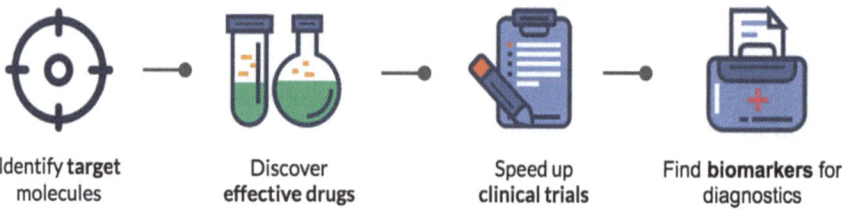

| Identify **target** molecules | Discover **effective drugs** | Speed up **clinical trials** | Find **biomarkers** for diagnostics |

Fig. 2 Drug development phases [27]

range of sources of data and then the detection of relevant patterns is indeed a challenge in traditional algorithms. ML techniques could analyze all accessible information faster, and can also learn to automatically recognize successful targeted proteins [27].

ii. **Discover Drug Candidates**:

Here it is required to discover a compound which might interact in the desired manner with the identified target molecule. This includes screening a wide range of potential compounds-sometimes several thousands, and even millions-for their impact upon the targets. These may be natural, artificial and bio-engineered compounds. Though, existing software is still unreliable and creates a huge amount of poor recommendations, hence it consumes a lot of period to limit it to the appropriate drug candidates. Here ML techniques may learn to predict a molecule's suitability dependent on molecular descriptors and structural fingerprints Then, they burn via thousands of possible molecules and then screen those all with minimum adverse reactions to the best choices. In drug design this winds up saving a significant amount of time.

iii. **Speed Up Clinical Trials**:

It is difficult to identify appropriate candidates for the clinical experiments. When wrong candidates are selected, trial will be prolonged, costing a tremendous amount of resources and time. ML will facilitate the layout of clinical experiments by mechanically selecting appropriate candidates and guaranteeing proper allocation for experiments participant classes. Techniques could assist to determine patterns which distinguish good and bad candidates. They may also serve as an early alert mechanism for clinical experiment that does not yield definitive outcomes, enabling earlier intervention by researchers and possibly saving the drugs development.

iv. **Finding Biomarkers for Disease Diagnosis**:

The patients may be treated for a disease once diagnosis is assured. A few methodologies are quite cost effective and require complex laboratory equipment's and specialist knowledge, like sequencing of the whole genome. Biomarkers are molecules found in bodily fluids which provide absolute confirmation whether or not a patient has a disease. They make the process for diagnosing a disease safe and affordable. They may also be utilized to detect disease progression, making it very easy for doctors to select the best medication and track if the drug is effective. But it is hard to discover suitable Biomarkers for a particular disease. This is one more expensive, time-consuming method which requires sampling of thousands of possible candidates for the molecule. AI could automatize and speed up a substantial part of human activity. The algorithms categorize molecules into good and bad candidates, enabling clinicians concentrate on analyzing the best opportunities.

The biomarkers may be utilized to recognize:

- Biomarker for Diagnosis: Existence of a disease as soon as possible.
- Biomarker for Risk: A patient's stake of evolving the disease.

- Biomarker for Prognostic: Probable disease progression.
- Biomarker for Predictive: If a patient is responding to a drug.

Biopharmaceutical companies are rapidly becoming aware of the effectiveness, precision and information which AI could offer because of advancements in technology. One of the largest drug discovery AI advancements happened in 2007, when investigators entrusted a robot called Adam with functions for yeast research. In public databases, Adam searched hundreds of millions of datasets to postulate regarding the activities of 19 genes inside yeast, identifying 9 latest and reliable postulates. Adam's robot companion, Eve, exposed that Triclosan, a primary component in toothpaste, could battle parasites that are based on malaria [28].

- **BioXcel Therapeutics (AI in Biopharmaceutical Development)**

It utilizes AI to predict and discover different medicines in the field of Neuroscience and Immuno-Oncology. In fact, the drug renovation study at the organization implements AI to identify potential uses for current medicines or to recognize the new patients. This research in drug discovery based on AI has been recognized as one of the "Most Creative Healthcare AI Innovations of 2019."

- **Berg Health (Treating Rare Disease with AI)**

BERG is a clinical-stage, AI centered biomedical system which maps diseases to promote innovative drug innovation and growth. By integrating its "Interrogative Biology" method with traditional research and development, BERG is capable of developing more effective drug candidates to combat rare diseases. At the Neuroscience 2018 conference, BERG, in recent times, introduced its research on the treatment of Parkinson's disease, using AI to identify interactions among chemicals in the body of human which were not known previously.

- **Xtalpi (AI, Cloud-based Digital Drug Discovery)**

XtalPi's ID4 platform incorporates AI, cloud, and quantum physics to predict the chemical and pharmaceutical properties of small-molecule candidates for drug design and development. In fact, the company says its predictive crystal structure technology predicts complex molecular structures in days rather than weeks or months.

- **Deep Genomics (Finding Better Candidates for Developmental Drugs)**

Deep Genomics AI platform is helping researchers identify candidates for neuromuscular and neurodegenerative disorder-related developmental drugs. Identifying the perfect candidates during the production of a drug has significantly improved the probability of passing clinical trials successfully, while also reducing the time and expenditure to market. Deep Genomics also works on "Project Saturn" that analyzes more than 69 billion different cell compounds and gives feedback to researchers.

6 Selection and Extraction of Features Using AI

The problem of variable selection has been extensively studied for various reasons, like classification, clustering and function approximation, becoming the subject of several research works in which hundreds and thousands of variables can be found in datasets. The possible input variables sub-set can be described by two distinct methods:

- Feature Selection: Selection of features helps to reduce the dimension by choosing a subset of the actual input variables.
- Feature Extraction: Extraction of features transforms the actual variables to produce more important features.

When the data under consideration have a huge amount of features, it's beneficial to decrease those to enhance the study of the data. For severe cases, the amount of variables may greatly surpass the amount of samples accessible, resulting in the curse of dimensionality problem that tends to a reduction in the precision of the learning technique whenever there is an increase in the number of features. The key justification for trying to reduce data involves the necessity to decrease the computation time of the provided learning technique, enhance its accuracy, and as well as to improve the information and understanding of the challenge under consideration by figuring out the aspects that directly influence it [29].

6.1 Feature Selection

By discovering the greatest minimal subset without transforming data into a new set, the feature selection method minimizes the dimension of a data-set of variables possibly related to a given process. Selection of feature highlights all of the input data which affect the process under discussion and is a significant pre-processing stage for data in various areas like data mining, ML, medical data and pattern recognition as well as many others. Selection of feature has also been extensively spread in platforms like classification, estimation and clustering of functions [29].

The complexity in removing the more appropriate variables is primarily because of the huge size of actual set of variables, the associations among the input data that cause duplication and finally the existence of variables that do not impact the phenomenon considered and therefore do not have any predictive power, for example when implementing a model which is trying to predict the outcome of a given system. The following main factors must be taken into consideration when selecting the correct subset of input variables:

- Relevance: The amount of variables selected has to be verified to prevent the likelihood of having fewer variables that don't communicate useful details.
- Efficiency in Computation: When the amount of variables considered for inputs is large, the computation complexity rises. This is apparent while performing

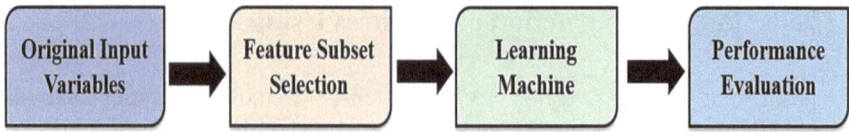

Fig. 3 Filter method generic scheme

ANN. In addition, the process of training an ANN is more complex, comprising inappropriate variables, since inappropriate variables create noise and slows down network training.

- Improving knowledge: Optimized choice of input variables leads to a broader knowledge of the behavior of the procedure.

To summarize, optimum input variables set should include the smallest amount of variables required to characterize the action of the system or process under consideration with minimal duplication and informative variables. If the optimum set of input variables is determined, then it is possible to develop a precise, effective, cheaper and easier to interpret model. Feature selection approaches are divided into three types: Filter, Wrapper, and Embedded approaches.

6.1.1   Filter Method

This method is perhaps a preprocessing step, irrespective of the learning technique used for adjusting as well as constructing the model which utilizes the variables selected as inputs. The filters are mathematically efficient but could get impacted by the issues of overfitting. Figure 3 illustrates a standard method.

The appropriate variables subset is obtained by estimating input -output relationship of the method being considered. When considering statistical tests, all input variables are categorized based on their importance to the target. The key benefit of this method is the low computation complication that ensures efficiency for the system. Key drawback of the filter method is that this approach could not modify the preferred system in the training machine, independently of the algorithm being used adjust or develop the model that is provided as inputs with variables selected. The prevalent methods for filtering are: Chi-square, Correlation and Information Gain methods.

6.1.2   Wrapper Method

Wrapper methods treat ML as a black box for selecting variables subsets dependent on their prediction ability. The general concept would be to utilize a given learning machine's predictive efficiency or classification accuracy to estimate the efficacy of a chosen features subsets. Figure 4 illustrates the general system regarding the Wrapper method.

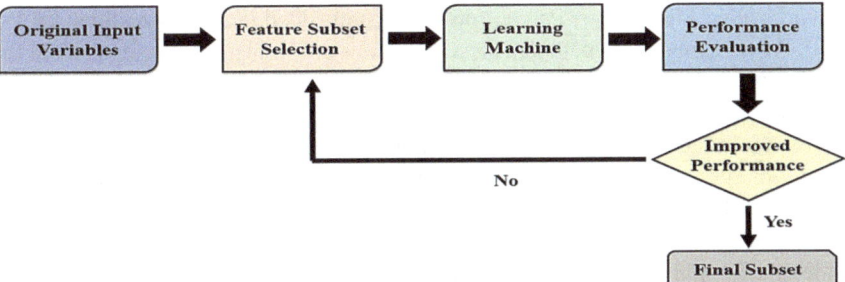

Fig. 4 Wrapper method generic scheme

Wrapper approach is computationally more costly than filter method, which could be perceived as an alternative to brute force. Wrapper approaches are simple and universal, considering the learning machine to be a black box. If the amount of variables becomes too large, the comprehensive search is impossible to afford. The commonly used wrapper methods are: Genetic algorithm method and Greedy Strategy.

6.1.3 Embedded Method

During the training phase, the variables are selected, thereby decreasing the computational expense and enhancing the effectiveness during selection of variables. The distinction amongst embedded method and wrapper method may not be apparent at all times, however the key fact is that embedded approach needs repetitive modifications as well as the development of model parameters is dependent on the models results. In addition, the wrapper method treats just the output of the chosen set of variables as model. Figure 5 demonstrates a common embedded solution scheme.

The learning machine and the feature selection must be implemented in embedded approaches, the structure of the functions considered plays a significant part. For example, the significance of a variable is evaluated via a restriction which has a logical meaning for classifiers based on SVM. An innovative model of the neural

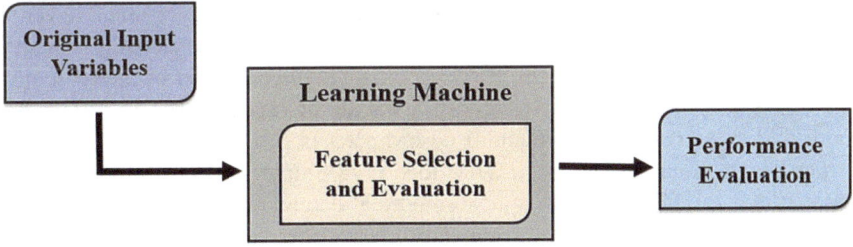

Fig. 5 Embedded method generic scheme

network called Multi-Layer Perceptron's uses Embedded Feature Selection (MLPs-EFS). As an Embedded method, selection aspect of the feature is integrated in the learning process. W.r.t traditional Multi-Layer Perceptron's this method incorporates a preprocessing step in which a scaling factor multiplies each variable.

Whenever the scalable variable is minimal the features are deemed as unnecessary whereas the features are appropriate when large. The major benefit is that most optimal techniques utilized for Multi-Layer Perceptron's are suitable for Multi-Layer Perceptron's uses Embedded Feature Selection as well. When comparison is made against additional current approaches like Fisher Discriminant Ratio (FDR) connected with Multi-Layer Perceptron's or Support Vector Machine with Recursive Feature Elimination (RFE), the authors show the efficacy of the proposed method. Results indicate that the MLPs-EFS is outperforming the other approaches considered. Another positive outcome of this method lies in its generalization that enables it to be extended to other neural networks [29].

6.2   Feature Extraction

Extraction of features is a method which by applying certain mapping, converts high-dimensional data into low-dimensional feature space. A major challenge in the investigation on NN, as well as in many additional fields involved in the area of AI is seeking a suitable depiction of multi-variate data. In this context, feature extraction is utilized to minimize complication as well as to provide simplified interpretation of the data, depicting every factor as linear combinations of the actual input variables in the feature space. If the extracted features are chosen correctly, then a simplified dataset can be used to perform with that of the related details from input data. Principal Component Analysis (PCA) is the most widely known technique for extraction of features, but several other alternatives have been introduced in the last years [29].

6.2.1   Principal Component Analysis (PCA)

PCA is unsupervised technique and comprises of an orthogonal transition that transform illustrations of related variables into illustrations of unrelated linear features. The newest features are considered as principal components and are much fewer or equivalent to the original variables. When the data is distributed usually, the principal components become independent. It converts data mathematically by applying it to a particular co-ordinate system for acquiring the initial largest variance on the initial coordinate and so on for the remaining co-ordinates [29].

The key justification for using PCA is that it is a simpler nonparametric approach that is utilized in extracting the utmost important details from a collection of noisy data. This approach decreases the amount of accessible variables by removing the principal components that are last, which won't contribute meaningfully to the detected variation. It is also a linear data transition, which reduces redundancy and significantly increases information.

6.2.2 Linear Discriminant Analysis (LDA)

LDA is a widely known supervised technique that is commonly utilized in Computer Vision, ML, Pattern Recognition, as well as additional relevant areas. It carries out an optimum prediction by increasing the distance among classes as well as at the same time, minimizing the distance among samples within every class. This method reduces dimensionality, retaining as much as possible class discriminatory data. The key drawback of this method is that it can generate small amount of feature predictions. When there is need for more features some other approach should be used. When using LDA, the input data is assumed to follow a Gaussian distribution, so using LDA to non-Gaussian data may lead to poorly categorized results.

Furthermore, LDA is a parametric approach but it loses when the biased data doesn't lie in the average value however lies in the data variability. LDA is not a suitable approach when data dimensionality overwhelms number of illustrations, which is recognized as the issue of singularity. In such circumstances the dimensionality of the data could be minimized by implementing the PCA prior to LDA technique. This method is known as PCA + LDA. Other methods addressing the issue of singularity include Null-Space LDA (NLDA), Orthogonal Centroid Method (OCM), Regularized LDA (RLDA) and Uncorrelated LDA (ULDA).

6.2.3 Latent Semantic Analysis (LSA)

LSA was presented as a variation of the PCA idea. Initially, LSA was introduced as technique of text analysis whenever the features were described by words that appear in the manuscript in consideration. LDA is subsequently used for audio analysis, image analysis, music analysis and video data. The LSA process's main purpose is to generate a mapping into a Latent Semantic Space (LSS) also known as Latent Topic Space (LTS). LSA identifies co-occurrence of words in records to offer a mapping into the LTS in which records could be linked if they include some common words regarding the actual space.

Sparse-LSA chooses hardly a limited pertinent terms for every subject offering a compressed depiction of the relations between subject and word. The key benefit of this method resides in the computation productivity as well as in the lower memory needed to store matrix of the projection. When comparing Sparse-LSA with LDA and LSA via experimentation on various real-world datasets, the results show that Sparse-LSA has comparable output w.r.t LSA however it is much more accurate and effective in computing the prediction, storage and best describes the relationships of the subject-world.

6.2.4 Independent Component Analysis (ICA)

ICA method aims in identifying linear representations of non-Gaussian data and statistically independent of the components calculated. It is a linear dimensionality reduction approach which takes a combination of independent components as input data and targets to accurately describe each component by removing all unwanted noise. When both their linear and non-linear dependence is equivalent to zero, two input features could be considered independent.

ICA could be utilized to extract input space features which find independent directions. This method is much more complicated than using the PCA method, because in PCA, the variability of the information along the path may be computed instantly and maximized by PCA alone, whereas there is no direct metric for measuring the individuality of the input space direction. Neural network algorithms have recently been implemented to remove the individual components. ICA is popularly used in medical applications like EEG and fMRI analysis to differentiate useful signals from inappropriate ones.

7 Disease Diagnosis with AI

It requires years of medical training to accurately diagnose diseases. Diagnosis is indeed a complex, time-consuming method even then. In several disciplines specialist demand far exceeds the supply available. This tends to put doctors under pressure and stress and quite often delays patient diagnosis that will save lives. AI, particularly DL techniques have achieved huge improvements recently in diagnosing the diseases automatically, making diagnosis affordable as well as more accessible. AI techniques will learn to see patterns in a same manner to doctors. A major difference is that in order to learn, algorithms need a lot of specific samples. And then these examples have to be digitalized smoothly because machines cannot read amid the lines in the textbook. AI is especially useful in fields where the medical details that a physician analyses has already been digitized [27].

Examples include:

- Lung cancer and strokes are detected based on CT scans.
- Evaluating the danger of unexpected cardiac demise or even other cardiac illnesses based on ECG and cardiac MRI images.
- Classification of skin conditions in images of the skin.
- Diabetic Retinopathy signs could be found in the images of eye (Fig. 6).

As abundance of quality data is accessible in these situations, diagnostic techniques are becoming as efficient as specialists. The variance is that, techniques could derive the results within a couple of seconds, and could be replicated quickly and efficiently throughout the globe. Soon everyone is going to get access towards the identical standard of best radiology diagnosis specialists worldwide, and even at a reduced price.

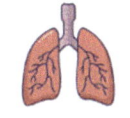 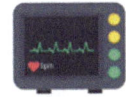 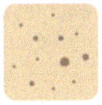 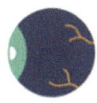

Detecting **lung cancer** from CT Scans   Assess **cardiac health** from electrocardiograms   Classify **skin lesions** from images of the skin   Identify **retinopathy** from eye images

Fig. 6 Disease diagnosis examples [27]

AI is just beginning to be implemented in disease diagnosis—many ambitious systems include integrating several sources of data (CT, Genomics, MRI, patient records, Proteomics and even hand-written documents) to determine a disease and its progress. The specialist would use AI systems to identify potential malignant lesions or risky heart patterns, enabling the physician to concentrate on interpreting those signals.

A research released by Lancet Digital Health recently examined the success of DL which is a form of AI in the identification of diseases through medical imaging against healthcare specialists, using a systematic literature review conducted between 1 January 2012 and 6 June 2019. The study reported that AI has become much more effective in these images in recognizing disease diagnosis over the past few decades, and it has become a more reliable source of diagnostic knowledge. In addition, when assessing the diagnostic efficiency of the AI relative to that of healthcare professionals, the researchers analyzed two results: specificity and sensitivity. "Sensitivity" describes the probability that a diagnostic test would have a favorable result in people with the disease. Specificity refers to the precision of the diagnostic test that enhances the measure of sensitivity. As per the researchers, the diagnostic output was found to be equal for 14 studies that examined deep learning techniques and healthcare professionals within the same sample [30, 31].

Most precisely, the study showed that AI would accurately diagnose diseases in 87% of cases, however detection by healthcare professionals provided an efficiency rate of 86%. The accuracy for deep learning techniques was 93%, relative to 91% for humans.

With advances in AI, over the next several years, deep learning can become much more effective in recognizing diagnosis. Bayer, a pharmaceutical company, recently partnered with technology companies to build software which helps to diagnose complex and unusual disorders as well as assist to invent new medicines for treating these diseases. They have also been collaborating with hospitals and researchers to identify what else AI needs to examine in order to better understand how to identify the medical status of the patient. The data the AI absorbs comes from a variety of factors that come from symptoms data, causes of disease, test results, medical images, physician reports and much more.

The aim of AI is to make computers most efficient in resolving challenging problems of healthcare as well as by making use of computers, data acquired through diagnosis of different chronic diseases such as Alzheimer's disease, Cardiovascular disease, Diabetes and numerous kinds of cancer such as Breast cancer, Colon cancer, etc., can be analyzed. This enables the detection of various chronic diseases that minimize the financial burden and disease progression. Different computational systems and devices like Arterial Spin Labeling (ASL) Imaging, ASL-MRI, Biomarkers, Brain-Computer Interfaces (BCIs) and numerous different techniques assist eliminate errors and track the progress of diseases. Computer aided decision support systems, diagnostics, experts systems as well as software integration can help doctors reduce the variance of inter and intra observers [32].

In order to simplify the diagnosis procedure, AI approaches especially ANN and Fuzzy method could be applied to manage various types of medical data. Artificial Neural Networks method detects the concealed connections as well as patterns in medical data and is efficient in scheming clinical support systems. AI application helps facilitate high-precision and speed interpretation of the results. Cardiovascular diseases, cancers, chronic respiratory diseases and diabetes are the four primary categories of non-communicable diseases or chronic diseases. Efficient identification of any non-communicable diseases will be of great help in reducing disease compilations. This assists in determining strategies for the treatment. There have been numerous protocols for identification and treatment that validate that AI is a boon to healthcare. The aim of AI is just to make computers most effective in resolving the problems of healthcare and by making use of computers, data acquired through diagnosis of different chronic diseases can be analyzed.

7.1 AI in Breast Cancer

Breast cancer is the main source of concern world-wide. This is the most regularly identified cancer among females, but may happen in males as well. It grows as cells expand and increase uncontrollably, that creates a neoplasm or tumor. Cancer may be identified at an early phase, using screening tests. Mammography is perhaps the greatest powerful method for identifying this cancer at its earlier and curable phase. AI has built devices which accurately understand mammogram data, instinctively convert the charts of patients into diagnosis data that estimates the danger of breast cancer accurately. The advent of digital mammography is considered to be the greatest development in breast imaging [32].

Techniques which rely on the principles of smart systems, like Computer-Aided Design techniques, Decision Trees, Fuzzy Logic method, Linear Programming methods, NN and Nearest-Neighbor methods. Presently, Curemetrix technique, Genes to Systems Breast Cancer Database (G2SBC), iT Bra, NLP software and Triple Negative Breast Cancer Database intelligent systems are being utilized for detecting the breast cancer.

- Computer-Aided Diagnosis (CAD) systems utilize digital technology to identify mammograms irregularities, also radiologists use these outcomes for identification, which plays a significant part. The output of CAD may vary from individual state since certain tumors are much harder to identify than the others, since they may possess identical properties to usual mammary tissues.

- Increased breast density generally suggests greater likelihood of malignant tissue being present. Without the knowledge of their overall brightness, a human spectator could differentiate diverse structures. In the automated classification of breast density, it's necessary to make the decision as to which factors offer the greatest partition among groups.
- Cycardia Health has created a smart, wearable monthly breast scanning device called iTBra. It might be a significant AI technique for early detection of breast cancer. These breast patches are equipped with detectors that monitor variance temperature variations over times that are assumed to be a circadian cellular transition induced by decreased PER1 (Period Estrogen Receptor) and Protein expression of PER2 in the existence of breast cancer. The Cyrcadia predictive algorithmic production shows an unusual metabolic pattern of variant when the tissue is healthy. The varying pattern of metabolic behavior is condensed in the case of cancer or reveals much like a straight lined pattern in tissue-infused tumors.
- Curemetrix technique identifies what projection of the breast has already been developed and also generates a specific "breast health score" for every image that can contribute to better interpretation of medical image and quantification of anomalies.
- G2SBC is a resource that incorporates data on transcripted genes and altered protein in breast cancer cells. This database symbolizes a systemically biologically focused approach to data integration dedicated to breast cancer.
- ANN is used to classify cancerous and non-cancerous images. Their capacity to learn from past examples has prepared them to be a very appealing analytical technique in healthcare, analyzing nonlinear data, handling inaccurate details and simplifying the model's application to independent data.
- Fuzzy logic is being used for predicting survival of breast cancer patients. An intelligent technique for helping in the breast cancer diagnosis as well as for the second opinion, utilized to process and organize the data acquired from fine needle aspirate breast mass smears.
- NLP software techniques for mammographic image characteristics as well as mammogram reports offer the clinical decision support system with an automated way to assist in data extraction and analysis.

7.2   Management of Alzheimer's Disease with AI:

The utmost prevalent neurodegenerative disease till date, without much treatment or preventive therapy, is Alzheimer's disease. It is the foremost cause of mental deterioration, resulting in significant memory loss, multiple cognitive function impairment and changes in behavior affecting a large population worldwide.

Use of AI can aid in early identification of this incurable disease. Usage of various automated systems and techniques such as Arterial Spin Labeling Magnetic

Resonance Imaging (ASL-MRI), Brain Computer Interfaces (BCIs), Electroencephalogram (EEG), Positron Emission Tomography (PET), Single Photon Emission Computed Tomography (SPECT) scans and numerous algorithms assist in reducing error, detect early and control progression of the disease. Usage of various AI algorithms in brain MRI scans provides a blueprint for distinguishing among early phases of this disease.

- ASL-MRI is pledging functional biomarker which produces maps of perfusion that identify patterns of blood perfusion in different parts of the brain that help detect various phases of Alzheimer's disease. MRI combined with ASL might interrupt or delay the progression of disease from subjective mental impairment to slight mental impairment to Alzheimer's disease. Usage of automatized ML approach has possible usage in Alzheimer's disease administration.
- BCIs assist Alzheimer's disease patients communicate simple opinions by transmitting instructions to an exterior origin from the brain.
- Electroencephalograms (EEG) have been used in research and diagnosis of AD as a reliable tool. It is a technology for brain imaging that is simple, noninvasive, and possibly portable. EEG does have a higher spatial resolution and hence can include essential details regarding irregular brain processes in patients with AD. Three main consequences of AD on EEG were observed: EEG stagnation, decreased EEG signal complexity, and EEG synchrony disturbances.
- PET scan is a practical technique in brain imaging which offers knowledge regarding brain physiological and biological mechanisms. PET scan tests the incremental and associated cerebral metabolic rate of glucose with AD. Flurodeoxyglucose (FDG) PET metabolic tracer is extensively used in Alzheimer's disease. FDG PET gives a successful biomarker of disease development, glucose consumption in Alzheimer's disease, and Flurodeoxyglucose becomes damaged in the brain. PET is being utilized in identifying the individuals at danger for Alzheimer's disease well in advance of the indications begin which serves as an important initial diagnostic tool.
- SPECT is a technique in molecular imaging that can have an understanding of the regional cerebral blood flow. Most SPECT research have found the hypoperfusion pattern in the area of the temporal and parietal cortex. Such variations in SPECT perfusion arise in normal brain areas, and disease helps to detect AD early.

Early identification of AD through AI assists in the early beginning of AD treatment that delays the development of the disease, increases the patient's life quality, and thereby decreases the economic cost responsible for managing healthcare.

7.3 Management of Diabetic Complications Using AI

Diabetes is a progressive, non-communicable metabolic disease defined through increased blood glucose. Rise in blood glucose is found because of pancreatic β-(Type I) destruction or insulin resistance (Type II) cells. Development of the disease tends to severe complications of the micro or macrovascular, such as cardiomyopathy, nephropathy, neuropathy, as well as retinopathy.

One of the early phases of diabetic neuropathy is amputation of the foot. To track and for early identification, a team of researchers from the Hebrew University of Jerusalem and the Hadassah Medical Center created SenseGO, a washable intelligent sock, capable of tracking changes in pressure on the patient's foot. It includes numeral pressure sensors which gather data about pain, improper position, over-exertion, and unfitting shoes-the factors that are accountable for foot ulcers. Furthermore, it transmits the collected data to the smartphone application.

For diabetic patients, peripheral diabetic neuropathy is the main source of impairment. Morphometric parameters of the corneal nerves may allow an early diagnosis. Ferreira and colleagues proposed a fully automated algorithm for the extraction of morphometric parameters and the segmentation of the corneal nerves. They intensified the corneal images via phase shift analysis, Hessian matrix computation performed the structure classification and then morphological approaches were used to create nerves. The algorithm developed provided better outcomes for nerve search as well as measuring the length of the nerve.

An independent forecaster of cardiovascular disease and diabetic nephropathy is Microalbuminuria (MA). Microalbuminuria identification is indeed a very significant screening device for identifying diabetic nephropathy. Marateb and colleagues proposed a Fuzzy MA classifier model for predicting Microalbuminuria without urine albumin measurements. They typically utilized clinical factors tracked in patients with Type II diabetes. Implementation of the law was achieved by optimization of the particle swarm. Multiple logistic regressions were performed with statistical features. As input parameters were used Age, BMI, Bs2hpp, CHOL, DD, FBS, Gender, HbA1c, HDL, LDL, Systolic BP, and TG. MA classifier performance was evaluated using ten-fold cross-validation. The suggested fuzzy classification scheme with the removal of the feature had a minimal Accuracy, Precision, Sensitivity, and Specificity of 92%, 84%, 95%, and 85%, respectively.

Among diabetic patients, deterioration in kidney functioning is variable; therefore, determinants of diabetic nephropathy are hard to predict. Cho and colleagues implemented different ML techniques like Feature Selection approaches and Support Vector Machine classification, and created a new visualization method that makes use of a nomogram method. The suggested technique will anticipate the occurrence of diabetic nephropathy approximately 2–3 months in advance to actual diagnosis. In addition, the visualization method gives doctors insightful knowledge for the study of risk factors.

Sanchez and colleagues assessed the results of a robust CAD system for diabetic retinopathy screening, by means of a freely accessible retinal image database, and contrasting its results with those of human specialists. They implemented a recently established CAD system for 1200 digital fundus color photographs. Under the ROC curve, the system has attained a region of 0.876 to efficiently distinguish normal images by those with DR, with the Sensitivity of 92.2% at a Precision of 50%.

7.4   ANN in Diagnosis of Cardiovascular Diseases

Substantial data is provided about cardiovascular disorders varying from details of indications to various kinds of biochemical data and outcomes of imaging devices to promote clinician diagnosis. ANN is a computational or mathematical model motivated by biological neural networks' functional and structural characteristics. ANN requires the comprehensive utilization of science and technology. This has also been used in the prediction of pathology disease probability. It has also proved its use in the study of leukemia detection, diabetes diagnosis and tuberculosis, radiography, and the image analysis of living tissue. The most significant use of this approach is in cardiovascular disease diagnosis. Based on the details available on different risk factors like age, alcohol consumption, cholesterol, cigarette smoking, diabetes, history of the family, high and physical inactivity, obesity, this technique could predict heart diseases.

For 331 elderly patients with anterior chest pain, Baxt et al. utilized ANN for the diagnosis of myocardial infarction and contrasted the precision and accuracy of the diagnosis with that of the clinician attending the patient. ANN was used in the analysis utilizing the available clinical information of 351 hospitalized patients for MI and subsequently the ANN method that examined the data on 331 patients with anterior chest pain. The research findings have shown that ANN can be a valuable diagnostic aid for myocardial infarction. In some other studies, the method used conventional and genetic factors to diagnose coronary heart disease. The research implicated the use of data fed into the system from the angiographic coronary, clinical, functional, laboratory, and single nucleotide polymorphism. The system was then utilized for diagnosing 487 patients resulting in accuracy up to 64% of accurate coronary heart disease diagnosis. Also, it is successfully utilized for the diagnosis of heart valve situations in the classification of cardiac sound signals measured by a stethoscope. Even with ischemia in myocardial perfusion imaging, the outcomes with substantial diagnosis accuracy have been very encouraging.

8   Medical Image Processing with AI

Medical image processing can be referred to as handling the images by the use of a computer. It includes several kinds of methods and processes like image gaining, storing, presenting, and communicating. Medical imaging is the method of producing graphical images of the body's inner structures for scientific and medical research, treatment, and care, and also a clear view o f he internal tissue function. Because of advances in image processing methods, like image analysis, improvement and recognition, medical imaging is growing quickly. Image processing enhances the proportion and volume of tissues identified. The image is a function which means the measurement of characteristics like light or color of a seen sight. Image processing technique is the use of computer for digital image manipulation [33].

For several years, doctors have employed medical imaging methods for treating diseases such as cancer. Furthermore, AI has the ability to expand this technology further and enhance potentials for medical imaging, including higher efficiency and improved productivity. AI could enhance processes of medical imaging such as image processing, and aid with the diagnosis of patients. With several implemented AI solutions as well as many other AI applications demonstrating successful scientific test outcomes, it is expected that the market for AI in medical imaging will increase substantially over the coming years [34].

AI-based medical imaging depends on a wide variety of medical case data to train its algorithms to determine patterns in images and to recognize different anatomical markers. By rigorously analyzing patterns in a provided digital image, the imaging techniques are able to extract metrics and performance which complement the radiologist's analysis which could be beneficial for rapid diagnosis. Through specialized equipment which can process more than 100 high-resolution diagnostic images incredibly fast, radiologists are now able to create distinct measurements and pinpoint information which are very difficult to capture with a naked eye [35].

AI-based medical imaging has led to significant advancements in economy, precision, and safety of patient care. In addition to allowing perfect diagnosis or timely treatment contributing to improved health outcomes, it also facilitates efficiency and quality control in the radiological workflow. Also, it offers automatic risk stratification, which could be an effective tool to classify high-risk patients so that personalized and optimized medical care can be received. AI-based medical imaging will certainly not replace radiologists but will increase them in clinical care and support for clinical decisions, thus helping to minimize the error and cost of professional misconduct.

Key Segments in AI-based Medical Imaging:

8.1 Breast Imaging

AI has proven useful for radiologists in the diagnosis of different medical situations allowing healthcare services around the globe to give their patients quality breast care. Complicated and innovative imaging techniques like Digital Breast Tomosynthesis (DBT), commonly known as 3D mammography, has enhanced visualization of the tumor and offered a remarkable degree of specificity when it refers to tumor analysis. DBT integration with ultrasound and MRI has improved precision in clinical diagnosis, thereby reducing the errors or recalls. This also assists in early breast cancer detection and possible mammographic abnormalities quickly and more effectively. AI systems may also assist radiologists to categorize patients depending on various data points, like breast density, individual medical background, and risk, thus directing patients to the correct interpreting radiologists, enabling efficient workflows.

8.2 Cardiovascular Imaging

Presently, AI-based medical imaging is playing a crucial role in Cardiology. A detailed cardiac analysis can now be accomplished using extremely integrated and devoted software which contains the necessary MRI tools for such processes. It has enabled the avoidance of invasive diagnostic procedures such as angiography, cardiac catheterization, and surgical examination. For example, Artery's cardiac MRI can automate the processes involved in a complicated cardiovascular study, through machine learning and trained models. HeartVista, a platform for developing and running state-of-the-art MRI applications, is composed of many highly developed MRI methods which produce images with high quality much faster than conventional imaging methods. All these systems are instances of how AI helps to advance rapidly and perhaps a more accurate diagnosis of cardiovascular diseases.

8.3 Lung Imaging

Lung Imaging is another area which has greatly benefitted from AI. Doctors now use AI technology to screen and examine detailed images of the lungs such as the lung parenchyma, airways, and vasculature. This technology enables for an efficient and high-resolution examination of the lungs enhancing efficiency in the screening of lung cancer. As a result, the efficient and effective detection of lung cancer features and lesions is increased. An organization leading in the development of AI is a start-up of AI called Infervision, whose enhanced CT screening solution (AI-CT) can accurately comprehend suspicious lesions of lung cancer in CT scans. This technology is helping in the early detection and diagnosis of lung cancer.

8.4 Neurological Imaging

It is also known as Neuroimaging or Brain Imaging. It is the usage of diverse approaches for generating images of a brain structure and function of the brain or some other parts of the nervous system. AI plays a key role in the detection and diagnosis of brain injury and the trauma with which he diagnoses certain diseases. This technology is integrated with Computerized Axial Tomography or Computerized Tomography (CAT or CT) and Magnetic Resonance Imaging (MRI) to achieve detailed visualization of the central nervous system [35].

AI is a key factor in medical imaging market growth. Signify Research has released a prediction stating that by 2023, AI in medical imaging will become a 2 billion dollar industry [34, 36] (Fig. 7).

World Market for AI-Based Medical Image Analysis Software by Algorithm Type
Revenue Forecast ($m)

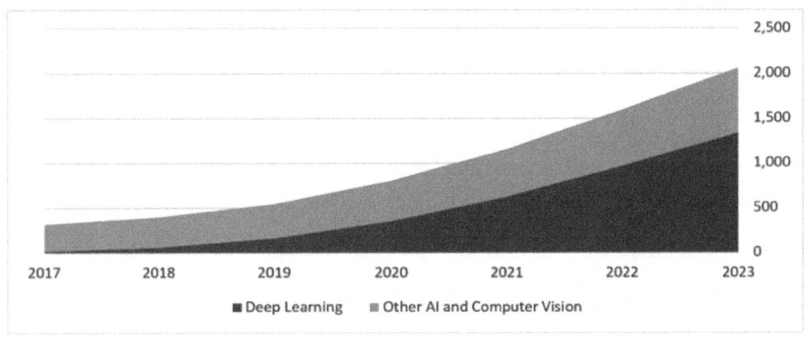

Source: Signify Research   Jul-18

Fig. 7 Revenue forecast for global medical image analysis software (signify research) [34, 36]

9   Patient Care and Treatment with AI

Patient care is perhaps the most key aspect of any hospital, and patient care technology is implemented in hospitals should be important in enhancing the quality of care and treatment. New advanced technology will be used in future smart hospitals, an environment of platforms and staff willing to redesign the care and treatment process and effectively meet patient needs using the latest technologies. The smart hospital environment can also be expanded to digital homes after discharge. This environment enables the continuous tracking, storage, and analysis of patient data. AI and Robotics are already evolving as important patient care and disease management technologies, particularly in the European Union, where new health and safety regulations are in effect [37].

AI has been transforming the healthcare field including guidelines for diagnosis and treatment, patient contact, and coordination of care. Numerous AI applications are available which can enhance patient care and help save lives. These applications include recognition of patterns, robotics, and NLP, including speech recognition and translation [38]. Increasingly, healthcare organizations embrace machine learning as well as other aspects of AI to enhance patient experience, care, and treatment results. Developing mobile apps to evaluate patient issues, away from standard medical terminology, to better understand the state of the patient, and eventually prescribe treatment and care options.

Some instances of the new tools leveraging AI as well as its subgroups to extend the numerous medical and healthcare industries, such as:

- **Virtual assistants**

This AI-driven platform may support people suffering from Alzheimer's disease with their everyday jobs. For instance, 59-year-old Brian Leblanc, who had been diagnosed with Alzheimer's early-onset disease in 2014, began to use Alexa on his Amazon Echo Dot for reminders to eat, bathe, and take medicine. This helps him to have more control over his life [38].

- **MelaFind**

This technology evaluates pigmented lesions using infrared light. Dermatologists can examine abnormal moles using algorithms, and diagnose severe skin cancers like melanoma. This technology can help to give an early identification.

- **Robotic-Assisted Therapy**

Bionik Laboratories in Toronto and Watertown, Mass., are using robots and AI to help patients recover from their strokes. A robotic arm and hand use computer algorithms to identify and direct movements which patients may not be able to perform during therapy. It will also assist patients to perform more recorded motions per hour than they would have if they were working with a physical therapist alone.

- **Caption Guidance**

This AI-powered technology has been approved by the Food and Drug Administration that can assist medical experts to capture echocardiographic images of a patient's heart which are of appropriate diagnostic quality without any advanced training. ML trains the software to identify and even capture video clips of high-quality 2D ultrasound images of the heart, thereby improving the way cardiovascular disease is diagnosed.

Molly a virtual nurse that tracks the status of people who have been previously treated for a long time or suffering from chronic diseases. This application was developed to structure data based on the person's state, submit it to an expert and provide suggestions. This system is also able to remind the time to take medicine and the need to see a doctor [39, 40].

In rural areas, AI is used to connect patients with available resources and care. Examples include:

- **Provide Customized Healthcare Advice to Patients**

Sage Bionetworks has initiated mPower as a study utilizing surveys and mobile sensors to monitor Parkinson's disease symptoms. The outcomes could assist patients, doctors and caregivers understand better overtime changes and the impacts of exercise and medication. Using AI, mPower data can also be used to establish particular suggestions for patients regarding healthcare [41].

- **Creation of Virtual Care Services for Chronic Patients**

Verily Health's Onduo project, which integrates a smart device and a smartphone application, provides online care for Type 2 diabetic patients. Onduo could even measure blood sugar levels, and provide nutrition and medication management information. This application also provides a counseling aspect which recognizes lifestyle habits and gives feedback to patients to enhance their health.

- **Increasing Treatment Access for Rural Populations**

AI has the ability to enhance and expand access to treatment in rural areas and other resource-constrained areas through voice assistants and chatbots. There is growing proof that chatbots driven by AI can resolve routine patient questions and assist doctors to interact with patients regarding their diagnosis and risk assessments.

Recent developments in ML and AI develop predictive systems and derive real-time conclusions for reasons like warnings, risk classification, and estimating the duration of stay from a diverse population of patients. Many of these methods are based on intensive care, utilizing physiological data which are regularly collected in ICUs. For instance, an intensive care monitoring and tracking model has been established to simulate the important indications of individual patients and to create patient-specific systems and alarm levels. Neural networks and Decision trees have been utilized for generating patient state binary classifiers and determining when and how to issue an alert.

A physiological test ranking for premature babies, utilizing time-series data collected from the first 3 h of the newborn's life, and a Bayesian hierarchical model, the subject model of the time-series. This method allows healthcare professionals to predict reliably the likelihood of a newborn's risk of such serious complications as cardiopulmonary infections. Physiological factors such as temporary variation in respiratory and cardiac levels demonstrated significantly larger predicting capacity than intrusive laboratory research, highlighting the opportunities for new and least intrusive perinatal care.

10 Conclusion

Artificial Intelligence systems are being promoted as one of the main innovations that contribute to a genuine advancement in healthcare. This chapter discussed the importance of AI in healthcare, the relationship between AI and healthcare, healthcare data collection and storage system, medical data pre-processing, AI algorithms for healthcare, AI methodology for medical and medicinal diagnosis, selection and extraction of features using AI, disease diagnosis with AI, medical image processing with AI, and patient care and treatment with AI. The application of AI algorithms in the field of medicine and healthcare would assist doctors to establish improved approaches and treatment strategies for patients. AI will continue to improve the efficiency of research in the coming years and enhance the abilities to accurately diagnose the disease, take decisions for the treatment and prognosticate.

References

1. Artificial Intelligence. https://www.talkyblog.com/artificial-intelligence/
2. Jake Frankenfield (2020) Artificial Intelligence. https://www.investopedia.com/terms/a/artificial-intelligence-ai.asp
3. Rong, G., Mendez, A., Assi, E.B., Zhao, Bo., Sawan, M.: Artificial Intelligence in Healthcare: Review and Prediction Case Studies. Elsevier, pp. 291–301 (2020). https://doi.org/10.1016/j.eng.2019.08.015
4. Artificial Intelligence. https://builtin.com/artificial-intelligence
5. Hintze, A.: Understanding the Four Types of Artificial Intelligence (2016)
6. The Importance of Health and Healthcare (2008). Economic report of the president, pp. 97–113
7. What is Healthcare. https://www.collegechoice.net/faq/what-is-healthcare/ (2020)
8. Healthcare. https://en.wikipedia.org/wiki/Health_care
9. Furnell, A.: The Importance of Healthcare in the Society (2017)
10. Chen, M., Decary, M.: Artificial Intelligence in Healthcare: An Essential Guide for Health Leaders. The Canadian College of Health Leaders. Health Management Forum, pp. 1–9 (2019). https://doi.org/10.1177/0840470419873123
11. Lauren Paige Kennedy. How Artificial Intelligence helps in Healthcare.
12. Le Nguyen, T., Do, T.T.H.: Artificial intelligence in healthcare: a new technology benefit for both patients and doctors. In: Proceedings of PICMET'19: Technology Management in the World of Intelligent Systems (2019). https://doi.org/10.23919/PICMET.2019.8893884
13. Reddy, S.: Use of Artificial Intelligence in Healthcare Delivery. eHealth-Making Health Care Smarter. InTechOpen, pp. 81–97 (2018). https://doi.org/10.5772/intechopen.74714
14. Uma, K., Hanumantappa, M.: Data collection methods and data pre-processing techniques for healthcare data using data mining. Int. J. Sci. Eng. Res. **8**(6), 1131–1136 (2017)
15. Patient Data Collection. https://www.usfhealthonline.com/resources/key-concepts/patient-data-collection/
16. What is a Health Information System. https://digitalguardian.com/blog/what-health-information-system
17. Healthcare Data 101 (2018), Data across Sectors for Health, pp. 1–17
18. Understanding the different types of Health Information Technology. https://www.officepracticum.com/blog/understanding-the-different-types-of-health-information-technology
19. Top AI Algorithms in Healthcare. https://rubikscode.net/2020/03/16/top-ai-algorithms-in-healthcare/ (2020)
20. Top 6 AI Algorithms in Healthcare. https://analyticsindiamag.com/top-6-ai-algorithms-in-healthcare/ (2020)
21. Top AI Algorithms for Healthcare. https://medium.com/sciforce/top-ai-algorithms-for-healthcare-aa5007ffa330 (2019)
22. Revolutionary Medical Advances through AI Medical Diagnosis. https://www.osplabs.com/ai-medical-diagnosis/
23. Machine learning for Medical Diagnostics - 4 Current Applications. https://emerj.com/ai-sector-overviews/machine-learning-medical-diagnostics-4-current-applications/
24. AI in Medicine. https://www.mendeley.com/careers/article/artificial-intelligence-in-medicine/#:~:text=AI%20in%20medicine%20refers%20to,of%20patients%20who%20require%20care (2018)
25. AI in Medicine. https://vocal.media/futurism/artificial-intelligence-in-medicine
26. How AI Technologies Accelerate Progress in in Medical Diagnosis (2020)
27. AI in Medicine. https://www.datarevenue.com/en-blog/artificial-intelligence-in-medicine
28. Dely, S.: Surgical Robots, New Medicines and Better Care: 32 Examples of AI in Healthcare. https://builtin.com/artificial-intelligence/artificial-intelligence-healthcare (2020)
29. Cateni, S., Vannucci, M., Vannoocci, M., Colla, V.: Variable selection and feature extraction through artificial intelligence techniques. In: Multivariate Analysis in Management, Engineering and the Sciences. INTECH, pp. 103–118 (2013). https://doi.org/10.5772/53862

30. Martin, N.: Artificial Intelligence is Being used to Diagnose Disease and Design New Drugs. AI and Big Data (2019)
31. AI Just as Good at Diagnosing Illness as Humans. https://www.medicalnewstoday.com/art icles/326460#AI-on-a-par-with-healthcare-professionals
32. Mishra, S.G., Takke, A.K., Auti, S.T., Suryavanshi, S.V., Oza, M.J.: Role of artificial intelligence in health care. BioChem. Int. J. 11(5), 1–14 (2017)
33. Abdallah, Y.M.Y., Alqahtani, T.: Research in medical imaging using image processing tech- niques. In: Medical Imaging-Principles and Applications. IntechOpen, pp. 1–16 (2019). https:// doi.org/10.5772/intechopen.84360
34. AI in Medical Imaging. https://missinglink.ai/guides/deep-learning-healthcare/ai-medical- imaging/#:~:text=AI%20in%20Medical%20Imaging%20Applications&text=Medical%20i mage%20analysis%E2%80%94this%20technology,medical%20images%20better%20than% 20doctors.&text=Automated%20AI%20can%20be%20used,risk%20detection%20and%20l ess%20misdiagnosis
35. The Best AI-based Medical Imaging Tools in 2020
36. AI in Medical Imaging: Global Market Outlook. https://medium.com/syncedreview/ai-in-med ical-imaging-global-market-outlook-ffeb96767e85
37. Shah, R., Chircu, A.: IoT and AI in healthcare: a systematic literature review. Issues in Inform. Syst. 19(3), 33–41 (2018)
38. Castelo, M.: The Future of Artificial Intelligence in Healthcare (2020)
39. Kharkovyna, O.: Artificial Intelligence and Deep Learning for Medical Diagnosis (2019)
40. Artificial Intelligence in Medicine. https://vocal.media/futurism/artificial-intelligence-in-med icine
41. Sharing and Utilizing Health Data for AI Applications: U.S. Department of Health and Human Services. The Center for Open Data Enterprise, pp. 1–20 (2019)

Data Collection and Processing in Health Care

S. R. Mani Sekhar, Tilak Singh, and Amit Doegar

Abstract Data collection and processing are used to gather information and enables one to answer the relevant questions. There is a need for collecting and processing data in every field like humanities, social science, engineering, business, etc. They play an important role in health care services as well. The volume of data in the health care sector increases exponentially day by day, hence the collection of data becomes not only important but also a tedious job as well. The data collection and its storage is a bigger problem for health sector organizations since it is huge and costly. These organizations take needful efforts in collecting the data by applying different methods and store them in their database, which can be shared with other organizations or to the government under few conditions. After the collection and maintenance of data, the processing step takes place which has its own pros and cons. The data collected has to be processed in order to get the analysis for that particular set of data. Based on the analysis, different steps could be taken by the health organizations in order to achieve their task. Every year millions of dollars are spent on data collection and processing in order to keep the system up to date. One can simply predict how arduous and gruesome data collection and processing in the healthcare sector can be. This chapter provides the overview of various concepts used for data collection and storage.

Keywords Health care · Data collection · Data storage

S. R. Mani Sekhar (✉) · T. Singh
Department of Information Science & Engineering, Ramaiah Institute of Technology, Bangalore, India
e-mail: manisekharsr@gmail.com

A. Doegar
National Institute of Technical Teachers Training and Research, Chandigarh, India

1   Introduction to Data Collection

Data collection can be defined as the continuous analysis, and interpretation of health data necessary for designing, implementing, and evaluating public health prevention programs [1, 2]. Collecting of data may vary but the goal of analyzing it and coming up with a formulated answer for a query is achieved. The data collection in health services involves the collection of different categories of data, which is essential in analyzing the patient to avoid unnecessarily squandering of the time or harming the patients by making treatment mistakes. It creates a comprehensive view of patients, personalize treatments, advance treatment methods, improve communication between doctors and patients, and hence enhances the health outcomes.

1.1   Importance of Data Collection

Some of the importance of data collection in the field of health care is as follows:

- The collected data of a patient will lead to an improved decision made by doctors or any other specialists for the treatment, hence improving the overall quality of the healthcare industry.
- The analysis of the data will make it easy to explicate the problems and it is a source that needs remodeling or correction.
- It will lead to the building of advanced technology that will overall increase the quality of the healthcare industry itself. The generation of this advanced technology will help patients by providing them with the treatment they need.
- The collected data can be stored securely and can be tracked for particular patients overtime to warn them for the future whenever their health might be at risk.

1.2   Challenges in Healthcare Data Collections

Data collection improves the results of the research, they help in analyzing the data and suggest suitable steps to take for a particular scenario [3, 4]. Despite being the foundational block of the data analysis, there are certain challenges in collecting data. Some of the challenges in the fields of healthcare are as follows.

- Cleaning: Data cleaning is the central part after collecting the data and challenging too. It is very important to keep the data clean so that the data consistency and accuracy are maintained. After the data is cleaned, it is processed to analyze, so data cleaning is important to get the correct and relevant results as well. In the healthcare sector, there is a huge amount of data that needs to be maintained but only limited storage is available, hence it becomes a tedious task to clean the data and keep only those fields that are necessary for the research purposes.

- Storage: As discussed earlier, another challenging factor in collecting the data is its storage. There is a large volume of data in health care that keeps on growing exponentially day by day. The cost of storing these volumes of data is very high. The additional cost of maintaining these data makes it challenging too for any healthcare organization.
- Security: Data security is the primary concern for any healthcare organization. The stored data needs to be checked and reviewed regularly to avoid any leaks to protect the patient's data. Different threats to data security are like Phishing, Data leakage, Hacking, etc.
- Updating: The healthcare data are not static, they keep on changing from time to time. Hence, to make it dynamic, the organization needs to update the data of every patient for each field required. The organization must also look for the duplication in the data to avoid inconsistency.

2 Types of Healthcare Data

The clinical data are usually collected during the ongoing treatment or sometimes during the formal clinical trial program [5]. The collected data falls into six different types which are as follows [6]:

- Electronic Health Record (EHR).
- Administrative Data.
- Claims Data.
- Patient/Disease Registries.
- Health Surveys.
- Clinical Trials Data.

2.1 Electronic Health Record (EHR)

Often referred to as the purest form of data, EHR is a systematic collection of patient's details as a digital format. These can be shared across healthcare settings. These are not shared with any outsiders for any research purposes. The fields of EHR include a wide range of data, from medical history to any allergies to patients, etc. EHR was built to store the patient data from time to time and track down their medical history to treat them correctly and avoid inaction. Due to its digital comportment, it becomes easy to access the patient's medical data from the past and predict the outcome.

2.2 Administrative Data

The administrative data are collected from the healthcare organization and are directly reported to the government to maintain health insurance for a particular patient. This helps to analyze the current trend and predict overtime information. There are a few disadvantages as well, like, sometimes the data are missing or are restricted to certain users.

2.3 Claims Data

Claims are another type of healthcare data. These are on a much bigger scale and collect information on millions of doctor's appointments, bills, insurance information, etc. Claims data describe the interaction between the insured patient and the healthcare delivery system. It can be obtained from the government or the commercial healthcare organization. Since the data are large, hence the researchers can easily analyze the patients with rare illnesses and can maintain data for that too. A few of the downsides of this healthcare type are the illegal billing and since the data is very huge the storage and cleaning of data becomes a problem sometimes.

2.4 Patient/Disease Registries

The registry contains the most extensive data. These are mainly used to store the secondary data of the patient like a diagnosis or certain procedure which plays an important role in post surveillance of the marketing or usage of specific drugs. It is very cost-effective. It is a very powerful tool to observe the disease and helps in understanding the variation in treatment and outcomes.

2.5 Health Surveys

Health surveys are conducted to get information about the health of an entire nation. The national health surveys are collected for research purposes, thus it is more accessible. It generally includes the measurement of the risk factor. The range of measurement is very wide, for example, Age, Gender, Race/Ethnicity, etc. [4]. The results after analyzing the data collected from surveys can be towards increasing mortality rate or proposal of the new policy in favor of the people of the nation.

2.6   Clinical Trials Data

The clinical trials are used to check the effectiveness of any particular medication. There is a database dedicated to this. The medications are applied on different samples and based on the outcomes the data are grouped and organized for future use or study. These are proven to be life-saving. There are two types of clinical data—interventional and observational. Intervention trial is used to find out about the particular intervention. Whereas observational tries to figure out what happens to people in different scenarios. The phases of clinical trial are named, Phase 0, Phase I, Phase II, Phase III, Phase IV. The data of clinical trials can be accessible.

3   Introduction to Data Processing

Data processing can be described as the collection, aggregation, cleaning, and updating of data so hospitals and other health systems can make use of it to come up with a strategic decision [7–9]. There are mainly five different ways for data processing: data acquiring, combining data, crosswalk, cleaning data, and quality assurance (Fig. 1).

3.1   Importance of Data Processing

Once the different types of data are collected through different methods, the data processing operation is applied. After the processing of the data, it is analyzed after which the keys decisions are taken for the treatment. Some of the other importance of data processing includes follows:

- More focus on patients is maintained. The in-depth analysis helps the health organization to treat the patient well according to their past medical history.
- It is cost-effective. Since the processing of data creates the report which can be referred to give the specific treatment to the patient rather than spending money on non-essential treatment procedures.
- It is reliable. It can be used for research purposes as well.

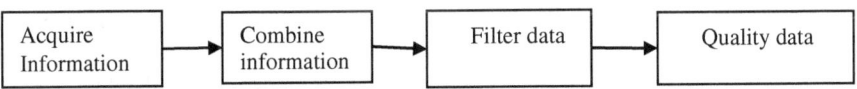

Fig. 1 Data processing technique

3.2 *Factors Affecting Data Processing*

To get an accurate result after data processing, there are various factors and levels. A few of the factors in data processing are data validation, data organization, data integration, etc. The most important is to verify the data. Data verification is the process to verify the consistency or inconsistency in data before evaluating the report. The validation ensures that the data which is being processed is correct, clean, and useful. Besides human errors, there may be a different type of errors as well, like System error, etc. There can be multiple points of data failure, few of them are wrongly entered data, duplication, inaccurate information, interface issue, etc.

To validate data the following steps can be taken into consideration.

- Identify that the data needs validation.
- Refer to the data source from where the data has been contributed.
- Create workflow and observe how that data is used in clinics
- Identify the errors in mapping and then fix it.
- Re-test the data.

After the data has been validated, the next thing to perform is to organize that data. Data organization is important since it creates a holistic view o f he patient. It enhances the involvement of the patient in the analysis. Since it is stored in a database, it can be useful for the future as well. A most common problem involving the organization of data is that there is a certain limit to organizing beyond which an organization is unable to store. After validation and storing the data from different sources the data need to be integrated, hence, the next factor before processing data is data integration where the work is mainly based on unifying data. Unifying data helps improve a healthcare organization's view of patient data. The goal of integrating is, it just needs to compile all the data of different formats into a single format file that can be read and performed on. But, the integration of the data is really complicated. Since the data is increasing exponentially day by day, it becomes really important that data integration is implemented to avoid massive storage of data.

4 Conclusion

Data collection and processing is the important task in healthcare industry. As the volume of data in the healthcare sector increases exponentially day by day, collection and processing of the data becomes a challenging task. In this chapter author has discussed the different methods related to data collection and procession. They also presented the various types of healthcare data and its use. Finally, the chapter presents the different ways of data processing and its importance.

References

1. Zhou, L., Song, Y., Alterman, V., Liu, Y., Wang, M.: Introduction to data collection in multilevel research. In: The Handbook of Multilevel Theory, Measurement, and Analysis, pp. 225–252. American Psychological Association (2019)
2. Sapsford, R., Jupp, V. (eds.): Data Collection and Analysis. Sage (1996)
3. Haluza, D., Jungwirth, D.: ICT and the future of health care: aspects of health promotion. Int. J. Med. Informatics **84**(1), 48–57 (2015)
4. Nerenz, D.R., McFadden, B., Ulmer, C. (eds.): Race, Ethnicity, and Language Data: Standardization for Health Care Quality Improvement. National Academies Press (2009)
5. Birnbaum, E.B.D.: Application of data mining techniques to healthcare data. Infect. Control Hosp. Epidemiol. (2004)
6. Data Resources in the Health Sciences. https://guides.lib.uw.edu/hsl/data/findclin
7. Reichertz, P.L.: Future developments of data processing in health care. Methods Inf. Med. **21**(02), 55–58 (1982)
8. Stratasan.   https://stratasan.com/data-processing/#:~:text=%22Data%20processing%22%20r efers%20to%20the,to%20make%20informed%20strategic%20decisions
9. Quah, S.R.: International Encyclopedia of Public Health. Academic Press (2016)

Healthcare Analytics

Sensor Data Analytics for Health Care

Minal Moharir, Nikitha Srikanth, and K. R. Pavan

Abstract This chapter deals with sensor data analysis for health care. Sensor technology and the increasing popularity of smart systems have paved the way for it to be integrated into every part of people's lives. Taking advantage of this could prove to be very useful in the domain of healthcare. Various sensor technologies have been explored in this chapter with two case studies to emphasize the importance of combining the forces of health care with sensor technology and data analysis.

Keywords Sensors · Data analysis · Healthcare · ECG · PPG · Heart rate variability

1 Introduction

Recent advancements in sensor technology and embedded devices have revolutionized the healthcare field. Its contribution to healthcare has aided in improving the quality of life. The constant attention of doctors and paramedics is no longer necessary with the advent of sensor technology in medicine. It can also provide constant monitoring during the daily lives of people to provide efficient early warning systems when physiological indicators measured by the sensors deviate from normal. This has also improved the early diagnosis of ailments and their treatment [1]. The insights gained from analyzing data from sensors can be used to understand the course of any health issue, right from the onset of symptoms to recovery post-treatment. This could also help researchers better understand the effects of a particular ailment on

M. Moharir (✉) · N. Srikanth · K. R. Pavan
RV College of Engineering®, Mysore Rd., RV Vidyaniketan, Post, Bengaluru, Karnataka 560059, India
e-mail: minalmoharir@rvce.edu.in

N. Srikanth
e-mail: nikithasrikanth.cs18@rvce.edu.in

K. R. Pavan
e-mail: pavankr.cs18@rvce.edu.in

© The Author(s), under exclusive license to Springer Nature Singapore Pte Ltd. 2021   97
K. G. Srinivasa et al. (eds.), *Artificial Intelligence for Information Management: A Healthcare Perspective*, Studies in Big Data 88,
https://doi.org/10.1007/978-981-16-0415-7_5

the body, and identify important features and indicators that are hidden in the vast intricacies of data. It is thus important for people to understand the sensor technology used and methods that can be employed to analyze the data from these sensors. This can be used to develop smarter systems that can work in conjunction with healthcare experts [2].

This chapter talks about the recent advancements in monitoring devices and sensors, highlighting some of the novel technology based on remarkable principles. Then, two case studies on ECG and PPG sensors are taken up describing the sensor technology and sensor data analysis [3], which could potentially prevent and predict cardiac diseases.

2 Identification and Sensor Technology

2.1 Blood Pressure Monitor

Hypotension and hypertension are some of the risks associated with blood pressure, which necessitates continuous monitoring when required. There are many instances during which continuous blood pressure monitoring is required. Ambulatory blood pressure monitoring enables the patient to be kept under BP monitoring throughout the critical period. The BP variations caused in the patient helps in providing better insight into the patient's condition [4].

Traditional measurements require the BP monitor device (Sphygmomanometer) to be used which is not only uncomfortable and can be inaccurate sometimes, but also less portable. Several invasive methods for monitoring of BP proposed in recent years based on Pulse Arrival Time (PAT), Pulse Transit Time (PTT), Pre-Ejection Period (PEP), Pulse Wave Velocity (PWV). Other methods include the volume clamp method and arterial tonometry used to measure BP. More recently a technique using radar sensors has been developed, using the Continuous Wave Doppler radar. This technique called the CWR, which can also detect heart rate without requiring skin contact that can act as a method of Continuous Systolic Blood Pressure Monitor. The CWR from the sternum along with PPG and the ECG sensor on the chest is used. Further processing of the signal generated involves wavelet transformation and an adaptive filter.

The CWR consists of a transmitter that emits high-frequency wave signals and a receiver at the sternum. The PPG sensor is used to record the PAT parameters. It is placed next to the earlobe as signals measured are clear and minimum noise created when movement. ECG on the chest to collect R-peaks, and thus all the 3 devices collect data in a synchronized manner. The signals are passed to filters to remove noise and interference. The heart rate is obtained from PPG data and used for analysis. Wavelet transformation is used in order to preserve timing information of the CWR signal [5]. Data relating to PEP is measured from the CWR as the difference between the R-peak of ECG and the foot of the CWR signal.

The CWR sensors are able to observe movements in the body. This proposes a simple CWR-based system that could be used in wearable devices, which can monitor both PEPs and PTTs.

2.2 Smart Bone Plates

Bone fracture injuries are quite common disabling conditions. During the treatment, the healing of the fracture becomes an important factor in making clinical decisions. When a bone fracture is treated by physicians, there is no definite method to assess the healing of the bone. Conventional methods such as X-ray scanning or physical assessment are not of much help in the early stages of healing. X-ray imaging gives better knowledge but is limited in use because of the radiation dose and cost factor.

Recent research in the monitoring of bone fracture healing has mostly focused on measuring the mechanical strength of the bone. In this method, electrical techniques are used to quantify fracture repair [6]. Here the bone is modeled as a combination of resistance and reactance. The iron-rich membrane in the intracellular and extra-cellular materials conducts charges and hence offers resistance. The cell membrane which opposes the flow of charge behaves as a capacitance thereby contributes to the reactance of the net impedance.

This method uses Electrical Impedance Spectrum (EIS) to monitor and quantify the healing of the fracture. In this method, a microscale ESI sensor is implanted in the fracture gap. It is made sure that this doesn't prevent the bridging of the bone. It is based on the observation that the frequency spectrum of electrical impedance of the bone changes sharply with the healing of the bone fracture [7]. The sensor design involves a pair of electrode pins of a few μm thickness, made of electroless nickel immersion gold, placed 0.5 mm apart.

To quantify bone repair, the impedance data throughout the healing was mapped to equivalent electrical circuits by the method of curve fitting, and the dominant electrical property varying with the bridging process was empirically determined. Thus, electrical impedance spectroscopy can be potentially used in clinical scales to monitor fracture healing and help in the early detection of nonunion fracture [8].

2.3 Degradable Sensor for Blood Flow Monitor

In medicine, post surgeries a procedure called Vascular Anastomosis is carried, which is the process of reconnecting vessels that were cut. Procedures like bypass surgery, hemodialysis, organ transplant, treating damaged arteries, and reconstruction after cancer require an immediate anastomosis procedure to be done to allow blood flow [9].

Vascular Anastomosis faces risks like anastomosis leaks especially if the patient is obese or drinks excessively, has a blockage in another vessel, or if surrounding vessels are damaged. Currently, the monitoring technique used is the Doppler system and manual evaluation by the color of the skin, within the clinic, and mostly none after the discharge. This necessitates the use of a smart continuous monitoring device easy to use and can be used outside the clinical environment [10].

Recently implantable Hall-effect sensors were proposed, but due to the composition of the sensor, it requires another surgery to be removed. This method developed by a group of researchers from Stanford University proposes using a biodegradable sensor that is operated wirelessly and without a battery.

The sensor consists of a fringe field capacitive sensor and a bilayer coil structure that is used for communication via radio signals [11]. The blood flow leading to a change in diameter during the formation of reconnection is sensed by the capacitive sensor leading to a change in frequency of the circuit which is monitored wirelessly using inductive coupling. The sensor is fabricated with Mg for electrical connection, polyglycerol sebacate for the dielectric, polyoctamethylenemaleate anhydride citrate, and polyhydroxybutyrate/polyhodroxyvalerate for packaging, and polylactic acid for the bilayer coils. With these materials, which are well known to be biodegradable this method proves to be a promising technology for future applications in the monitoring of vascular anastomosis [12].

2.4   Continuous Glucose Monitoring

These sensors continuously track glucose levels in the body at regular intervals and can act as effective warning systems if glucose levels fall below or above a certain threshold, and are extremely useful for diabetic patients [13].

This differs from self-blood glucose testing sensors, which rely on the patients performing tests themselves several times during the day. Self-blood glucose monitoring kits are more complex and come with needles for extracting a few drops of blood, which is then tested for glucose levels. The blood is applied onto a testing strip which is inserted into a reflectance photometer for an automated reading. The testing strip reacts with the glucose in the blood and the product of this reaction produces a characteristic change in color. The photometer measures the amount of light reflected from the product of the reaction. With the help of small computational units, the reflectance is converted to blood glucose levels in mg/dL, using reference values that relate it to a function of the reflectance for the reagent used [14]. This method is highly dependent on the user taking measurements at the prescribed time and is also very time-consuming. Further, nothing can be said about glucose levels at other points during the day.

Continuous Glucose Monitors (CGM), on the other hand, are convenient, do not require manual testing, and provide real-time, continuous insights. Further, along with the glucose content, they can also provide the direction of change at a given instant, i.e., whether it is decreasing or increasing. CGMs that are electrochemical based, usually rely on measuring electrochemical signals generated at the electrodes due to a reaction between glucose and an enzyme such as glucose oxidase. The longevity and reliability of these sensors depend on the stability of the enzyme over time and the build-up of by-products surrounding the sensors. Some sensors are optical based, which are embedded in the subcutaneous tissue of the skin. The part in contact with the skin is coated with a polymer that binds to glucose [15]. An LED in the sensor emits light which is used to excite the glucose-dependent polymer. Photodiodes measure the intensity of fluorescence exhibited by the polymer. There are antennas inside the sensor that can communicate and receive power wirelessly through an externally worn transmitter.

Several non-invasive sensors also shine a light on the skin or clip onto the ear.

After sensing has taken place, the transmitter receives data wirelessly which is then transferred to a computational device through Bluetooth, or NFC which can then derive insights from the readings [16]. Sometimes data is also sent to a cloud storage system through a Wi-Fi module, where data can be remotely accessed and stored.

Mean glucose values over some time can be tracked and this can be used to describe the overall control of glucose in the body. Further, average before and after a meal can be computed to understand the effects of consumption of a particular product [17]. The percentage of time spent above and below a certain threshold can be analyzed to provide an insight into the fluctuation of glucose content. Target limits can also be established, and deviations from the target can be measured.

2.5 Medication Adherence Monitors

A lot of deaths and complications are caused due to patients failing to adhere to their medicine intake schedules. This can indeed be avoided with a warning system when a person does not comply with their medication regimen [18].

There are several types of sensors that can monitor medicine intake. There are some sensors worn on the neck that sense the activity of swallowing and train machine learning algorithms or neural networks to identify when the pill is swallowed. These sensors use piezo-electric sensors that translate the mechanical stress on the skin due to swallowing to voltage values that can be recorded. However, this would require some training of the model with user-specific data, and there is still quite a lot of research to be done in this area to improve the accuracy of the models.

Similar models that rely on machine learning and neural networks are wrist sensors. These are devices that contain models that are trained on the activity of the wrist when the medicine container is opened and the intake gestures while the pill is consumed. The activity of the wrist is measured by sensors that use accelerometers and gyroscopes to detect motion in a 3D coordinate system. However, this also requires some more in-depth research and development before it can be reliably used. Certain ingestible sensors activate once they come in contact with acid in the chamber of the stomach. Once activated, they transmit a code to a receiver outside the body. This code can help identify which medicine was taken and keep a log of medicinal intake [19]. However, due to the ingestible nature of these sensors, they pose ethical concerns and must adhere to standards on several levels ranging from non-toxicity, electrical safety, mechanical safety, etc.

The classic medication adherence monitoring technique is using smart pillboxes. These could be equipped with plungers that detect the opening of the lid of a compartment in the pillbox. This then triggers a switch to a microcontroller. Data is then wirelessly transmitted to a nearby computer that keeps records of medicine intake patterns. It can also be equipped with Wi-Fi modules to send it to a cloud server, which can enable remote monitoring by doctors. Another approach that has been proposed in literature includes 3D printed pill bottles that come with magnetic switch sensors and accelerometers. The switch senses the opening of the pillbox and activates the accelerometer. This then records the movement of the pill bottle and captures the activity of pouring the pill onto one's hand [20]. Once the bottle is placed back, the accelerometer is deactivated with the switch again. When the cap is closed, a load sensor is activated that measures changes in weight that can indicate that the pill has indeed been taken.

2.6 Surgery Recovery Monitors

Surgeries can cause drastic changes that take away normal functioning and bring about drastic changes in lifestyle. Especially for people who undergo total knee replacement or hip replacement surgery [21], constant monitoring of recovery can be a source of understanding how efficient the results of the surgery will be in the long term, and also discover early if patients are not able to regain the range of functionality and motion, and provide the required assistance and health services. There exist visual tracking systems in the literature that rely on cameras, feature extraction, and image processing models to determine different stages of recovery. These tend to be limiting in terms of the area that the patients need to be in for the camera to track their progress. These devices mainly use accelerometers, barometers, magnetometers, temperature sensors, and gyroscopes to sample motion data continuously and obtain daily progress. These sensors are strapped on to the back as well as on the side of the thigh and shin [22]. The range of motion of the knee is calculated using the sensor data post a series of exercises and walking. The correlation between the collected range of motion data and body mass index was studied. This is because the weight of the person is directly applied to the post operated knee. Its correlation with anesthetic and other drugs consumed for blood coagulation was also analyzed. Further, other descriptors about pain and ease of movement are taken from the patient [23].

For total hip replacement surgery, the device is attached to the back of the non-operated thigh, and also has sensors like accelerometers to measure the time that can be spent standing upright and the sit-to-stand transition time. The longest upright time managed in a day is also regularly updated to get a better understanding of the restoration of normal functioning. This can also be used to understand the effects of age, blood pressure, and an analysis of mean, median, interquartile, minimum, and maximum values for different people correlated with other physiological indicators.

All of this data is used to track the recovery over time and identify which conditions better help with recuperation [24].

3 Case Studies

In the following two case studies, basic analysis techniques that have been used in literature are described, for data obtained from ECG and PPG sensors, both of which measure heart rate.

The major advantage of understanding data processing and analysis from scratch is the ability to create custom techniques to derive measurements relevant to the purpose of research. Thresholds can be set for accuracy, unnecessary patterns can be smoothed out, and the important ones can be highlighted. This can further be used to develop analysis packages for any purpose. ECG and PPG sensors have been largely integrated into wearables and other smart devices, and are one of the most popularly used sensors in the domain of health care, integrated with personal devices. This means that these can be used for efficient real-time health monitoring, and it can thus prove useful to understand the basics of what these sensors measure, and how they can be interpreted [25].

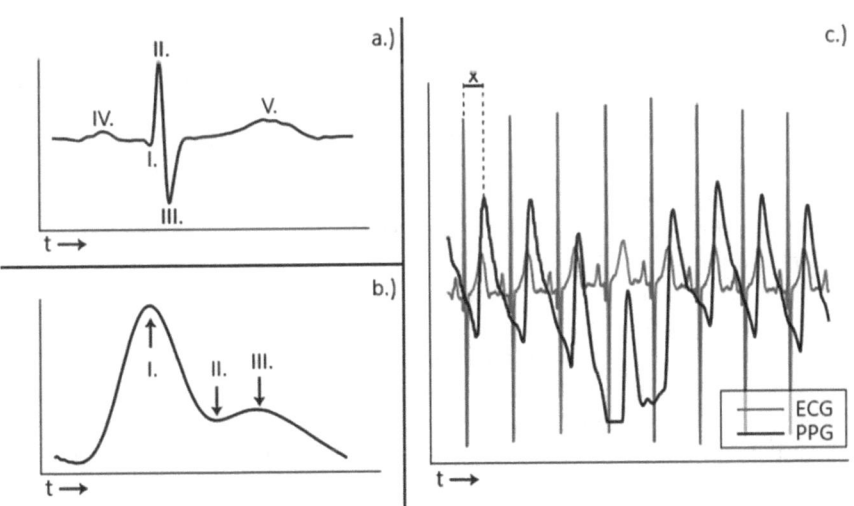

Fig. 1   a One cycle of ECG signal, with I-III being QRS complex, IV. P-wave, V. T-wave; **b** One unit of PPG signal, with I. Systolic Peak, II. Dicrotic Notch, III. Diastolic Peak; **c** ECG and PPG signal over time

The methods that have been outlined for both are largely similar, but the outcomes of the visualization are slightly different, as shown in Fig. 1, and the ease of obtaining the required metrics may slightly differ.

3.1 Background

A healthy, normally functioning heart usually displays a wide range of variability in response to various stimuli [26]. This ensures that the body is being responsive and active. However, in case of certain problems such as cardiovascular diseases and viral infections, heart rate variability reduces, which reflects the body's inability to respond to the changes, and could be a sign of mortality as well.

3.1.1 Heart Rate Variability Metrics

Heart rate variability metrics are based on the time interval between two successive heartbeats, and how this interval changes over time. These are mainly analyzed with time-domain measures and frequency-domain measures [27].

Time-domain measures include those that are derived using statistical methods from peak-to-peak intervals. In all the metrics below, NN intervals indicate normal intervals, from which artifacts have been removed. In general, these are referred to as R-R intervals to indicate the distance between R-peaks in the QRS complex [28]. These measures are used to measure the variability in the time interval between successive heartbeats. Some of the common measures of variability in R-R intervals are described.

BPM. Beats Per Minute (BPM) is one of the most basic measures of overall heart rate. It is simply the average number of contractions of the heart in one minute. Each contraction generally forms one beat.

IBI. Inter-Beat Interval (IBI) is the mean value of all the R-R intervals in a given time interval.

SDNN. This is the standard deviation of a measurement's R-R intervals (or NN intervals) and is often calculated over 24 h. This longer duration of observation enables the measurement of the heart's reactions to a wider range of environmental triggers and changing workloads. This is generally an indicator of the body's sympathetic activity. Sympathetic activity is the activation of the body's involuntary responses to dangerous and stressful situations. Stable or increasing levels of SDNN could mean signs of recovery and normalcy.

RMSSD. This is the Root Mean Square of Successive Differences between each heartbeat. It can capture fast changes in the instantaneous heart rate and is thus a measure of parasympathetic activity. Parasympathetic activity involves the body's rest and recovery system, which explains how well the body is resting and recovering in response to stressors. Similar to SDNN, stable or increasing rMSSD values are generally a sign of normalcy and recovery.

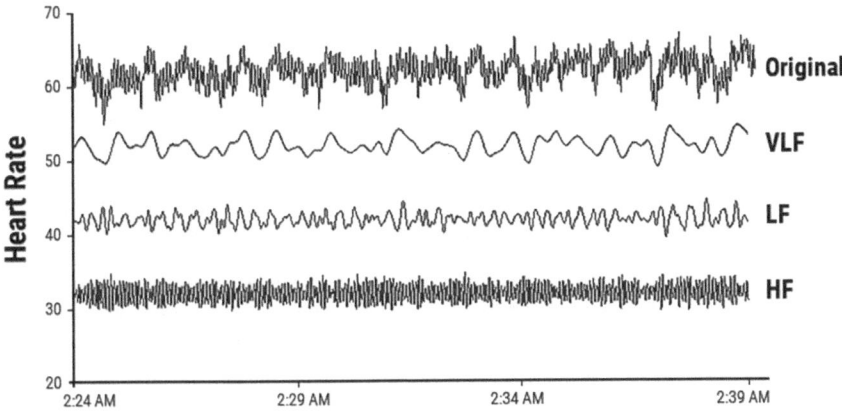

Fig. 2 Signal decomposed into its constituent frequencies

pNN50. Percentage of adjacent R-R intervals (or NN intervals) that differ from each other by more than 50 ms. This could be a reliable measure of parasympathetic activity for short intervals.

PNN20. Percentage of successive NN intervals (peak-to-peak) whose difference is greater than 20 ms.

A time-series or time-domain graph shows changes in a signal over time. However, the same series can also be visualized in the frequency domain. This can be done by analyzing the individual frequencies that make up the signal, or what proportion of the signal lies in a particular frequency band, as shown in Fig. 2.

LF. The low-frequency band (0.04–0.15 Hz) corresponds to modulations with periods occurring between 7 and 25 s. LF is usually affected by slow and controlled respiration rates. It is also associated with sympathetic activity in the body.

HF. The high-frequency band (0.15–0.4 Hz) corresponds to periods occurring between 2.5 and 7 s. This is usually associated with parasympathetic activity and largely influenced by the respiratory cycle. This is highly correlated with PNN50 and RMSSD measures.

3.1.2 Sensors Used

ECG Sensor. In the upper right chamber of the heart is a special tissue called the sinoatrial node (SA node), the pacemaker of the heart. It produces electrical pulses around 60–100 times a minute which then travels through the conduction pathway causing the heart to contract and pump out blood. These are more than just beats and can describe a lot more about one's mental and physical health. These signals causing the heart's activity can be captured through the skin by placing electrodes to record the small changes in voltage. An electrocardiogram is a plot of this signal voltage with time, which reads the rate and rhythm of the heart. ECG is a non-invasive

Fig. 3 ECG heart rate signal

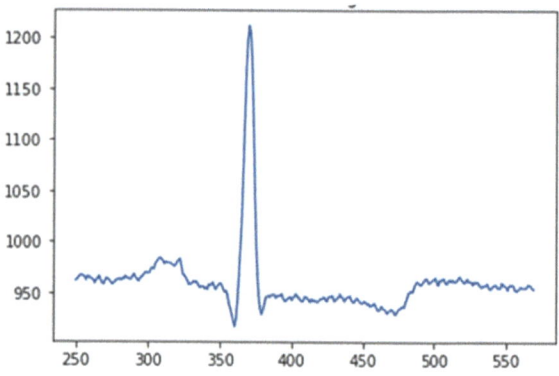

method of diagnosis and is often used for many common heart problems in people of all ages. In an ECG each beat is defined by a QRS complex, which is the subject of this analysis. A typical ECG signal is shown in Fig. 3. Tracing the ECG signal, the P-wave is observed around 40 ms after the SA node fires during which atrial contraction occurs [29]. This is followed by ventricular polarization. Then, the QRS represents the electrical signal traveling through the electrical path, first through the AV node then the interventricular septum, and finally the ventricles. The S-T segment represents quick repolarization. In the end, the T-wave represents the electrical reset of the heart and preparation for the next cycle.

PPG. As blood is pumped into various parts of the body by the ventricles of the heart, the volume of blood in the blood vessels increases. This is the systolic phase. During the diastolic phase, blood flows into the auricles and the blood vessels relax, blood pressure in them decreases. A plethysmogram is a device that measures changes in volume within an organ. A photoplethysmogram (PPG) is a device that accomplishes this using light. Apart from the regular cardiac cycle, blood flow due to several other physiological factors can be used to monitor breathing, loss of salt in the blood vessels, and much more. A typical PPG sensor consists of a light source or photoemitter and a photodetector. Light is incident on the skin and passes through tissues and blood vessels. As the volume of blood changes in the blood vessels, the light detected by the photodetector also changes. The changes in light received are translated into voltage signals over time and thus forms the basis of a PPG detected signal [30]. Typically, the light source is an LED and the detector is a photodiode that conducts electricity when light is incident on it. The sensor can operate in two modes.

Transmission mode. The emitter and detector are placed on diametrically opposite sides of the skin, so the light passes through absorbent substances, such as the skin pigmentation, bone, and arterial and venous blood, and is then received by the photodetector on the other side. These generally use red or infrared light as they can penetrate through the tissue and can be detected on the other side.

Reflective mode. The emitter sends light which is reflected by the skin, and received by the detector on the same side. This mode is applied mainly in body parts where transmission of light is impractical due to thicker skin (for example, wrist and forehead). These use green light as the maximum component of the reflected light that describes pulse is detected at wavelengths close to that of green.

The light reflected onto the photodiode produces a small current through the circuit. This current is too small and thus amplifiers are used to increase the amplitude of the current versus the time signal produced. This is then converted to a voltage versus time signal so it can be fed into ADC. The ADC converts it into a digital form that can be used for computation. The hardware necessary for the entire setup is very simple and not very expensive. Due to its ease of use and convenience, it is being widely used in wearable sensors. The PPG signal generally has three critical points-systolic peak (point of highest blood pressure), dicrotic notch (closure of aortic valve closes), diastolic peak (blood begins to rush into the heart).

3.2 Analysis Overview

It is important to ensure that the sampling frequency of measurements is fairly constant throughout the time period of data collection, which is true for any signals that are measured. Thus, it is important to check standard deviations of the consecutive time intervals to ensure that the measurements were made at approximately regular intervals. In the case of irregular measurements, a better sensor must be procured for studies. Further, the raw signal must be filtered to remove non-heartbeat signals. Several filtering techniques can be easily employed with scientific and statistical libraries.

Moving average. This is a very simple technique where random portions of noise are effectively removed by smoothing out short-term fluctuations and highlighting long-term trends or cycles. This is done by creating a series of averages for small subsets of the given set of data. Initially, a small subset is taken, and its average is calculated. Next, the first value is discarded and the subset is shifted forward to include the next value in the subset, creating an average that moves.

Adaptive filtering. This is another technique that can be employed, which uses a reference signal that has a strong correlation with either the useful part of the signal or with the artifacts. This reference signal must be obtained with additional hardware such as an accelerometer that senses motion. The unwanted part is removed from the actual signal by subtracting the noise or retaining the useful parts as per the reference.

Butterworth filter. Noise created due to the environment, DC component, and other artifacts can be handled with the help of a bandpass filter, which chooses the lower and upper limit for the frequencies required.

In particular, the Butterworth bandpass filter has a uniform response to all frequencies in the specified range but also does not completely reject the unwanted signals. It suppresses frequencies more as they move away from the thresholds.

After filtering, the peaks are identified in both ECG and PPG signals. The distance between the peaks is used to calculate different time-domain measures such as BPM, RMSSD, SDNN, IBI, PNN50, PNN20, etc. These involve calculating mean, standard deviation, differences, squared differences, and other simple statistical measures, which can be easily accomplished through mathematical libraries. There are several ways to transform the signal into its frequency domain, such as wavelet transforms, Laplace transforms, and Z transforms, but in this case study, the Fast Fourier transform was used.

3.3 ECG Analysis

The dataset is obtained from the MIT-BIT database, which is a repository of ECG data from 47 individuals from a mix of inpatients and outpatients. It is measured with a resolution of 11 bits and a range of 10 mv. For this case study, Python and its modules are used. The flow of analysis is shown in Fig. 4.

The ambulatory ECG obtained is typically noisy. No sensor is perfect and hence produces some noise. The ECG can also pick up noise from the power line of the monitoring device. Muscle contractions produced in the subject is also a source of noise [31]. The QRS complex can be observed to be abnormal when the conduction of the electrical pulse takes a detour. This makes the QRS complex widen and frequency is attenuated.

Noise can be removed by using filters like the Butterworth filter by determining the frequency of the signal. Also, the baseline wandering problem occurs due to the respiration and muscle contractions produced in the subject. This can bring errors in the detection of R-peaks. This can be removed by using a notch filter around a small frequency range which removes the baseline wandering problem and preserves the disposition of R-peaks in time. Once the baseline-corrected ECG is obtained, it can be used for the diagnosis of ECG, which can be in the time domain or frequency domain.

For analyzing the ECG signals, as the first step, the R-peaks have to be identified. To determine these peaks, methods like curve fitting followed by x-maxima, finding

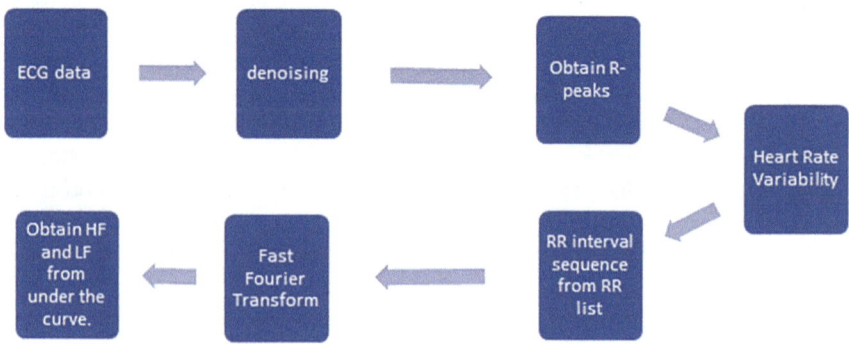

Fig. 4 ECG analysis

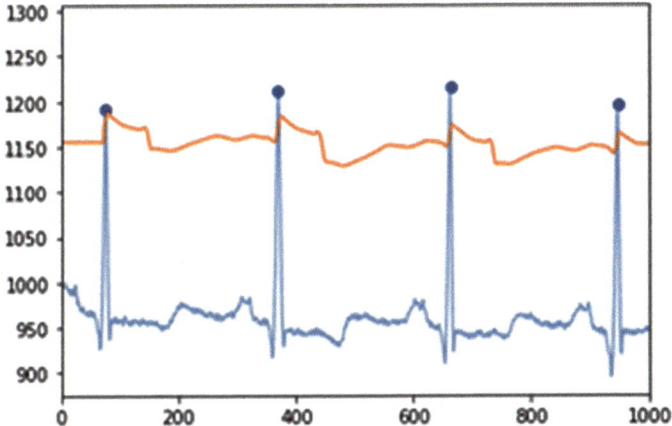

Fig. 5 Detection of peaks in the signal

the slopes to determine the point where the slope changes sharply and determining local maxima within the ROI of the individual QRS complex can be used. The exact mathematical solution can be obtained by the method of curve fitting, but it comes with a greater computational cost. For the method of maxima, a moving average is drawn to the graph. A rolling mean is used as a finite impulse response filter which effectively deals with the fluctuating sequence. Then, all the points lying above the mean line are marked as the ROI. Within this region, the point of maximum x coordinate is detected as the R-peak. The R-peak detected using moving average is represented in Fig. 5.

After detecting the R-peaks, calculating Beats Per Minute is straightforward, which is the average rate of peaks per minute. Followed by that, the standard deviation of R-R intervals sequence is calculated. From this, the R-R pair differences and their squared differences are calculated in the time-domain heart rate variability measures. Fast Fourier Transformation is used to convert a signal from the time domain to the frequency domain. It is used to break up a signal into several sinusoidal waves of constituent frequencies. By applying Fourier transformation over the R-R interval sequence approximated to a sinusoidal wave, the frequencies that make up the signal can be derived.

From Fig. 6, it can be observed that the R-R interval sequence has a pattern. The continuous function is interpolated to map the R-peaks to the R-R intervals. By applying FFT the frequencies of the sine waves that make up this pattern can be derived. The comparison of interpolated and the original signal is shown in Fig. 7.

Now the LF and HF frequency peaks can be observed from the frequency spectrum. To determine the LF band and HF band, the area under the peak with the limits as (0.04, 0.15) Hz for LF and (0.15, 0.40) Hz for the HF must be found. This can be further used to analyze the signal (Fig. 8).

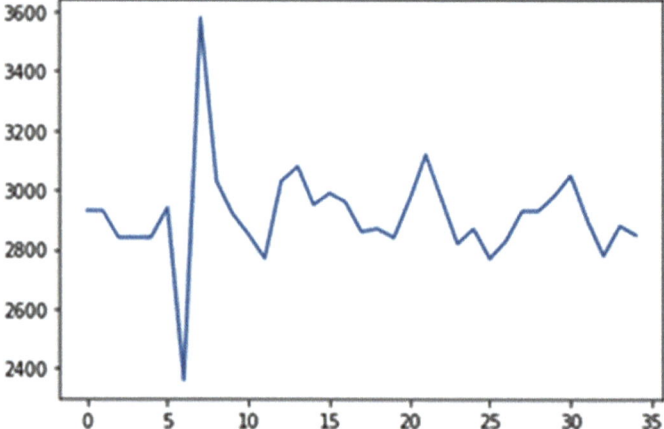

Fig. 6 R-R interval sequence

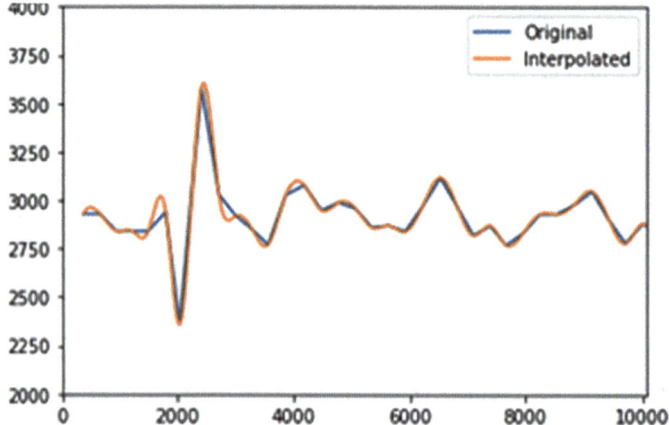

Fig. 7 Signal interpolation

3.4 PPG

PPG heart rate data was obtained from the BIDMC dataset of 53 critically ill patients taken at a hospital. This data was recorded at a sampling frequency of 125 Hz. Sometimes, the sampling frequency of the sensor that was used is not known. One way to check the sampling frequency is to find the total time period during which the observations are made and divide by the number of observations. This approximately gives the total time passed between two successive measurements and thus the sampling frequency of the sensor [32].

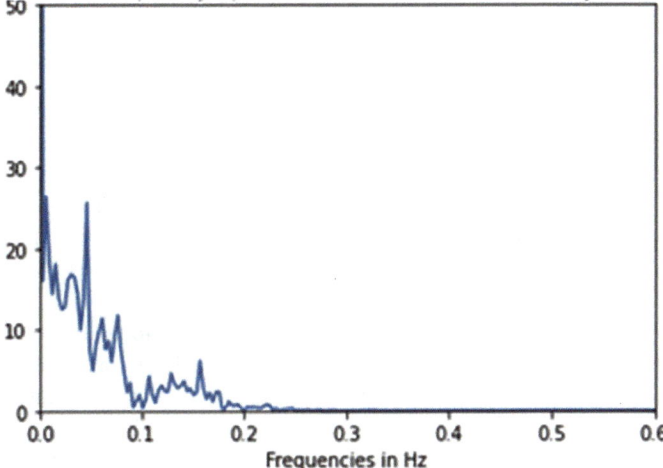

Fig. 8 Frequency spectrum of heart rate variability

It is important to ensure that the sampling frequency of measurements is fairly constant throughout the time period of PPG data collection, which is true for any signals that are measured. Thus, it is important to check standard deviations of the consecutive time intervals to ensure that the measurements were made at approximately regular intervals. In case of irregular measurements, it is important to obtain a better sensor for studies.

Since the data was collected from critically ill patients in a hospital, measurements were taken while lying down on a hospital bed, and motion artifacts are largely eliminated.

The rest of the noise can be removed using the Butterworth filter. The comparison of the original and filtered signal obtained using the Butterworth bandpass filter can be seen in Fig. 9a, b.

The most common method used for analyzing PPG values is to detect systolic peak values in the signal corresponding approximately to systolic phases of the cardiac cycle and find the time passed between successive peaks. How this time

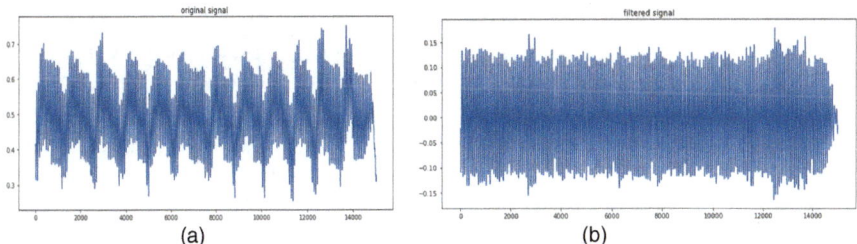

Fig. 9 a Original raw PPG signal; **b** Filtered PPG signal

interval between successive peaks changes forms the basis of heart rate variability. Time-domain and frequency-domain heart rate variability metrics can subsequently be easily derived once these peaks and the intervals between them are identified.

To detect peaks, the maximum value in the points that comprise a cycle must be found. However, it is enough if the maximum point in the systolic phase is identified. Most points in the systolic phase tend to have larger amplitudes and hence tend to be greater than the average. Hence the moving average can act as a good threshold as to which points can be considered to be a possible peak value and find the maximum from them. In Fig. 10, the moving average (shown in green) fitted over the actual signal (shown in blue) can be seen.

Small windows or regions of interest can be created periodically every time the signal crosses the moving average limit in that region. Each region of interest consists of all values greater than the moving average. Once a value lesser than the moving average is encountered, the maximum of the points in the already obtained region is marked to be the peak. A new region of interest is opened when the value moves above the moving average again. In Fig. 11, it can be seen that the detected peaks are marked in red, while the moving average (green) is fitted over the signal (blue).

Fig. 10 PPG signal (blue), moving average (green)

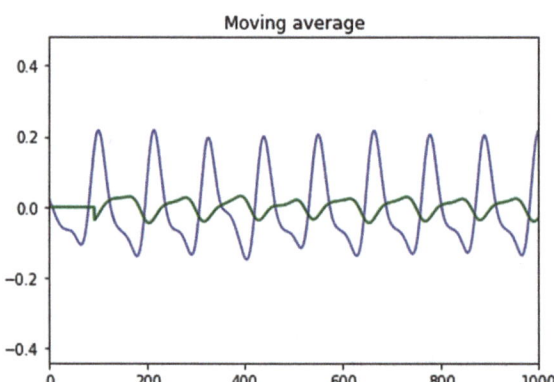

Fig. 11 Detected peaks (red), moving average (green), signal (blue)

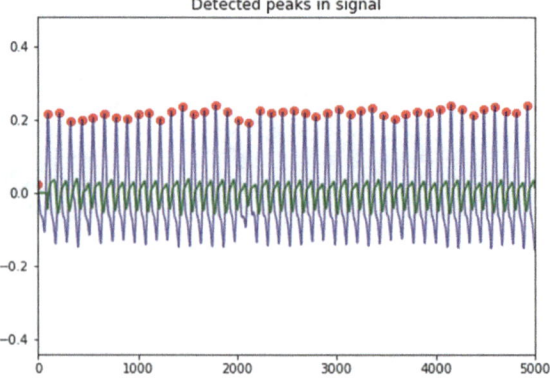

Fig. 12 Interpolated signal
fit over original R-R intervals
versus peak list graph

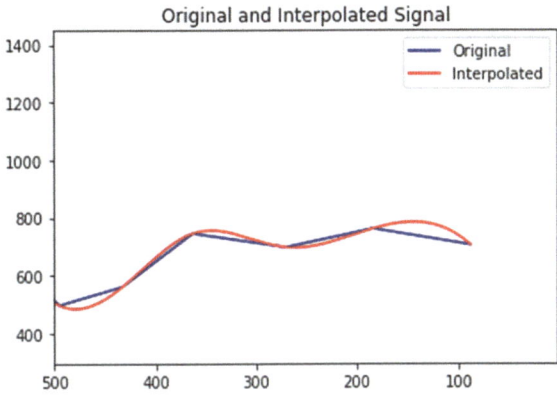

From the peaks obtained, the distance between successive peaks is used to calculate different time-domain measures. Since the analysis of the variability produced in the lengths of the peak-to-peak intervals is desired, a continuous function that maps the position of peaks to the length of the intervals between the peaks must be interpolated. This becomes the new time-series signal. In Fig. 12, the interpolated signal can be seen (in red), approximating the function that maps the position of peaks (x-axis) to R-R intervals (y-axis).

The Fast Fourier transform is applied to this function, which can also be obtained as a method through certain libraries. A sample spacing converted to frequencies is also calculated to plot the final frequency-domain curve. The LF, HF power can be calculated by finding the area under the curve of the frequency-domain signal, shown in Fig. 13, for the corresponding frequency band.

Finally, this is successfully able to reproduce a filtered signal that can be used to derive the heart variability metrics. Each patient's PPG data consisted of 8-min recordings. These were then split into intervals of about 64 s each, and 8 whole intervals were obtained. For each interval, the HRV metrics were calculated and plotted to show the changes over the 8 intervals, as shown in Fig. 14a–d. The average BPM for most patients was about 90 BPM, which would be typical of critically ill patients.

3.5 Results and Discussion

Similar methods can be used to analyze data from sensors that measure heart rate. ECG and PPG sensors both have disadvantages and advantages, but both can be used fairly well as long as constant measurements with reliable sensors are taken. While a healthy heart must show significant variability in heart rate, each metric and the way it changes is specific to the person, as well as underlying health conditions.

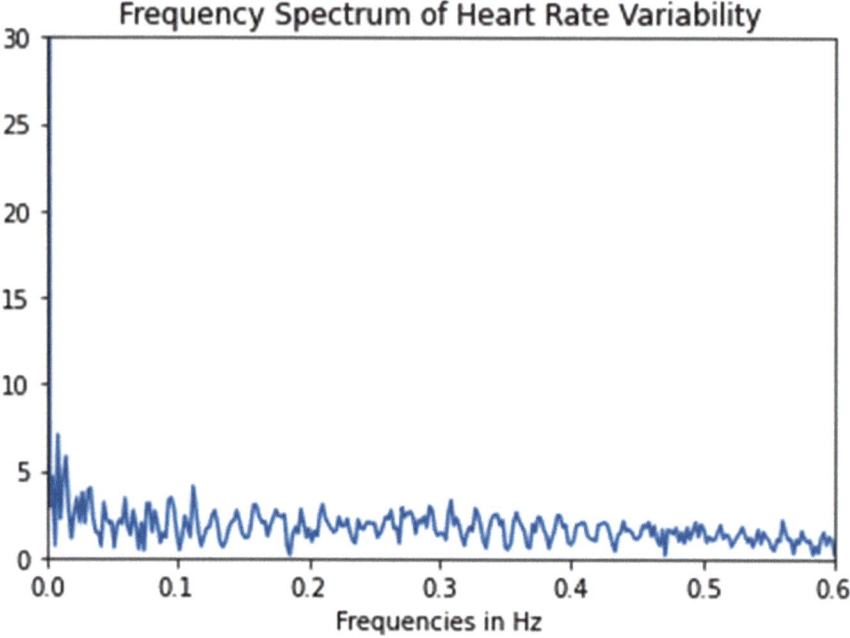

Fig. 13 Frequency spectrum of PPG signal

The analysis methods that have been used in the above case studies are some simple exploratory methods described in the literature that can be used to understand how these metrics are derived, and what the data looks like. Data from all sensors do not come under similar formats, and might not always have continuous measurements. With the ability to explore, clear, and process the metrics, from scratch, custom datasets can be created by data analysts and healthcare professionals, to use for further research, without relying on APIs and libraries that require data that in standard formats. Additional analysis and processing techniques can be employed keeping the basic idea behind heart rate analysis in mind. This acts as a foundation for using the data for machine learning and deep learning models that can be employed along with sensors to provide real-time insights about health. Health experts and data scientists can work together to understand the implications of the results obtained as well.

4 Conclusion

For any computation to be efficient, accurate data is required. With data accuracy, a better understanding of the data at hand is necessary, to understand where the results are coming from.

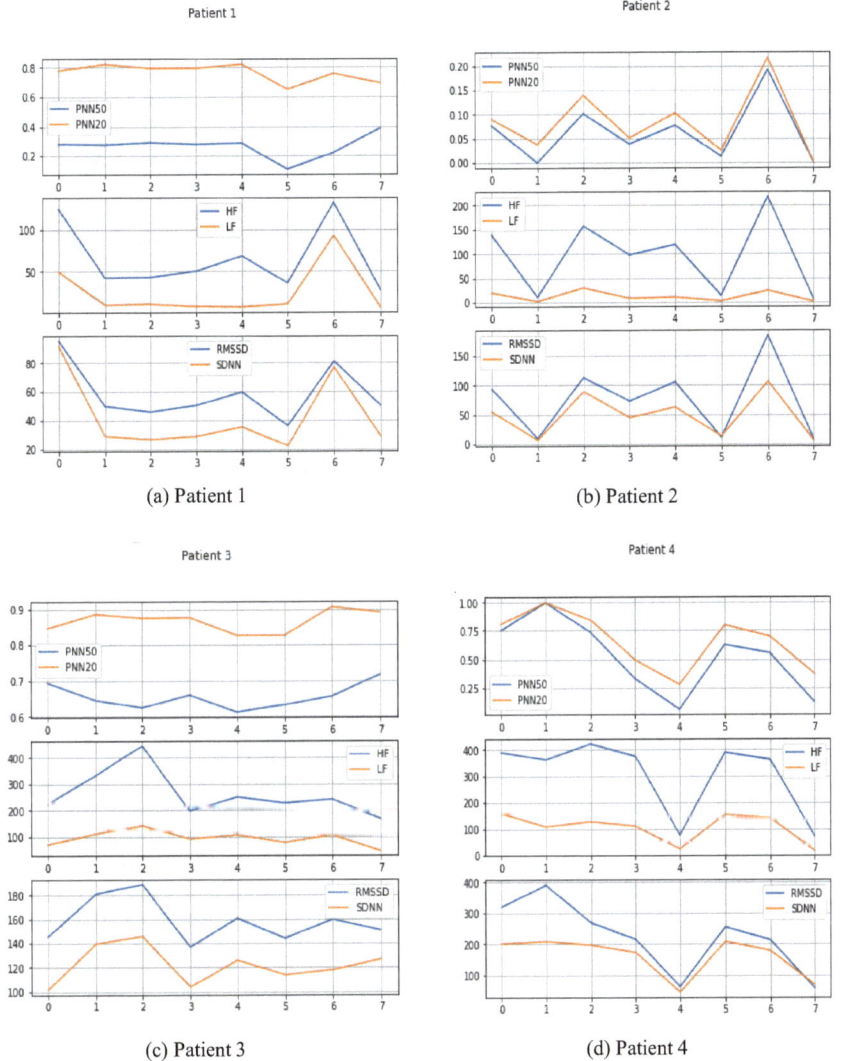

Fig. 14 **a** Patient 1. **b** Patient 2. **c** Patient 3. **d** Patient 4

In the domain of health care, data can prove to be very valuable in the form of providing a better understanding of one's health. Analysis of data from sensors is an extremely promising tool that can be used as effective warning systems, enabling the early prognosis of health issues. Continuous, real-time monitoring can save many lives, as well as expenses that are incurred due to late diagnosis.

References

1. Kawasaki, D., Rozan, H.A.B., Bertoncini, J.V., Romano, V.D., Spatti, D.H.: Arrhythmia classification through characteristics extraction with discrete wavelet transform & machine learning. Maedeh Kiani Sarkaleh and Asadollah Shahbahrami
2. Pour Ebrahim, M., Heydari, F., Wu, T., et al.: Blood pressure estimation using on-body continuous wave radar and photoplethysmogram in various posture and exercise conditions. Sci. Rep. **9**, 16346 (2019)
3. Lin, C.-H.: Frequency-domain features for ECG beat discrimination using grey relational analysis-based classifier. Comput. Math. Appl. **55**(4), 680–690 (2008)
4. Joshi, S.L., Vatti, R.A., Tornekar, R.V.: A survey on ECG signal denoising techniques. In: 2013 International Conference on Communication Systems and Network Technologies, Gwalior, 2013, pp. 60–64. https://doi.org/10.1109/CSNT.2013.22
5. Pour Ebrahim, M., Heydari, F., Wu, T., Walker, K., Joe, K., Redoute, J.M., Yuce, M.R.: Blood pressure estimation using on-body continuous wave radar and photoplethysmogram in various posture and exercise conditions. Sci. Rep. **9**(1), 16346 (2019). https://doi.org/10.1038/s41598-019-52710-8
6. Markx, G.H., Davey, C.L.: The dielectric properties of biological cells at radiofrequencies: applications in biotechnology. Enzyme Microb. Technol. **25**, 161–171 (1999)
7. Chiang, C.Y., Chen, K.H., Liu, K.C., Hsu, S.J., Chan, C.T.: Data collection and analysis using wearable sensors for monitoring knee range of motion after total knee arthroplasty. Sensors (Basel) **17**(2), 418 (2017). Published 2017 Feb 22. https://doi.org/10.3390/s17020418
8. Bahadori, S., Immins, T., Wainwright, T.W.: A review of wearable motion tracking systems used in rehabilitation following hip and knee replacement. J. Rehabil. Assist. Technol. Eng. **5**, 2055668318771816 (2018). Published 2018 Jun 18. https://doi.org/10.1177/2055668318771816
9. Alqaraawi, A., Alwosheel, A., Alasaad, A.: Heart rate variability estimation in photoplethysmography signals using Bayesian learning approach. Healthc. Technol. Lett. **3**(2), 136–142 (2016). Published 2016 Jun 13. https://doi.org/10.1049/htl.2016.0006
10. Elgendi, M., Fletcher, R., Liang, Y., et al.: The use of photoplethysmography for assessing hypertension. NPJ Digit. Med. **2**, 60 (2019). https://doi.org/10.1038/s41746-019-0136-7
11. Pimentel, M.A.F., Johnson, A.E.W., Charlton, P.H., et al.: Toward a robust estimation of respiratory rate from pulse oximeters. IEEE Trans. Biomed. Eng. **64**(8), 1914–1923 (2017). https://doi.org/10.1109/TBME.2016.2613124
12. Choi, J., Gutierrez-Osuna, R.: Removal of respiratory influences from heart rate variability in stress monitoring. IEEE Sens. J. **11**, 2649–2656 (2011). https://doi.org/10.1109/JSEN.2011.2150746
13. Ram, M.R., Madhav, K.V., Krishna, E.H., Komalla, N.R., Reddy, K.A.: A novel approach for motion artifact reduction in PPG signals based on AS-LMS adaptive filter. IEEE Trans. Instrum. Meas. **61**(5), 1445–1457 (2012). https://doi.org/10.1109/TIM.2011.2175832
14. Tamura, T., Maeda, Y., Sekine, M., Yoshida, M.: Wearable photoplethysmographic sensors—past and present. Electronics **3**(2), 282–302 (2014)
15. Scholkmann, F., Boss, J., Wolf, M.: An efficient algorithm for automatic peak detection in noisy periodic and quasi-periodic signals. Algorithms **5**(4), 588–603 (2012)
16. De Hennis, A., Mortellaro, M.: CGM sensor technology (2020). https://doi.org/10.1016/B978-0-12-816714-4.00006-5
17. Aldeer, M., Martin, R.P., Howard, R.E.: PillSense: designing a medication adherence monitoring system using pill bottle-mounted wireless sensors. In: 2018 IEEE International Conference on Communications Workshops, ICC Workshops 2018 – Proceedings, pp. 1–6. Institute of Electrical and Electronics Engineers Inc. (2018). https://doi.org/10.1109/ICCW.2018.8403547
18. Jeldi, A.J., Grant, M., Allen, D.J., et al.: Upright time and sit-to-stand transition progression after total hip arthroplasty: an inhospital longitudinal study. J. Arthroplasty **31**(3), 735–739 (2016). https://doi.org/10.1016/j.arth.2015.09.024

19. Aldeer, M., Javanmard, M., Martin, R.: A review of medication adherence monitoring technologies. Appl. Syst. Innov. **1**, (2018). https://doi.org/10.3390/asi1020014
20. Benjamin, E.M.: Self-monitoring of blood glucose: the basics. Clin. Diabetes **20**(1), 45–47 (2002). https://doi.org/10.2337/diaclin.20.1.45
21. Clarke, W., Kovatchev, B.: Statistical tools to analyze continuous glucose monitor data. Diabetes Technol. Ther. **11** (Suppl 1), S45–S54 (2009). https://doi.org/10.1089/dia.2008.0138
22. Moraes, J.L., Rocha, M.X., Vasconcelos, G.G., Vasconcelos Filho, J.E., de Albuquerque, V.H.C., Alexandria, A.R.: Advances in photoplethysmography signal analysis for biomedical applications. Sensors (Basel) **18**(6), 1894 (2018). Published 2018 Jun 9. https://doi.org/10.3390/s18061894
23. Shaffer, F., Ginsberg, J.P.: An overview of heart rate variability metrics and norms. Frontiers in Public Health. **5**, 258 (2017). https://doi.org/10.3389/fpubh.2017.00258
24. Sachin, M.U., Nagaraj, R., Samiksha, M., Rao, S., Moharir, M.: 2nd International Conference for Convergence in Technology (I2CT), 7–9 April 2017, pp. 236–239. https://doi.org/10.1109/I2CT.2017.8226127
25. Aimie-Salleh, N., Ghani, N.A.A., Hasanudin, N., Shafie, S.N.S.: Heart Rate Variability Recording System Using Photoplethysmography Sensor, Autonomic Nervous System Monitoring - Heart Rate Variability, Theodoros Aslanidis, IntechOpen (2019). https://doi.org/10.5772/intechopen.89901
26. Van Gent, P., Farah, H., Nes, N., Arem, B.: Heart Rate Analysis for Human Factors: Development and Validation of an Open Source Toolkit for Noisy Naturalistic Heart Rate Data (2018)
27. Maiya, P., Moharir, M.: Statistical Modelling and Machine Learning Principles for Bioinformatics Techniques, Tools, and Applications, pp. 63–74. Springer, Singapore (2020)
28. https://www.paulvangent.com/2016/03/15/analyzing-a-discrete-heart-rate-signal-using-python-part-1/
29. https://www.paulvangent.com/2016/03/21/analyzing-a-discrete-heart-rate-signal-using-python-part-2/
30. https://www.paulvangent.com/2016/03/30/analyzing-a-discrete-heart-rate-signal-using-python-part-3/
31. https://www.heartmath.org/research/science of the-heart/heart-rate-variability/
32. https://github.com/paulvangentcom/heartrate_analysis_python

Social Media Analytics for Health Care

K. Aditya Shastry, H. A. Sanjay, and Manoj Kumar

Abstract The increase in health-related communication due to Social Media (SM) has significantly contributed to the rapid progress of the healthcare industry. SM allows for 2-way communication among the patients, health experts, and third parties. It has become a major platform in which the public searches for information related to health care. Hence, the SM has developed as the largest source of discussions related to health care worldwide. Rich healthcare content is generated daily by the large network of healthcare stakeholders such as patients, doctors, pharmaceutical companies, organizations, government agencies on these Social Media platforms (SMP). Valuable knowledge can be extracted from this huge healthcare data if proper techniques are adopted. If this healthcare data related to SM is mined effectively, then the majority of the patient needs may be satisfied. In view of these aspects, this chapter describes how Social Media Analytics (SMA) is being applied in the domain of health care. The chapter focuses on the different SMA approaches used in health care, followed by certain recent case studies of SMA in health care. The research areas that can be explored for SMA in healthcare are also discussed along with certain drawbacks.

Keywords Social media analytics · Health care · Techniques · Applications · Research

K. Aditya Shastry (✉) · H. A. Sanjay · M. Kumar
Department of Information Science & Engineering, Nitte Meenakshi Institute of Technology, Yelahanka, Bangalore 560064, Karnataka, India
e-mail: adityashastry.k@nmit.ac.in

H. A. Sanjay
e-mail: sanjay.ha@nmit.ac.in

M. Kumar
e-mail: manoj.kumar@nmit.ac.in

1   Introduction

Several SM tools such as sites sharing media, platforms related to social networking, gaming and virtual reality along with blogs and microblogs aid the Health Care Professionals (HCPs) [1]. These tools can be employed to enhance care and education of patients, promotion-related activities of organizations, networking of professionals and education along with programs associated with public health. Nevertheless, certain potential hazards due to the improper usage of these tools that can adversely impact the HCPs includes the generation of information that is of poor quality, damaging the professional image, issues related to privacy of patients, misuse of personal and professional information along with the issues related to licensing and law [2]. In the following subsections, we briefly discuss the definition of SM and how HCPs participate in SM.

- *What are Social Media:*

"Social Media" definition is very broad and is continuously changing. Broadly, it refers to tools linked with the Internet that permits communities and individuals to communicate in a group for sharing ideas, messages, images and other information. It also allows the collaboration of individuals or organizations in real time [3]. "Web 2.0" or "social networking" is another name for SM [4]. A variety of features are provided by SM that serve the individual users for different purposes [5].

SM participation by the general public has enhanced rapidly over the recent decade [6]. Since 2005, the proportion of adults participating in SM has enhanced from 8 to 72%. There is no age restriction on SM usage and is prevalent around the world [7]. For instance, the users of Facebook (FB) during 2012 surpassed 1 billion people globally representing one-seventh of the global population [8]. Also, every single day 100 million Twitter (TWTR) users send more than sixty-five million tweets. Similarly, approximately 2 billion videos are watched on YouTube (YT) [9]. Significant political and social events are associated with SM. One of the drawbacks of SM is that it has significantly reduced the attention span of individuals leading to the reduced usage of print media [10].

- *Participation in SM by Health Care Professionals:*

The HCPs utilize SM for several tasks such as sharing health-related information, debating about policies related to health care, promoting healthy habits, interacting with people, and in educating students, patients, colleagues [11]. The utility of SM by HCPs aids in improving health outcomes, development of professional networks, enhancing the awareness related to the latest research developments and drug discoveries, motivating the patients and deliver authentic health information to the medical community [12].

HCPs usually participate in online communities so that they can be updated about latest health-related news, hear what medical experts have to say, get updates regarding any recent research developments in health care, or discuss patient issues with colleagues on a global level [13]. Doctors can share their case studies or ideas, provide referrals to patients, publicize their research, advertise their best practices, or involve in promoting health products [14]. Certain physicians utilize SM for direct consultation with patients for providing online healthcare [15].

A study done by SM site QuantiMD discovered that out of the 4,000 surveyed doctors, 90% of them utilized SM for personal activities and around 65% of them utilized SM for activities related to their profession [16]. Around, one-third of the doctors conveyed that they are using social networks [17]. This clearly indicates that the SM is being used by the physicians for both professional and personal reasons [18].

Conversely, the usage of SM by pharmacists has been slower when compared to physicians. However, social networks dedicated to the pharmacy are being created and used [19]. Studies have demonstrated that pharmacists are mostly making use of FB [20]. Even though FB is being used for personal communications, it has been observed that greater than 90 pages have been dedicated to the pharmacy profession like Cynical Pharmacist, etc. But TWTR is being used by only 10% of pharmacists while there are around 538,628 profiles related to Pharmacists in LI [21, 22].

The rest of this chapter has four sections. The second section highlights the different methods that can be employed for performing SMA in health care. The third section describes some real-world applications of SMA in the domain of health care. The fourth section analyses the numerous research domains related to SMA in Healthcare that can be beneficial to researchers and academicians. The conclusion of the chapter is described at the end.

2   Approaches for Analytics in SM for Health Care

In this section, we discuss certain commonly utilized techniques for analyzing the data from SM in the field of health care.

Recently, there is a surge in SM activities related to healthcare in which various stakeholders of medical professionals such as patients, doctors, etc., are involved. Health-related problems along with the possible treatments are discussed in these online communities leading to a better understanding of health-related benefits. The major reasons for this upsurge are that detailed discussion about the health-related topics can be carried out between the stakeholders as opposed to the brief question and answer sessions between doctors and patients. Several health-related benefits will be the consequence of this. The topics of health care can be effectively analyzed in order to process medical text content. Earlier, the analysis of the healthcare topics was based on mining the text associated with medical prescriptions and the medical texts. However, recent analysis of user-created medical contents on SM such as scientific logs of web, Q&A related to health, and online health care groups are being done [23].

Due to the rapid competition in health care and high expectations from healthcare providers, SM is gaining rapid attention for developing stronger bonds between patients and physicians. SM enables doctors in responding quickly to patient queries which may get delayed when interactions are done face to face due to a shortage of time [23].

Popular SMPs like FB, LinkedIn (LI), TWTR, and YT aids the doctors in the promotion of their services in an online fashion. Some of the top strategies for SM in the healthcare industry are highlighted below [24]:

- *Analyze the target audience for marketing the SM content*: Different platforms of SM have different types of users. For instance, the kind of people using FB and TWTR are quite different from those using LI. Hence, exclusive campaigns must be designed for diverse SMPs and not go with a common campaign for all.
- *Handling Queries of Patients*: Queries or grievances from patients can be handled via online communities and forums of discussion on FB. For example, in the "Just Ask" campaign of Apollo Hospital, the doctors answered queries regarding specific ailments using the comments section on FB [24].
- *Deliver Health Information*: Using SM various tips of doctors, health quotes, and live medical procedures can be shared via images, videos of YT, infographics on Pinterest, Flickr, and FB. Blog posts can also be shared via these SMPs. Queries related to health can be effectively answered using platforms such as Quora. An active community is connected via correct answers, which in turn enhances the ranking in the search engine. Hangout sessions like webinars and chats can be easily created via platforms such as Google+ in which medical specialists can interact with patients. For example, a live video of knee surgery performed by the Medical Center of the Raritan situated in New Jersey was posted on YT and the surgery details were posted on TWTR. The objective was to educate the medical details about the finer specifics of knee surgery.
- *Starting, Creating, and Branding trends and SM campaigns*: Online contests can be scheduled to promote brands associated with health care. Effective, valuable information can be found from quizzes constructed out of healthcare topics. The names of brands can be included as hashtags to promote awareness of brands (For e.g., #Ask [BrandName]). Apart from TWTR, hashtags can be utilized in Instagram and FB as well. An initiative of FB and TWTR called #MonsoonMantra provided useful health tips for monsoons. Similar campaigns such as Donation of Organs have been started by Fortis which has resulted in around 2.6 K TWTR followers [24].

Individuals not having brands can tweet the latest topics related to health care. These tweets can be complemented with supporting images. For example, when the #WorldCancerDay was trending on TWTR, @MaxBupa which is a health insurance company performed this task.

- *Building of Brands along with Management of Reputations*: Significant role is played by SM Marketing (SMM) in managing the online reputations. The testimonials of patients help in improving the branding and reputation of the healthcare industry. Reviews of the customer can be shared by medical insurance organizations, hospitals, and doctors via SM. The activities of Customer Social Responsibilities (CSR), engagement of customers offline, and campaigns for creating awareness can be promoted online. Certain popular regional personalities can be included in a campaign if the business is local which can aid in enhancing the visibility of brand both online and offline [24].

- *Building Loyalty with patients and creating long lasting relationships*: Generation of new leads is not the only task involved in SMM. Sustaining good relationships with prevailing employees along with developing trustworthiness between patients also form major tasks in SMM. In such a scenario, customers who are satisfied and happy with the business will spread word of mouth which can help in expanding the customer base. For instance, a campaign called Fit2Run was launched by Institute related to Heart located in Asia (AHI), which is a center for cardiac care situated in India. The campaign talked about the benefits of getting treated in AHI and how normal cardiac condition can be achieved. The runners who participated in marathons conducted by AHI posted personal quotes that acted as a marketing strategy for AHI [24].
- *Establish Online Communication Protocols*: Each organization must have a well-planned policy for communications that are online in nature. Appropriate care and precision should be inculcated in the employees of an organization for using the SM. Employees can also be provided incentives for using SM. However, employees should be prohibited from breaching the privacy and ethics of customers while utilizing SM. Health experts must verify the health tips or any medical information before the content is published online since wrong information related to health can cause considerable damage to the customers and the organization. Monitoring of competitors' feedback on online behavior is necessary along with a professional response.
- *Search Engine Optimization (SEO) Through SM*: Google+, FB are certain major SMPs on which profiles of doctors and hospitals can be found when they are searched. Similarly, Quora, YT are the major sites in which health-related queries with answers can be found. In such cases, if a company wants to appear higher in a search then SEO of content and profile needs to be performed. Several phrases such as disease names, related symptoms, remedies, etc. can be included in names of profiles, description of owner, and any other shared material for a company to appear higher in internet searches. To obtain direct traffic, link can be provided to the organization's website from these accounts.

As most people utilize SMPs it acts as an ideal place on the web for interaction purposes. Well-thought-out campaigns can get more weightage by sharing the competencies of SM. Hence, SM needs to be used in a smart way for connecting with patients and keeping them loyal. The section on comments comprises questions that can be shared to a wider range of people in order to obtain quick answers.

3 Real-World Applications of SMA in Health Care: Case Study

This section discusses certain real-world applications of SMA in health care in the form of case studies. Following are the case studies that are discussed in this section.

3.1 Navicent Health SM Case Study: [25]

Navicent Health is one of the premier providers of health care in Georgia, USA. The hospital provides solutions that are multidisciplinary in nature, apart from having a deeper bond with the community. The organization plays a major leadership role in Georgia due to its well-planned local initiatives and partnerships with reputed universities. The organization recruited an SM campaigning company called Captivate for implementing its SM strategy.

Navicent Health desired for an effective, consistent, and multilayered SMM strategy that would inform the public about issues related to health care, increase the access of patients to services, manage issues related to public relations, create awareness, and assist the employees in growing their social network.

The key plan was to strengthen the ties among providers of health care and the patients. The SMM company Captivate established an effective strategy that was centered on the overall goals of Navicent. Captivate also provided customized strategies to meet the services, demands, and target audiences of Navicent.

The key components in the hospital's SM strategy comprised of the following:

- To develop the calendar for editorial containing interesting contents, the keyword research, and hashtag trends were analyzed.
- Executing the proven process for effective community management and the periodic evolution of engaging content.
- Regular analysis and reporting to identify crucial areas for the optimization and growth opportunity.
- Utilizing the streams of Hootsuite keyword search, response to time-sensitive messages can be quick.
- Training the medical personnel on the management of SM and development of interesting posts on each channel.
- Generating the custom imagery and infographics on a regular basis that aligns with the editorial calendar that was approved.
- Campaign development for sharing testimonials of employees and patients.
- Developing a campaign to share patient and employee stories and created a new process for campaign content curation helped to implement the new process at the hospital.

Currently, good progress and efficiency were observed by Navicent since it employed effective SM strategies for marketing purposes. Currently, captivate leads the management and development of the SM strategy of Navicent with precision which is measurable and targeted. This generated a swift growth of Navicent in numerous platforms related to SM like Instagram, TWTR, YT, FB, and LI [25].

3.2   St. Louis Hospital Case Study: [26]

tSunela is an organization specialized in SMM strategies. It was approached by a leading hospital in the St. Louis area that consisted of 2,500 medical professionals for SEO and assistance regarding SM. The hospital wanted to spread consciousness about health and the services provided through SM.

The key issues that tSunela had to resolve were to design a social strategy for marketing the hospital. Firstly, the client had to be educated about the SM domain which itself was a great challenge. Awareness had to be created for the hospital about the return of investment that can be got if SM is used for marketing the hospital. The hospital had to be made aware of the SM benefits for expanding the hospital's reach.

In this regard, an SM campaign called "Doctor of the Week" was used to highlight the primary care providers. Furthermore, videos and photographs related to health care were published on Flickr and YT. This content was then optimized so that the search related to the topic would rank higher when searched in search engines. Events related to health care such as screening of diabetes, learning expos, etc., along with spreading the press releases were done to promote the hospital's brand.

These SM strategies such as the "Doctor of the Week", SEO, and extensive distribution of outlets related to SM generated faster accomplishments. The monthly views of the hospital in YT enhanced by 161% (i.e., unique views increased to 445 from 170) and in Flickr image the viewers increased to 132 from 69 (i.e., enhanced by 94%). Furthermore, the active FB users enhanced to 150% (i.e., the viewers increased to 5,373 from 2,152) on a regular basis. On the website of the hospital, the webpage on "Doctor of the Week" ranks among the highest viewed pages on their sites.

The client hospital has now understood the importance of an exclusively dedicated campaign for SM and is observing a high return on the investment associated with digital marketing. The brand recognition and loyalty of the organization have been strengthened due to the high engagement of the target audience with the hospital.

Some of the domains that have utilized SM in health care are summarized from Sects. 3.3, 3.4, 3.5, 3.6, 3.7 and 3.8 [27].

3.3   Health Awareness

Several medical educational institutions are highlighting the future aspects of SM in healthcare by conducting training and workshops for physicians and patients [28]. For instance, the students of nursing are encouraged to create short YT videos of 3–5 min duration instead of the traditional pamphlet distribution [28].

Moreover, a current study confirmed that utilizing TWTR and FB as supplementary tools for delivering educational content can be an effective way to engage medical trainees [29]. Founded on a novel study, FB and YT were the most commonly utilized platforms by medical course participants, which amounted to 89% of 291 members that were polled [30].

To enable wider interaction among HCPs and physicians and report medical news, the professional medical societies like the oncology center located in the US (ASCO) are utilizing SMPs like TWTR [31]. Furthermore, it is observed that the use of SM has allowed cases to be reported on a live basis that led to better monitoring around the globe [32].

In general, physicians feel that using SM can ensure suitable distribution of medical information through scientific publications and educational videos to patients and HCPs [33]. SM is enhancing the accessibility and approachability of doctors by the patients. Patients feel that they are in more control as they can ask the physicians knowledgeable questions [34].

In real world, consultations are bounded by time. In such a situation, SM provides a platform in which patients can expand their medical information base. Additionally, SM provides support to existing relationships of patients with their doctors [35].

3.4 Professional Education

Education related to the medical field is being enhanced due to the communication capabilities provided by SM. It has been observed that the extensive usage of SM by individuals between the age of 18 and 29 years has led to the adaptation of clinical syllabi [3, 6]. Several studies have demonstrated that the SM has led to significant improvements in the understanding power, professionalism, communication, and ethics among the medical students. Students are being recruited by universities through SM for improving the academic library access, and for creating classrooms and office hours that are virtual in nature along with other different learning experiences [36].

SM has found its usage in the curriculum of UG pharmacy. Approximately, one-third of programs related to pharmacy are utilizing TWTR in certain ways. A survey conducted in the year 2018 found that about 47% of staff in pharmacy were utilizing FB for teaching purposes. The other half planned to use SM in future. In one instance, a faculty of geriatric pharmacotherapy course utilized FB for encouraging discussions in class and to link the students with senior members of society (participated voluntarily). This exercise not only enhanced the views of the students toward the senior citizens but also exposed the seniors to FB. In another instance, Faculty at the Auburn University created TWTR handles for the pharmacy students to discuss class-related topics anonymously. By the semester end, around 81% of the students realized that they were able to express their opinions more frankly using the TWTR handle. However, 71% also felt that TWTR had led to a certain amount of distraction [36].

With respect to nursing, online SM has influenced the way educational institutions work. A survey reported that around 54% of schools linked with nursing were utilizing SM tools. For instance, it has been found that the critical decisions to be taken by the nurses during critical scenarios have been enhanced due to the thorough usage of TWTR. The videos related to the clinical scenarios were seen by the clinical students, who in turn gave their observations through TWTR on the condition of the patient. The instructor then gave his/her feedback on the student's observations [36].

3.5 SM Utilization by Consumers

By means of SM, the users can meet their requirements, preferences, and needs. As per the survey conducted by the Institute of Research related to Health (HRI) of PricewaterhouseCoopers, around 42% of the users utilized SM for accessing reviews of HCPs [37]. According to this survey, around 20% took part in health forum activities, health cause was supported by approximately 30%, while health experience was posted by roughly around 25% [4]. Valuable experiences can be shared by the patients through the SM. Nowadays, terminology called e-patients has come that represents the patients who go online for searching health-related information, and illnesses. Apart from the younger people, the usage of SM is picking up among older people also. Furthermore, the tools offered by SM enable groups to be formed from individuals and communities from groups so that activities can be efficiently organized [4].

3.6 Patient Care

Slowly, the HCPs have started using SM directly for the care of patients. For instance, a platform known as Web View is provided by the Health Sciences University located in Georgia that permits the patients to interact with doctors by asking questions and requesting refills of prescriptions [38, 39].

Current studies demonstrated that physicians have started to involve more in SM interaction with patients [39]. The communication with patients is being improved due to the extensive utilization of SM like TWTR and FB by physicians [39]. Around 60% of physicians favored the utilization of SM for interaction with patients [39]. But other related work has demonstrated substantial resistance for utilizing SM by physicians for interacting with patients.

A study of 480 practicing and student doctors revealed that 68% felt that it was ethically wrong to interact with patients on SM regarding providing health-related solutions in the absence of in-person interactions with the patients [39].

3.7 Health Insurance Company Uses

The HRI survey for consumers demonstrated the fact that consumers prefer sharing information with healthcare providers such as physicians and hospitals through SM rather than sharing them with health insurance or pharmaceutical companies. However, certain health insurance organizations are utilizing SM to disseminate health-related information to their customers. For instance, certain tips linked to a fit lifestyle such as healthy diets, controlling smoking habits are offered to consumers by the health insurance establishments [39].

3.8 Pharmaceutical Company Uses

Even though consumer relies less on pharmaceutical companies, several of them utilize SM for marketing purposes. The product comments by patients and doctors on SM are monitored by pharma companies. Blogs/Medical sites contain comments/tips on the cure of a particular disease by a drug/device. But the key disadvantage is that certain off-label drugs may be endorsed by pharmaceutical companies through SM which may be potentially harmful to its consumers. Although physicians may prescribe off-label drugs, they cannot be prescribed by any drug companies without doctor consultation. Hence, drug manufacturers, now have a set of guidelines on the use of off-label drugs/device [40] (Table 1).

4 Research Areas Related to Analytics in SM (SM) for Health Care

Healthcare research is using websites of SM like LI, TWTR, and FB as tools. Novel prospects for research are emerging on topics related to health care such as the weight loss programs in mobile social networking. Despite efforts to establish guidelines for researching online health information, researchers are facing several challenges related to ethics that are still unresolved. This section deliberates detailed issues for doing research linked with SM. It also discusses ways to handle issues linked to privacy, confidentiality, and consent when tools related to SM are being used for research in healthcare [42, 43].

LI, FB, and TWTR are the 3 most frequently used websites for SM [44–46]. Students, public, and professionals use these sites to share and collect health-related information. For example, in the U.S.A, around 78% of the Internet users utilized sites associated with social networking in 2019 [47]. The patterns of communication are being changed by sharing information via SM [48]. Consequently, tools of SM are becoming prominent tools for doing research [49].

Table 1 SM website resources related to healthcare [41]

Name	Description	Website
33 Charts	Blog on medicine, health, and social media	www.33charts.com
Dose of Digital	Blog on digital technology and social media in pharma and healthcare social media wiki	www.doseofdigital.com
Geri Pal	Geriatrics, hospice, and palliative medicine blogs	www.geripal.org
iHealth Beat	Free, daily news digest reporting on technology's impact on health care	www.ihealthbeat.org
Kevin MD	Offers narrative of doctors on latest health bulletins	www.kevinmd.com
Mashable	Delivers the latest SM and Web technology news	www.mashable.com
Mayo Clinic Center for SM	Provides access to tools and resources on the use of SM in healthcare and hosts the SM health network service	www.socialmedia.mayoclinic.org
Pallimed	Blog on hospice and palliative medicine	www.pallimed.org
Project related to Pew Internet and life of Americans	Offers analysis of data on the internet influence on communities, health care, and lives related to civil & political activities	www.pewinternet.org
SM University, Global	Offers training in SM, particularly for communications, advertising, and community relations professionals	www.social-media-university-global.org
Symplu	Healthcare SM consultancy for possessing the project related to healthcare hashtag that focuses on making the TWTR usage available for health care	www.symplur.com

Numerous research prospects are being offered by channels of SM for performing research on topics like:

- The social networks influence apparent social aid for persons having chronic illness [50].
- The ways of gathering, distribution, and information exchange related to health by the users of social channels [51–53].
- The dissemination of fake information related to outbreaks of illness and to educate consumers about the strategies of health communication [54].

- Patient recruitment for trials related to medicine [55, 56].
- The impact of exposures associated with SM related to certain behaviors [57].
- The distribution of information related to public health such as awareness of cancer and the prevalence of specific behaviors like opioid misuse [58–60].

As can be observed from the above points, new interesting insights from health-related information can be extracted by utilizing SM channels as tools of research. However, there are certain risks associated when utilizing SM for research. This section discusses certain ways in which these issues can be handled by researchers. This section describes how issues related to ethics, privacy, confidentiality, and consent can be addressed while performing internet research using SM.

4.1 SM (SM) Websites and Ethical Challenges

The primary obstacle while doing research using SM channels is that all the information in it are public. This creates a major hindrance when doing research. The division between private and public online spaces can sometimes get vague leading to ethical related issues in research. Numerous ethical concerns particularly in research related to health can arise since SM channels are governed by a different set of rules than conventional research [61].

Specifically, conventional research practices are overseen by high standards of ethics comprising of integrity, and the professional conduct of researchers. Mainly, the privacy and confidentiality of research information is ensured in good research. However, when performing research utilizing SM, several challenges related to informed consent, privacy and confidentiality arises.

(i) *Privacy*: In SM, the boundaries linked to geography do not exist as compared to communications that occur face-to-face. Based on the settings of user's privacy, the personal profiles of users can be visible to unknown persons from diverse cultures and communities who are not known directly to the user. This leads to grave issues around the privacy of an individual using the SM [61]. For instance, the privacy settings in FB is reliant on the self-education of the user.

This concern related to privacy in SM is real and not imaginary. For example, a survey conducted by the Otago Medical School University located in New Zealand found that approximately one-fourth of the doctors using the FB was not aware of its privacy settings. This made their information publicly accessible. This led to the breaking of the protocol among patients and doctors (for instance, publishing photos of admitted patients on FB without consent from the patient). This study demonstrates an important fact that many users may not be aware or worried regarding the options of privacy when employing SM in their personal as well as professional life. Even if, the privacy options are used it may not full proof. For example, full privacy is not guaranteed by FB.

This poses challenges for researchers in medicine who are willing to use the SM as they could fail to obtain legal consent from the users [61].

(ii)   *Consent*: When users join FB, by default the user's information is made public and hence is widely accessible. Hence, when friends connect via FB, they can access information of all the others in the group [23]. For example, by analyzing the posts and activities of a medical intern, a researcher may understand whether the intern is exhibiting professional behavior or not. Researchers can access and mingle with associates in social networks without utilizing techniques that confirm whether a consent is truly informed/provided [62].

The paper [62] dealt with issues related to ethics that emerge when using SM. It provided valid evidence. Wide publicity was received by this paper due to the technique used. The newsfeeds of FB users were manipulated while the participants were unaware of this. The journal editor defended the publication by emphasizing that the author's work followed the guidelines of the Data Use Policy of FB. They went on to defend it by saying that prior to account creation in FB the authors were aware of this experiment. The trial was performed by FB for internal validations. As observed, this poses a serious risk to the user's privacy in which the user's data can be collected easily by SMPs such as FB.

4.2   Dangers of SM in Health Care

Certain hazards of SM in health care are summarized below:

1.   Poor Information Quality:

The key drawback of healthcare information prevalent on SM websites and other online platforms is the absence of reliability and quality. Unknown authors publish medical articles on SM and cannot be traced leading to unreliable health-related information being circulated throughout the web. Furthermore, the information related to medicine may not be referenced properly, can be incomplete, or not formal. Individual patient stories are given more preference on SM rather than evidence-based medicine, which relies more on scientific evidence. Because SM is interactive in nature, any user can upload any unreliable medical content on SM websites making it more dangerous than the classic online media. Explicit and implicit conflicts of interest may arise in SM, making the users of SM more vulnerable since they may find it hard to interpret [62].

2.   Risks associated with SM:

The following points highlights certain dangers that may be caused when new SMPs are utilized in health care:

- Control of Message:
  Compared to traditional media, messages in SM spread faster giving less time for reacting/thinking or controlling the situation. Hence, proper care must be ensured before posting any message on SM. It is better to take suggestion from communication experts if the user posting the message is unsure regarding the content, he/she is going to post on the SM.
- Breaches in Security and Privacy:
  Concerns associated with security and privacy form the primary concerns when information related to health is shared via SM [53]. Following precautions should be taken by providers of health care when SM is being utilized for distributing information [62]:

  - Personal content in SM can be secured by utilizing appropriate privacy settings.
  - The healthcare providers and stakeholders must regularly check their SM profiles and contents to verify whether the information is accurate and not modified. The reputation of the medical experts may get significantly damaged by undue or irresponsible online content posted by them.
  - Professional boundaries must be kept by doctors during online interaction with their patients. The patient data must be secured by ensuring proper safety and security [62].

- Damage to the professional reputation:
  Unethical comments posted by patients about doctors, medical institutions can seriously damage their professional reputations. A long-lasting impression is usually generated that reflects the type of personality, values, and priorities of the doctor based on the content that he/she posts on SM. Certain views of the person posting SM contents gets formed based on his/her profile, posts, comments, photos, friends, etc. [63]
- Weaknesses in Health Care:
  Internet restrictions may not be fully understood by some patients since no proper guidelines are established for handling information related to health on SM channels. Patients may be susceptible to fake health information circulating around the SM. The patients must know their medical history is not considered when online medical advice are provided via SM. Till now, no proper guidelines are available for online patient consultation by physicians. The accountability of online medical consultation is still not established. For instance, in the USA, the health information provided by AmericanWell.com via videoconferencing between patients of Hawaii and the U.S.A is available for all irrespective of their location [63].
  Several constraints are faced by HCPs for posting health stories of patients via SM. As per the Act associated with the Accountability and Portability of Health Insurance (HIPAA) established in 1996, the data of patients can be used without their agreement only for payment, treatment, and operations related to health care. This ensures the confidentiality of patients by HIPAA. Thus, the physicians are

required to obtain the prior consent of patients before their information is used in SM either publicly or on restricted networks [63].

- Legal Issues:

New legal complexities are rising due to the extensive SM utilization. Several rights of the constitution can be applied to SM usages like freedom of speech, right to confidentiality, and freedom from seizure and search. But these rights can be subjected to challenges. For instance, nursing students were expelled since they had posted vulgar messages on SM regarding their patient's race, gender, and beliefs. This expulsion was upheld by the District Court of U.S.A in 2009 since the nurses had violated the code of conduct of the school. The school's code of honor and confidentiality agreement specified standards of acceptable behaviors. During recruitment, signature on this document was taken from by all the nurses and hence the claim of the nursing students that their freedom of speech was violated was rejected by the court. Likewise, a student who posted drunken pirate pictures on SM was expelled [64].

As mentioned before, the discussions between patients and HCPs along with any personal information of the patient should not be posted on SM without the consent of the patient. If permission is given by the patient, then it should be mentioned clearly in the post. A disclaimer needs to be published in the post stating that the opinions that are posted are the self-views of the person posting and is not connected with the employer. Discussions on legal cases are prohibited in SM since the current law doesn't allow it [64].

- Barriers related to SM:

Numerous challenges exist in SM even though it represents an extremely beneficial tool. Some of the barriers are summarized below:

- Obstacles faced during return of investment:

As with other forms of marketing, the SM starts with the service line identification with surplus capacity and the strategy development to fill them. The benefit of utilizing SM tools for marketing is that most of them are free. However, substantial staff time is consumed for SMM. Also, related costs are incurred like the amount of staff time spent. But new and trustworthy patients can be attracted by using good strategies in SM projects. A study done by YouGov (a research organization) specified that 57% of clients were inclined to opt for a hospital that has a strong SM connection with them [65].

- Obstacles related to time:

Time is critical, mostly for HCPs and physicians. Responding/maintaining each and every update in FB or TWTR can consume a lot of time for the physicians. Instead of reading every update, the incoming information can be organized to create lists focusing on specific themes. For instance, organizing the messages based on priority level o r specialty can be a good idea [66].

Another guideline is addressing the societal needs that are critical to the physician and that motivate him/her. Additional responsibility is added for the HCP when using SM during their free time. Hence, it is better to focus on relevant issues that justify the effort put into it [66].

4.3 Guidelines Issued by Professional Organizations to Be Followed by HCPs When Using SM

Guidelines on how to use SM are being issued by several societies linked with HCPs. For instance, guidelines for SM usage by pharmacists was issued by the Pharmacists of the System of Health in the American Society (ASHP) in the year 2012. The pharmacists were advised by ASHP to follow professional standards such as [66].

- Providing clinical advice only when the complete case history of the patient is known.
- To identify which type of communication suits the needs of a patient.
- Accurate information to be delivered to the patient in a timely fashion.
- To invalidate any medical information that is misleading.
- Privacy of patient to be safeguarded.
- Maintaining the reputation of pharmacists when using SM anonymously or personally.

The establishment of procedures and policies for healthcare systems was recommended by the ASHP for balancing the benefits of SM along with its probable dangers and accountability issues.

In the year 2011, a document of guidance for the suitable usage of SM was published by the Boards of the State Medical Federation (FASB). This document stresses the following points [66]:

- Safeguarding the privacy keeping the information of patients discreet.
- Maintaining transparency and professionalism.
- Avoiding giving any medical advice via online as the information can be distributed endlessly.

The general rules/guidelines that must be followed by HCPs while using SM are illustrated in Table 2 [67].

5 Conclusion

SM has a vital role in the sector of health with a wider scope. However, several queries related to the analytics of data, confidentiality, expertise, and quality of information continue to be unanswered. The application of SM tools in an astute and sensible fashion can promote personal and public health along with professional progress and development. In this chapter, the participation level of healthcare professionals in SM is discussed along with various techniques employed for analyzing SM data in health care. Recent real-world case studies in the domain of SMA in health care have been described. The potential research areas, dangers of SM in health care have been discussed in detail. The chapter ends with the general guidelines to be followed for implementing SMA in health care.

Table 2 Guidelines for SM usage by healthcare workers [67]

Context	Concept
Credibility of contents	• Data from reliable sources should be shared • Disprove any imprecise material encountered
Issues related to law	• Authored materials may be discoverable • Laws of privacy related to nation and states need to be obeyed • Laws associated with copyright need to be followed
Concerns associated with licensing	• Laws related to professional licensing needs to be obliged
Networking guidelines	• Patients should not be contacted to join the SM networks • Patients willing to join the SM network must be guided on secure means of joining
Patient care	• Non-patients should not be given advice related to medicines • Disclosures should be made in a suitable manner and accuracy; privacy disclaimers should be published
Privacy related to patients	• Addressing particular patients should be avoided • Laws related to patient confidentiality need to be strictly followed • Consent of patients should be acquired wherever possible • Identity of patients should be protected • Patients should be addressed in a dignified manner
Personal privacy	• Stringent privacy settings that are available must be utilized • Professional and personal profiles must be separated
Professional ethics	• Remuneration received must be revealed • Illegitimate or pseudo claims must be avoided
Self-identification	• Identifying oneself on sites that are professional in nature is essential • Correct credentials must be stated • Employees should specify their employers and should not indulge in freelance advice

References

1. Ventola, C.L.: Social Media and health care professionals: benefits, risks, and best practices. P&T **39**(7), 491–520 (2014)
2. Grindrod, K., Forgione, A., Tsuyuki, R.T., Gavura, S., Giustini, D.: Pharmacy 2.0: a scoping review of Social Media use in pharmacy. Res. Soc. Adm. Pharm. **10**(1), 256–270 (2014)
3. Peck, J.L.: Social Media in nursing education: responsible integration for meaningful use. J. Nurs. Educ. **19**, 1–6 (2014)
4. Chauhan, B., George, R., Coffin, J.: Social Media and you: what every physician needs to know. J. Med. Pract. Manag. **28**(3), 206–209 (2012)
5. Lambert, K.M., Barry, P., Stokes, G.: Risk management and legal issues with the use of Social Media in the healthcare setting. J. Healthc. Risk Manag. **31**(4), 41–47 (2012)
6. Von Muhlen, M., Ohno-Machado, L.: Reviewing Social Media use by clinicians. J. Am. Med. Inform. Assoc. **19**(5), 777–781 (2012)

7. ASHP statement on use of Social Media by pharmacy professionals. www.ashp.org/DocLib rary/BestPractices/AutoITStSocialMedia.aspx
8. Dizon, D.S., Graham, D., Thompson, M.A., Johnson, L.J., Johnston, C., Fisch, M.J., Miller, R.: Practical guidance: the use of Social Media in oncology practice. J. Oncol. Pract. **8**(5), 114–124 (2012)
9. George, D.R., Rovniak, L.S., Kraschnewski, J.L.: Dangers and opportunities for Social Media in medicine. Clin. Obstet. Gynecol. **56**(3), 453–462 (2013)
10. Househ, M.: The use of Social Media in healthcare: organizational, clinical, and patient perspectives. Stud. Health Technol. Inform. **183**, 244–248 (2013)
11. Farnan, J.M., Sulmasy, L.S., Worster, B.K., Chaudhry, H.J., Rhyne, J.A., Arora, V.M.: Online medical professionalism: patient and public relationships: policy statement from the American College of Physicians and the Federation of State Medical Boards. Ann. Intern. Med. **158**(8), 620–627 (2013)
12. Bernhardt, M., Alber, J., Gold, R.S.: A Social Media primer for professionals: digital do's and don'ts. Health Promot. Pract. **15**(2), 168–172 (2014)
13. MacMillan, C.: Social Media revolution and blurring of professional boundaries. Imprint **60**(3), 44–46 (2013)
14. Pirraglia, P.A., Kravitz, R.L.: Social Media: new opportunities, new ethical concerns. J. Gen. Intern. Med. **28**(2), 165–166 (2012)
15. Fogelson, N.S., Rubin, Z.A., Ault, K.A.: Beyond likes and tweets: an in-depth look at the physician SM landscape. Clin. Obstet. Gynecol. **56**(3), 495–508 (2013)
16. Chretien, K.C., Kind, T.: SM and clinical care: ethical, professional, and social implications. Circulation **127**(13), 1413–1421 (2013)
17. Moorhead, S.A., Hazlett, D.E., Harrison, L., Carroll, J.K., Irwin, A., Hoving, C.: A new dimension of health care: systemic review of the uses, benefits, and limitations of Social Media for health care professionals. J. Med. Internet Res. **15**(4), e85 (2013)
18. Grajales, F.J., 3rd., Sheps, S., Ho, K., Novak-Lauscher, H., Eysenbach, G.: Social Media: a review and tutorial of applications in medicine and health care. J. Med. Internet Res. **16**(2), e13 (2014)
19. O'Hara, B., Fox, B.J., Donahue, B.: Social Media in pharmacy: heeding its call, leveraging its power. J. Am. Pharm. Assoc. **53**(6), 561–564 (2013)
20. Childs, L.M., Martin, C.Y.: Social Media profiles: striking the right balance. Am. J. Health Syst. Pharm. **69**(23), 2044–2050 (2012)
21. Medical Directors Forum. www.medicaldirectorsforum.skipta.com
22. Hasty, R.T., Garbalosa, R.C., Barbato, V.A., Valdes, Jr, P.J., Powers, D.W., Hernandez, E., John, J.S., Suciu, G., Qureshi, F., Popa-Radu, M., Jose, S.S., Drexler, N., Patankar, R., Paz, J.R., King, C.W., Gerber, H.N., Valladares, M.G., Somji, A.A.: Wikipedia vs. peer reviewed medical literature for information about the 10 most costly medical conditions. J. Am. Osteopath. Assoc. **114**(5), 368–373 (2014)
23. Surya, P., Sarojini, B.: Social Media networks in online health care for topic analysis and sentiment analysis using text mining techniques. Int. J. Pure Appl. Math. **118**(18), 2929–2934 (2018)
24. Effective strategies for Social Media marketing in health industry. https://www.fatbit.com/fab/8-effective-strategies-social-media-marketing-health-industry
25. Navicent health Social Media case study. https://www.captivateseo.com/social-media-case-stu dies/navicent-health-social-media-case-study.html
26. Leading St. Louis Hospital engages in Social Media marketing. https://tsunela.com/health-care/
27. Singh, S.P., Rai, A.K., Wal, A., Tiwari, G., Tiwari, R., Parveen, A.: Effect of Social Media in health care: uses, risks, and barriers. World J. Pharm. Pharm. Sci. **5**(7), 282–303 (2017)
28. Green, B., Hope, A.: Promoting clinical competence using Social Media. Nurse Educ. **35**(3), 127–129 (2010)
29. Bahner, D.P., Adkins, E., Patel, N., Donley, C., Nagel, R., Kman, N.E.: How we use Social Media to supplement a novel curriculum in medical education. Med. Teach. **34**(6), 439–444 (2012)

30. Wang, A.T., Sandhu, N.P., Wittich, C.M., Mandrekar, J.N., Beckman, T.J.: Using Social Media to improve continuing medical education: a survey of course participants. Mayo Clin. Proc. **87**(12), 1162–1170 (2012)
31. Chaudhry, A., Glode, L.M., Gillman, M., Miller, R.S.: Trends in Twitter use by physicians at the American society of clinical oncology annual meeting. J. Oncol. Pract. **8**(3), 173–178 (2012)
32. Dreesman, J., Denecke, K.: Challenges for signal generation from medical Social Media data. Stud. Health Technol. Inform. **169**, 639–643 (2011)
33. Singh, A.G., Singh, S., Singh, P.P.: You Tube for information on rheumatoid arthritis–a wakeup call? [Validation Studies]. J. Rheumatol. **39**(5), 899–903 (2012)
34. Stevenson, F.A., Kerr, C., Murray, E., Nazareth, I.: Information from the internet and the physician-patient relationship: the patient perspective: a qualitative study. BMC Family Pract. **47**, 1–8 (2007)
35. Culver, J.D., Gerr, F., Frumkin, H.: Medical information on the internet: a study of an electronic bulletin board. J. Gen. Intern. Med. **12**(8), 466–470 (1997)
36. Newbold, B.: Social Media in public health. National Collaborating Centre for Healthy Public Policy (2015)
37. PwC HRI SM consumer survey. Social Media. https://www.pwc.com/us/en/health-industries/
38. Social Media Healthcare. https://www.smhcop.wordpress.com/2012/01/05/the-fdas-firsts ocial-media-guidelineoff-label-is-on-the-mark/
39. Kristen Perosino, M.P.H.: Social Media and health care: implications for aging and advanced illness populations. Highlights from Duke University's—Health Care Gets Social‖ Forum Altarum Institute, August 2012, 6–7
40. Azer, S.: Social Media channels in health care research and rising ethical issues. AMA J. Ethics **19**(11), 1061–1069 (2017)
41. Twitter statistics directory. https://www.socialbakers.com/statistics/Twitter
42. Zephoria Digital Marketing. https://zephoria.com/top-15-valuable-FB-statistics/
43. DMR Business Statistics: 220 amazing LinkedIn statistics and facts. https://expandedramb lings.com/index.php/by-the-numbers-a-few-important-linkedin-stats/
44. LinkedIn Statistics. https://foundationinc.co/lab/b2b-marketing-linkedin-stats/
45. Statista Social Media statistics and facts. https://www.statista.com/topics/1164/social-net works/
46. Zhou, C., Zhao, Q., Lu, W.: Impact of repeated exposures on information spreading in social networks. PLoS ONE **10**(10), e0140556 (2015)
47. Adams, S.A., Van Veghel, D., Dekker, L.: Developing a research agenda on ethical issues related to using Social Media in healthcare. Camb. Q. Healthc. Ethics **24**(3), 293–302 (2015)
48. Patel, R., Chang, T., Greysen, S.R., Chopra, V.: Social Media use in chronic disease: a systematic review and novel taxonomy. Am. J. Med. **128**(12), 1335–1350 (2015)
49. Naslund, J.A., Aschbrenner, K.A., Marsch, L.A., Bartels, S.J.: The future of mental health care: peer-to-peer support and SM. Epidemiol. Psychiatr. Sci. **25**(2), 113–122 (2016)
50. Wells, D.M., Lehavot, K., Isaac, M.L.: Sounding off on Social Media: the ethics of patient storytelling in the modern era. Acad. Med. **90**(8), 1015–1019 (2015)
51. Shepherd, A., Sanders, C., Doyle, M., Shaw, J.: Using Social Media for support and feedback by mental health service users: thematic analysis of a Twitter conversation. BMC Psychiatry **15**(1), 1–9 (2015)
52. Fung, I.C., Fu, K.W., Chan, C.H., Chan, B.S., Cheung, C.N., Abraham, T., Tse, Z.T.: Social Media's initial reaction to information and misinformation on Ebola, August 2014: facts and rumors. Pub. Health Rep. **131**(3), 461–473 (2016)
53. Pedersen, E.R., Kurz, J.: Using Facebook for health-related research study recruitment and program delivery. Curr. Opin. Psychol. **9**, 38–43 (2016)
54. Valdez, R.S., Guterbock, T.M., Thompson, M.J., Reilly, J.D., Menefee, H.K., Bennici, M.S., Williams, I.C., Rexrode, D.L.: Beyond traditional advertisements: leveraging Facebook's social structures for research recruitment. J. Med. Internet Res. **16**(10), e243 (2014)

55. Becker, A.E., Fay, K.E., Agnew-Blais, J., Khan, A.N., Striegel-Moore, R.H., Gilman, S.E.: Social network media exposure and adolescent eating pathology in Fiji. Br. J. Psychiatry **198**(1), 43–50 (2011)
56. Xu, S., Markson, C., Costello, K.L., Xing, C.Y., Demissie, K., Llanos, A.A.: Leveraging Social Media to promote public health knowledge: example of cancer awareness via twitter. JMIR Pub. Health Surveill. **2**(1), e17 (2016)
57. Huesch, M.D., Galstyan, A., Ong, M.K., Doctor, J.N.: Using Social Media online social networks, and internet search as platforms for public health interventions: a pilot study. Health Serv. Res. **51**(2), 1273–1290 (2016)
58. Chary, M., Genes, N., Giraud-Carrier, C., Hanson, C., Nelson, L.S., Manini, A.F.: Epidemiology from tweets: estimating misuse of prescription opioids in the USA from Social Media. J. Med. Toxicol. **13**(4), 278–286 (2017)
59. Swirsky, E.S., Hoop, J.G., Labott, S.: Using Social Media in research: new ethics for a new meme? Am. J. Bioeth. **14**(10), 60–61 (2014)
60. Zhou, L., Zhang, D., Yang, C.C., Wang, Y.: Harnessing Social Media for health information management. Electron. Commer. Res. Appl. **27**, 139–151(2018)
61. Sekhar, S.R., Siddesh, G.M.: Introduction and implementation of machine learning algorithms in R. In: Rajput, D.S., Thakur, R.S., Basha, S.M. (eds.) Sentiment Analysis and Knowledge Discovery in Contemporary Business, pp. 126--147. IGI Global (2019)
62. Mani Sekhar, S.R., Siddesh, G.M., Manvi, S.S., Srinivasa, K.G.: Optimized focused web crawler with natural language processing based relevance measure in bioinformatics web sources. Cybern. Inf. Technol. **19**(2), 146–158 (2019)
63. Mani Sekhar, S.R., Tewari, S., Rahman, H., Siddesh, G.M.: Data collection in fog data analytics. In: Tanwar, S. (ed.) Fog Data Analytics for IoT Applications. Studies in Big Data, vol. 76. Springer, Singapore (2020)
64. Mani Sekhar, S.R., Siddesh, G.M., Tiwari, A., Robin, A.K.: Identification and analysis of nitrogen dioxide concentration for air quality prediction using seasonal autoregression integrated with moving average. Aerosol Sci. Eng. **4**(2), 137–146 (2020)
65. Mani Sekhar, S.R., Siddesh, G.M., Kalra, S., Anand, S.: A study of use cases for smart contracts using blockchain technology. Int. J. Inf. Syst. Soc. Change **10**(2), 15–34 (2019)
66. Mani Sekhar, S.R., Siddesh, G.M., Manvi, S.S.: Data visualization in R. Sentiment Analysis and Knowledge Discovery in Contemporary Business, pp. 205–222. IGI Global (2018)
67. Surani, Z., Hirani, R., Elias, A., Quisenberry, L., Varon, J., Surani, S., Surani, S.: Social media usage among health care providers. BMC Res. Notes **10**(1), 654 (2017)

Multi-modal Data-Driven Analytics for Health Care

Srinidhi Hiriyannaiah, Siddesh G. M., Mumtaz Irteqa Ahmed,
Kolli Saivenu, Anant Raj, K. G. Srinivasa, and L. M. Patnaik

Abstract In this day and age, Artificial Intelligence has crept into every domain of work. It is only fitting that it be made a part of the medical domain as well. With the vast amount of healthcare data available in various forms such as image, video, text, and due to emerging technologies and advancements in data science, tools are being created to ease the process of medical analysis and provide an efficient and accurate diagnosis of the patient. Such techniques save lots of human efforts and provide a rather accurate result. In particular, the chapter focuses on emphasizing the importance of multimodal system where instead of relying on a particular data source or a particular field of data analytics; one can combine multiple sources and apply multi-domain techniques to extract information to an even greater extent. The high-quality information retrieved from the analysis can be further used to determine and diagnose more symptoms and hence help in providing accurate solutions.

S. Hiriyannaiah (✉) · S. G. M. · M. I. Ahmed · K. Saivenu · A. Raj
Ramaiah Institute of Technology, Bengaluru, India
e-mail: srinidhi.hiriyannaiah@gmail.com

S. G. M.
e-mail: siddeshgm@gmail.com

M. I. Ahmed
e-mail: fareed2000ahmed@gmail.com

K. Saivenu
e-mail: ksaivenu2010@gmail.com

A. Raj
e-mail: anant.rj.421@gmail.com

K. G. Srinivasa
National Institute of Technical Teachers Training Institute, Chandigarh, India
e-mail: kgsrinivasa@gmail.com

L. M. Patnaik
National Institute of Advanced Studies, Bengaluru, India
e-mail: lalitblr@gmail.com

© The Author(s), under exclusive license to Springer Nature Singapore Pte Ltd. 2021   139
K. G. Srinivasa et al. (eds.), *Artificial Intelligence for Information
Management: A Healthcare Perspective*, Studies in Big Data 88,
https://doi.org/10.1007/978-981-16-0415-7_7

1 Introduction

There is a huge amount of data that is generated every day in the field of health care, which can be in the form of text such as tabular records, unstructured reports, etc., or images such as CT scan, ultrasound, etc., or video such as CCTV camera recordings. All this data can be processed and analyzed to improve the quality of diagnosis and minimizing errors in a decision-making process. The abundance of data and limited number of human resources also makes the manual diagnosis an issue, hence it is viable to use a machine learning or deep learning based analysis to help the physicians by saving their time and providing efficient and faster decision-making capabilities as well as providing the patients with accurate medical treatment.

The data sources mentioned above individually make a huge impact in the field of health care but a multimodal data-driven approach that combines the use of all these sources can add an even greater improvement in the quality o f dagnosis. With the continuous demand for data analysis and diagnosis and with the advancement and transformation of data science technologies, new techniques can be introduced to utilize the maximum of the available resources to provide a highly accurate and good quality diagnosis result which will benefit the physician as well as the patient.

This chapter talks in great detail about the kinds of data that can be analysed in the healthcare sector, its sources and the various analytical techniques that can be applied to the data. This chapter also talks about the popular frameworks that are currently in the market that is being used in the research field to perform analysis and prediction of healthcare data. The chapter finally concludes with a medical example that describes the process of analysis of text and image data for an accurate diagnosis of a health condition.

2 Multi-modal Data for Health Care

2.1 Textual Data

Text is one of the most primitive forms of data that can be extracted for analysis. Such data could either be in a particular language or it could also be numerical/textual data of various important health parameters. Some of the textual data types are discussed below.

Administrative Health Data. The administrative health data is a collection of all the de-identified records for a large population of citizens within the provincial health care system. The data in such a collection can include details about doctor visits, hospital discharge notes, PERS (Personal Emergency Response Systems), and pharmaceutical prescriptions, etc. This collective data can be used to study the distribution of diseases, physician practice and the quality of healthcare provided. Using such a dataset, other smaller datasets can be constructed which are more disease specific. Hence, such a dataset can act as a single source of information for various diseases and health conditions for domain experts to work on.

Characteristics of Administrative Health Data:

- It can capture the general health trends of the population of the area effectively.
- Each record is given a unique identifier to ensure the confidentiality of patients and doctors.
- Since such data is continuously collected over time, it is easier to track the changes in important health parameters over time and perform effective analysis.
- Such data can act as a source of information for various other datasets which can be disease specific.
- Such data is highly reliable and hence used extensively in research.

An example dataset is a MIMIC-III dataset, which stands for "Medical Information Mart for Intensive care". The dataset contains a vast amount of diverse medical data such as vital signs, medications history, laboratory/medical device measurements, length of stay in hospitals, and various other such health parameters of over 38,000 patients collected over a period of 11 years. Since it is a large and publicly available dataset, it is used extensively in medical informatics research [1].

IoT Devices. With various electronic gadgets such as fitness bands and smart watches in the market, this has opened up the gates to attain various other types of data such as the calories burnt, heart rate, etc., on the go which are numerical and continuous in nature. Various types of techniques such as time-series analysis can be done on the data collected to extract useful information and help in keeping the wearer healthy.

Social Media. Social Media can be another important source of textual data. The kinds of posts or blogs that patients write can be analysed using various Natural Language Processing Techniques and useful knowledge could be extracted out of it. Such data is useful in diagnosing psychological disorders such as depression and anxiety [2].

2.2   Image Data

In the field of health care, images account for at least 90% of all medical data sources and are also one of the most difficult to be analysed which calls for more exploration and advancements of deep learning technology in healthcare sectors as this huge amount of data is quite overwhelming for manual review and diagnostics.

The technique used to attain the visual representations of the body parts for clinical analysis and medical intervention is called medical imaging. This procedure is responsible for obtaining large amount of image data on a daily basis which is used for further analysis. The progress in medical imaging is observed because of development and improvement in image processing techniques. This method provides important information about the body's internal structure for analysis without using invasive procedures. The digital images generated by this technique are handled by computers. The processing includes several operations such as image collection, compression, storage, presentation and transmission. These digital images are easier to store, provide immediate quality assessment and adaptable manipulation. Some limitations are the need for fixed resolution for quality preservation, large storage memory, and an efficient and fast processor for handling and manipulating the images.

These digital images are mainly of two types. A raster image is the first one which consists of an arrangement of pixels. The image has fixed resolution due to their pixel size and on resizing process, digital images lose their quality. These include many formats such as Portable Network Graphics (PNG), Windows Bitmap (BMP), Paintbrush (PCX), etc. The second one is a vector format that is an object precisely defined by a computer with attributes like dimensions, line width, etc., and doesn't introduce any quality loss while scaling and is mainly used to create diagrams and designs.

Some of the major sources of the medical digital image dataset that is obtained for analysis purposes are the following.

- **MRI**. Magnetic Resonance Imaging is used for detecting problems in soft tissue areas. The Arterys Cardio AI deciphers the cardiac MRI images and does multiple layers of analysis which takes a very small time of 15 s compared to a manual analysis by a specialist which takes almost 30 min.
- **CT**. Computed Tomography scans detect life-threatening conditions such as tumors, internal brain injury, and so on. Zebra Medical Vision helps in calculating coronary calcium score based on chest CTs with the help of image analysis.
- **Ultrasound**. It scans body organs and looks for any kind of anomaly in them. This is considered one of the least invasive technique and is used to monitor fetal development progress.
- **X-Ray**. This technique identifies any type of abnormalities or damage to the body organ. The scans are classified and the potential problems are identified from X-Ray with the help of computer vision.
- **Nuclear Imaging**. It visualizes the structure and function of the tissues and the organs. This process involves the emission of a minimal amount of radioactive substance which is analysed after absorption by the body tissue based on which the radiologists make the assessment.

These are some of the most commonly used methods for generating medical images for analysis purposes. Digital images are a pictographic representation of medical data and their processing and analysis retrieve a lot of important information in a very less amount of time [3].

2.3 Video Data

Analysis of healthcare data which are in the form of videos for an accurate diagnosis is a relatively new field of research that is catching up over the years. Video analytics can provide more insights into the patient's symptoms and conditions, which would otherwise be difficult to extract verbally. One of the most important requirements for effective analysis of healthcare videos is the procurement of huge amounts of high-quality data which in itself is a difficult task because of labour and legal issues associated with it. Once the required data is obtained, robust artificial intelligence architectures should be designed to extract essential features and draw insights. The format of the video could be any of the widely used formats such as MP4, MKV, MOV, etc.

After obtaining the videos, there are multiple ways in which video analysis could be done. Two of the ways are listed below.

- One way could be to break up the video into images and use an Image classification architecture (such as Convolution Neural Networks) for analysis. Open-source tools such as ffmpeg can be used to extract images from a video at desired frames per second and each image could be passed as input to the image classification architecture to draw insights [4].
- Another way would be to again break up the videos into images and use Recurrent Neural Network architecture for analysis. One advantage this method provides over the previously mentioned method is that the recurrent neural network would be able to provide context to each image based on the previous images, hence it can be used in tasks such as video activity classification where it is imperative to consider a sequence of images for classification rather than just one image without any context [5].

Video data for healthcare can be of various forms and can come from various sources; some of the sources are described below.

- Emergency accident videos obtained from city CCTV cameras.
- Videos obtained from medical equipment like ultrasound, endoscopy, etc.
- Video footage of patients obtained from cameras at clinics/hospitals.

Video data is one of the most important aspects of analytics and as such certain challenges are encountered that are associated with healthcare video data. Some of them are:

- One of the most important requirements for video analysis is high-quality videos which could, when aggregated, take up space in terabytes or petabytes. Hence storage of such videos poses a stiff challenge.
- With such a huge amount of video data being generated continuously, transmission of such data in quick time also becomes a problem. For example, transmission of 4k (high resolution) videos would need bandwidths that are 100 Gbps in magnitude. A solution to such a problem would be to only select the part of the video that is useful for clinical diagnosis using some form of video analysis and discard the rest of the video.
- Video healthcare data can come in diverse modes such as endoscopy, ultrasound, and emergency videos that are usually obtained from CCTV cameras. Each category of mode can have subcategories within them, such as ultrasound could be of

cardiac related, femoral related, carotid related, etc. Each video mode has to be seen from a different lens for effective analysis which is a difficult task.

- The video obtained for analysis should be a high quality. Some compression algorithms can deter the quality of the video. Hence care should be taken to ensure that video compression is done without much loss of quality.
- Most videos obtained from hospitals and health clinics have unwanted elements called **noise** within them which could come in the way of effective analysis of the video. Hence making the video noise free is of utmost importance [3].

3 Multi-modal Analytics for Health Care

3.1 Textual Analytics

This section deals with the kind of analytics that can be performed on the textual data based on the form the data is in. The textual data can be mainly divided into two types, one is the raw textual data which consists of meaningful sentences of any language, which is mainly used in analysing psychological disorders. The other one is a tabular form where the data is arranged in rows and columns with each row giving information about a patient. Such data consists of attribute names as the first row and the subsequent rows would contain information about the patients which is denoted by the values of the attributes. Such tabular data is used in predicting both physiological and psychological health conditions.

Raw Text. Raw text such as text found in online blogs, social media posts, etc., could help in diagnosing various forms of mental disorders. One such case where it can be used is in diagnosing cognitive distortions which are basically irrational or exaggerated thoughts that could lead to other conditions such as depression or anxiety. To diagnose such a disorder, doctors usually analyse the journal that they maintained for the patient which has details of the interaction that happened between the two. Data can also be obtained from various social media sites, blogs, etc. Due to the vast amount of data present on the internet, the data can be filtered based on keywords such as "lonely", "sad" etc. Once the required amount of data is obtained, the data is labelled as "distorted" and "undistorted" by experts in the field. The data can then be analysed using LIWC software which stands for Linguistic Inquiry and Word Count. It is a piece of software that is used for language analysis. It can perform various tasks such as simple word frequency calculation, extraction of information from text such as sentiment, detection of part of speech, etc. Using LIWC, the data obtained is converted into a vector consisting of 93 dimensions which are the input attributes and 1 label. This data obtained will act as the dataset for analysis. Various machine learning algorithms can be used on this data for prediction. Apart from that, one could also perform dimension reduction techniques to decrease the size of the dataset which could sometimes give better accuracy [6]. Apart from the above technique, various deep learning techniques can also be applied to the text corpus directly. Various deep learning algorithms like LSTM (Long Short Term Memory) can be used for analysing the text corpus. The advantage that LSTM provides is that it can remember the context of the text corpus which is not possible by other algorithms; hence it provides much more accurate results when compared to other machine learning algorithms.

Text in Tabular Form. There are various health datasets out there, one such dataset is the UCI Heart Disease Dataset [7], which is a dataset used by a large number of Machine Learning researchers in the prediction of heart diseases. The dataset consists of various attributes of patients such as age, gender, cholesterol levels, blood pressure levels, etc. Various machine learning techniques have been applied to this dataset in the field of research. One such technique is using the J48 algorithm which is a decision tree algorithm. The model was trained using the dataset and once the decision tree rules were obtained, reduced error pruning technique was performed to reduce over-fitting. On similar lines various machine learning techniques can be performed on this or various other datasets in the healthcare domain for effective analysis and prediction [8, 9].

3.2 *Image Analytics*

The advancements in the field of image processing and analytics in the healthcare sector are still under progress and some commendable changes have been observed in the past few years. The performance of image-based analysis in the healthcare sector is observed to be enhanced with the addition of multiple cues and modalities. Automated analysis by deep learning based computer vision software provides fast and accurate results compared to manual analysis.

The involvement and evolution of machine learning and deep learning technologies in the healthcare sector can benefit the physicians as well as the patients in many ways. The number of physicians is not sufficient to cope up with the enormous amount of image data that is captured by X-rays, MRI, PET, etc., and is generated on a daily basis. Based on a report by 'Personnel Today', it was seen that in the United Kingdom, the workload of the radiologists was increased by 30% over a period of five years whereas only 15% of increase in the workforce was observed. The progress in the field of automated image analysis will save the time of physicians in image diagnosis and anomaly detection and they can rather focus on the diagnosis that requires more human intervention. The patients will also receive accurate and timelier diagnoses. Also, the decrease in a number of scans will reduce the effect of radiation on the patient's body.

There are some applications that will illustrate how automated medical image analysis can help the patients and physicians. The measure of various heart structures helps in identifying the risk of any cardiovascular disease or any severe issue that might require surgery. Automation in the area of abnormality detection in chest X-rays can give faster results and minimize diagnostic errors to a great extent. The availability of multiple AI tools can help in measurement automation for tasks such as carina angle measurement, aortic valve analysis and many others which help in providing target appropriate treatments for patients [9].

Artificial intelligence models also help in identification of dislocations, soft tissue injuries or even hard-to-see fractures. The detection of fracture type on standard images is often difficult but AI tools observe subtle variations in the image indicating instability in need of surgery. Image processing and analytics also help in the detection of Breast Cancer with the help of mammograms. There are errors during results interpretation using mammograms due to variation in image quality and expertise of the radiologist and image processing can reduce these errors to a great extent.

In case of retinopathy, a large set of retina images are processed, clustered and browsed with the help of a software tool called ImageScape. This tool allows clustering based on image features, context tags and also supports tagging the images in the user interface and is implemented as a set of web services. The availability of all these tools is to minimize errors and improve the quality and accuracy of the diagnosis result that is provided to the patient [10].

3.3 Video Analytics

In recent years, an extensive amount of research has been done within the discipline of video analysis for diagnosis and rehabilitation. Some of the examples and the method associated with them are discussed below.

Video Analytics in Psychology Cases. Video Analytics has great potential in the diagnosis of mental health conditions. An important aspect of diagnosing mental health conditions is analysing various body cues, which could give valuable insights into the underlying mental health condition. In one of the experiments done, the research team used machine learning techniques to analyse various bodily cues such as facial expression, posture shifts, gaze and tone of voice to make a more concise and accurate diagnosis. In the experiment, using interviews of more than 500 participants using a webcam and input from mental health clinicians, the research team was able to observe various behavioural patterns related to depression. Using video analytics and machine learning, 68 points on the face that are essential for human expression were detected and the minute changes in the muscles of the face that are responsible for expression change were analysed. This data was collected over time to accurately predict behaviour markers that are correlated to certain psychological traits. This kind of video analytics is very useful as mental health patients face difficulty in expressing their emotions verbally, hence in such cases, emotion, body language and micro-expression analysis and yield a lot of insights into the underlying mental health condition [11].

Video Analytics in Physiological Cases. One such research done in a physiological context is in assessing the impairment in the upper limb that occurs after a stroke. In this experiment, 5 keys points of the upper limb are chosen, which are cervical spine, shoulder, pelvis, elbow and wrist and these 5 points are continuously monitored and the 3 main joint angles are calculated which are

- The supplementary angle to the shoulder-elbow-wrist angle is represented using α.
- The pelvis–cervical spine–vertical angle is represented using β.
- Angle at the intersection of pelvis–cervical spine and shoulder–elbow lines represented using γ.

The 3 angles obtained from each frame are made to pass as input to a machine learning model and based on the output; the patient can be classified into various classes that denote how well the patient has recovered [12].

Video Analytics in Hospital Management. Video analytics is being used not just in diagnosis and rehabilitation but also in hospital management. Many video analytics software products are present in the market that are being used in hospitals to perform various activities such as monitoring recovering patients using AI/ML, preventing intruders from gaining access to unauthorized parts of the hospital, and also in keeping track of visitor movement for patients so as to ensure that the patient is not in a state of discomfort at any point of time [13].

4 Multi-modal Framework for Healthcare Analytics

In this section, two case studies of how data analytics can be used in the healthcare sector are discussed. One case study is in the domain of text analytics, where tweets are analysed and based on the emotion of the tweet; efforts are made to determine if the patient is suffering from any mental condition such as depression. Another case study is in image analytics, where efforts are made to determine if the patient has pneumonia or not based on the patient's chest X-Ray.

4.1 Data Collection

Image. The dataset used for image analysis is the Chest X-Ray Images (Pneumonia) dataset found on Kaggle [14]. It is a binary class dataset with images of 2 classes, healthy chest X-Ray and X-Ray of chest infected with pneumonia. The images were in JPEG format. The sample images of the dataset are shown in Figs. 1 and 2. The dataset contains a total of 5856 images, distributed as shown in Table 1.

Text. The dataset used for our sentiment analysis model is Sentiment140 dataset taken from Kaggle which has 1.6 million tweets [15]. These tweets can be retrieved from Twitter with the help of Twitter API. The tweets have been divided into two classes. They have been labelled as '0' for a negative tweet and the positive ones are

Fig. 1 Chest X-Ray of a
healthy patient

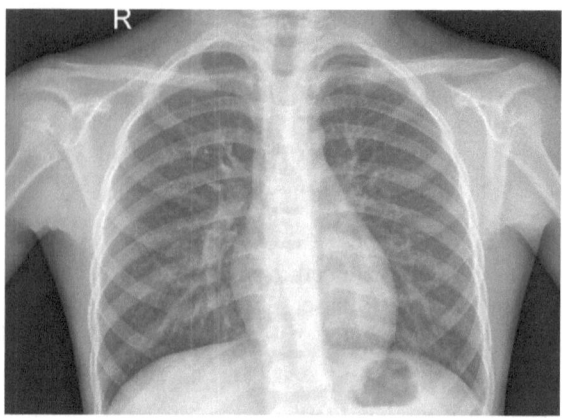

Fig. 2 Chest X-Ray of a
patient suffering from
pneumonia

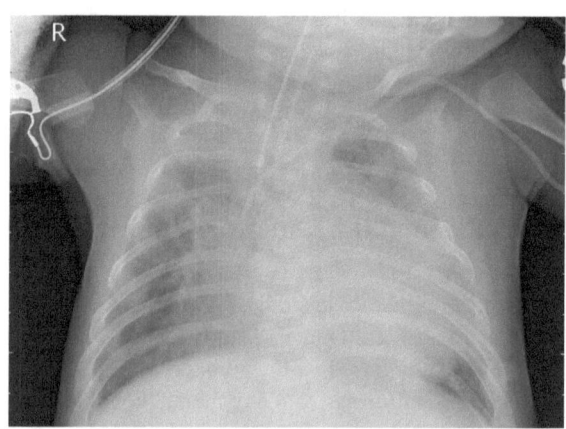

Table 1 Dataset class
distribution among training,
testing and validation images

	Training images	Testing images	Validation images
Normal	1341	174	68
Pneumonia	3875	282	116

labelled as '4'. The dataset has a total of 6 fields associated with the tweet. A sample
of the dataset is shown in Fig. 3.

	label	id	timestamp	na	na	tweet
0	0	1467810672	Mon Apr 06 22:19:49 PDT 2009	NO_QUERY	scotthamilton	is upset that he can't update his Facebook by ...
1	0	1467810917	Mon Apr 06 22:19:53 PDT 2009	NO_QUERY	mattycus	@Kenichan I dived many times for the ball. Man...
2	0	1467811184	Mon Apr 06 22:19:57 PDT 2009	NO_QUERY	ElleCTF	my whole body feels itchy and like its on fire
3	0	1467811193	Mon Apr 06 22:19:57 PDT 2009	NO_QUERY	Karoli	@nationwideclass no, it's not behaving at all....

Fig. 3 Snapshot of dataset

4.2 Pre-processing

Image. The following pre-processing was performed on the dataset.

- **Image Resizing**. Since a pre-trained VGG16 model is used which takes an image of size 224×224 as input, the images were scaled down from their original size to 224×224 dimensions.
- **Normalization**. Each pixel of the image can take a value between 0 and 255. To normalize the value of each unit of pixel, each pixel is divided by 255 to ensure that the value of each pixel lies in the range 0–1.
- **Data Augmentation**. To ensure that the model generalizes well to the real-world inputs, a technique called data augmentation is performed where multiple similar images are generated from the existing dataset by flipping the images, zooming on the images, adding a shear angle to the images, etc. Such a technique can help in generating more images for training and testing and help in training the model better [16].

Text. We need to convert our dataset in a format that can be feed to the neural network and analysis can be done. For that purpose, we have performed the following pre-processing.

- **Data cleaning**. All the words in the tweets are converted to lower case, the punctuations are removed and text is split into individual words. Unnecessary columns that were of no use for the purpose of analysis were dropped.
- **Encoding**. We need to create dictionaries where the words in the vocabulary are mapped to integers and after converting the reviews into integer based on the dictionary they can be passed as an input to our network. For this purpose, TweetTokenizer is used for encoding each word in a tweet and the labels are also encoded to '0' and '1' for negative and positive, respectively.
- **Outlier removal**. In this step, any review that was not of appropriate size (extremely long and extremely short) or was considered as an outlier for input to our network was removed. Also, the length of the reviews was made uniform by padding data to shorter ones and truncating from longer ones [17].

4.3 Framework and Architecture

Image. Convolution Neural Networks is a popular deep learning algorithm that is extensively used in image analysis. In such an algorithm, the input image passes through several layers of convolution layers with kernels and pooling layers and the features are extracted out of the image. Once the features are extracted, it passes through a fully connected network whose task is to classify the image (Fig. 4).

For this particular case study, a technique called transfer learning is employed. In transfer learning, a pre-trained model, i.e. a model that has already been trained on a larger dataset is used for training. New fully connected layers and an output layer, that is more suited to the current problem's needs, are added to the existing pre-trained model and the model is trained on the new data. One also has a choice to decide which layers to train and not train during the training phase of the model. Transfer learning takes less training time and has better convergence when compared to CNN architectures built from scratch, hence it is used here.

The pre-trained model that has been used here is the VGG16 model. It is a complex Convolution Neural Network architecture that is trained on the ImageNet dataset, which is the largest dataset of images currently available. The original fully connected and output layers of the VGG16 model were replaced with 2 dense layers each with 128 nodes that use ReLu activation function and an output layer with 2 nodes that use the softmax activation function.

The framework used in the case study is Keras, which is a robust and easy to use framework for beginners. It is a high-level machine learning framework that uses Tensorflow and Theano as its backend. Using the APIs provided by Keras, one can easily stack layers and create architectures without worrying about the backend's complex mathematical implementation. Using Keras, loading of the dataset, pre-processing, changes to the architecture, training were performed and the results were obtained [18, 19] (Fig. 5).

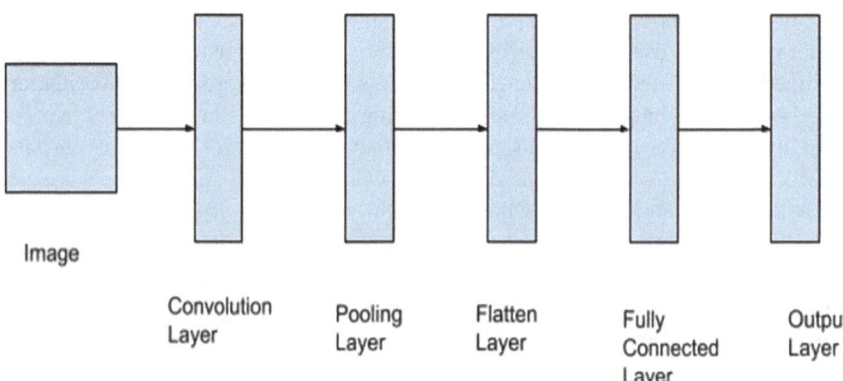

Fig. 4 Simple convolution neural net architecture

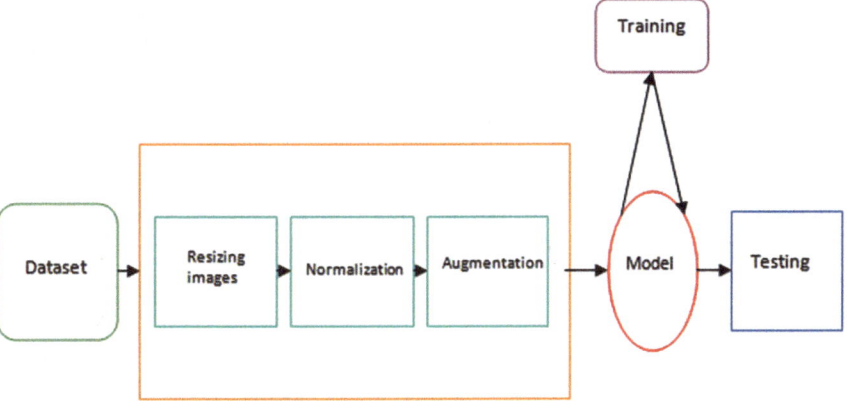

Fig. 5 Workflow of the process

Text. For our model, we have used an artificial recurrent neural network (RNN) architecture known as long short-term memory (LSTM) [5]. Unlike traditional neural networks, LSTM contains feedback connections that help it process sequences of data. The layers involved in our LSTM Network architecture are described below.

- Tokenize: It is not a layer but a compulsory step to convert the words into integers so that they can be fed to the network.
- Embedding Layer: It converts the tokens into required size embeddings.
- LSTM Layer: It is defined by a hidden_state size and the number of layers in the network.
- Fully Connected Layer: Based on the desired output size, this layer maps the LSTM layer output.
- Sigmoid Layer: This is an activation layer that turns the outputs into a value between 0 and 1.
- Output Layer: The last sigmoid output here is taken as the final output of the model [20] (Fig. 6).

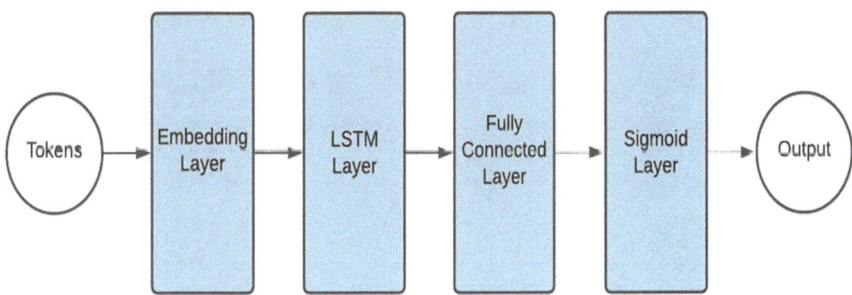

Fig. 6 LSTM network architecture

After the architecture was designed, the model class was defined. For training purpose, we used GPU as it is faster. The RNN model was defined and all the layers were set up. The model was instantiated with the following hyperparameters:

- vocab_size: range of values for the input tokens,
- output_size: number of classes we need to output,
- embedding_dim: size of embeddings,
- hidden_dim: number of units present in the hidden layers of LSTM cells, and
- n_layers: total number of LSTM layers used in our network.

4.4 Experiment and Results

Image. For the pre-trained model, only the fully connected layer and the output layer were made trainable. The loss function used for the model is the categorical cross-entropy function. The "adam" optimization algorithm is used as the optimizer for the model. A call back function is used to terminate the training process if the testing accuracy does not increase in 5 epochs and the model version with the highest accuracy will be considered. The model is trained for 15 epochs on the training images and once the training terminates, it is tested on the validation dataset. The accuracies, precision and recall are mentioned in Table 2.

The accuracy versus epoch graph is plotted and is shown in Fig. 7. The loss versus epoch graph is plotted and is shown in Fig. 8.

Table 2 Accuracies, precision and recall observed for the image analytics model

Training accuracy (%)	Test accuracy (%)	Validation accuracy (%)	Precision (%)	Recall (%)
97.51	86.18	94.56	89.70	95.31

Fig. 7 Accuracy versus epoch graph for CNN model

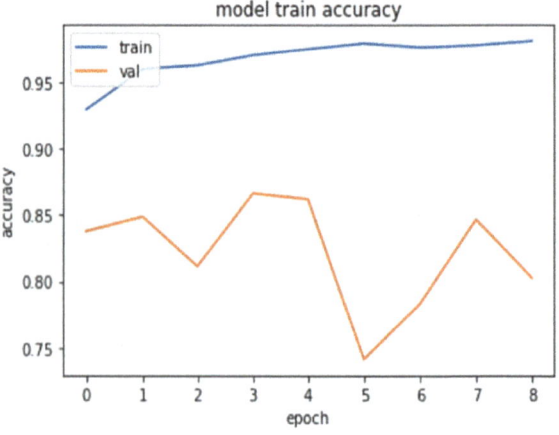

Fig. 8 Loss versus epoch graphs for CNN model

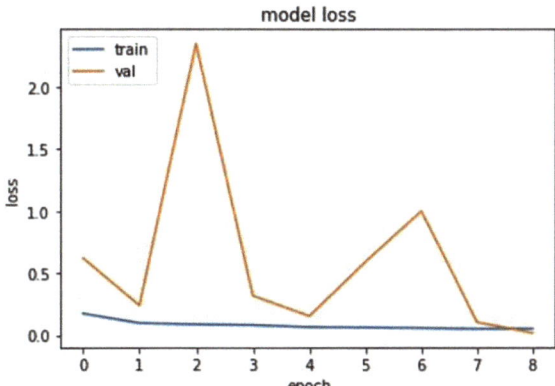

Text. We trained the mode with Binary Cross-Entropy loss as it works with single Sigmoid output and the loss is applied to a value in the range 0–1. The training hyperparameters used are mentioned below.

- lr: optimizer's learning rate,
- epochs: total number of times for iterating through the training set,
- clip: gradient value's maximum limit.

The model was trained based on optimal parameters on the training dataset. The test dataset was used to measure the performance of the model based on its accuracy. The model was trained for a total of 15 epochs and was tested on the validation dataset once the training was done. The train, test and validation accuracy are mentioned in Table 3.

The accuracy versus epoch graph is shown in Fig. 9.

The loss versus epoch graph is shown in Fig. 10.

It was noted that the training accuracy was 97.51%, testing accuracy was 86.18%, validation accuracy was 94.56%, precision was 89.70% and the recall was 95.31% pc. Further research could be done by trying out various other pre-trained models or a new architecture could be constructed from scratch. One can also experiment with the various loss functions and optimizers and see which one works best.

From the experimentation, the training accuracy was observed as 99.9%, validation accuracy was 56.0% and testing accuracy was 60.4%. It can be observed from the graphs that the model that we have developed was over-fitting. We can further try out a different architecture or can add more parameters to the model of the existing one which might provide us even better results from what we obtained.

Table 3 Accuracies observed for the text analytics model

Training accuracy (%)	Test accuracy (%)	Validation accuracy (%)
99.9	60.4	56.0

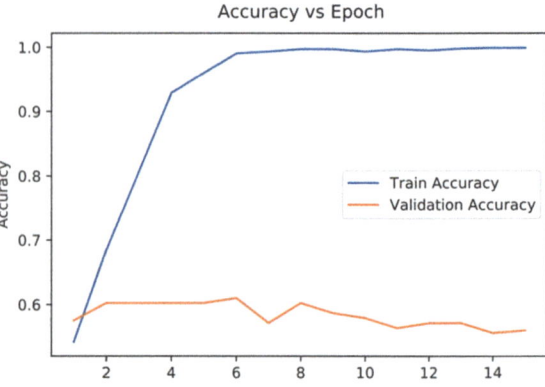

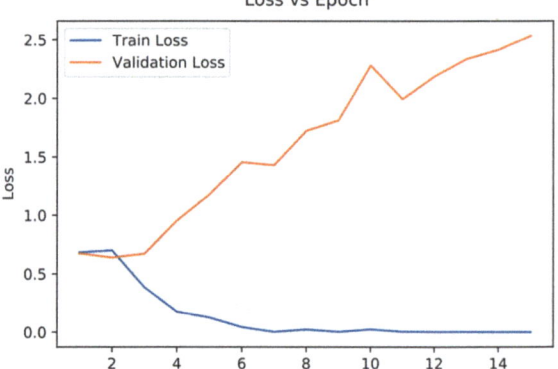

5   Conclusion

In this era of data, where data analytics is revolutionizing every field, it is only a logical step to be able to use these data analytic techniques in the field of health care. Such analytics make doctors smarter, hospitals safer and patients healthier. For this chapter, 3 important types of data that can be used for analytics were talked about, namely, text, image and video. The chapter starts with the explanation and examples of each data form, then moves on to the various analysis techniques that can be performed based on the scenario. It then explained two case studies, one for text and one for image analytics and it is described in detail the various stages of the analysis process such as collection of data, pre-processing, model compilation, training phase, testing phase, etc., and the final results of each of the case studies were observed.

References

1. Menegotto, A.B., Becker, C.D.L., Cazella, S.C.: Computer-aided hepatocarcinoma diagnosis using multimodal deep learning. In: International Symposium on Ambient Intelligence, pp. 3–10. Springer, Cham, June 2019
2. Mathews, S.M.: Explainable artificial intelligence applications in NLP, biomedical, and malware classification: a literature review. In: Intelligent Computing—Proceedings of the Computing Conference, pp. 1269–1292. Springer, Cham, July 2019
3. Panayides, A.S., Pattichis, C.S., Pattichis, M.S.: The promise of big data technologies and challenges for image and video analytics in healthcare. In: 2016 50th Asilomar Conference on Signals, Systems and Computers, pp. 1278–1282. IEEE, Nov 2016
4. Tian, H., Tao, Y., Pouyanfar, S., Chen, S.C., Shyu, M.L.: Multimodal deep representation learning for video classification. World Wide Web 22(3), 1325–1341 (2019)
5. Pang, B., Zha, K., Cao, H., Shi, C., Lu, C.: Deep RNN framework for visual sequential applications. In: Proceedings of the IEEE Conference on Computer Vision and Pattern Recognition, pp. 423–432 (2019)
6. Simms, T., Ramstedt, C., Rich, M., Richards, M., Martinez, T., Giraud-Carrier, C.: Detecting cognitive distortions through machine learning text analytics. In 2017 IEEE International Conference on Healthcare Informatics (ICHI), pp. 508–512. IEEE (2017)
7. Heart Disease dataset. https://archive.ics.uci.edu/ml/datasets/Heart+Disease
8. Patel, J., Upadhyay, T., Patel, S.: Heart disease prediction using machine learning and data mining technique. Heart Dis. 7(1), 129–137 (2015)
9. Amin, M.S., Chiam, Y.K., Varathan, K.D.: Identification of significant features and data mining techniques in predicting heart disease. Telemat. Inform. 36, 82–93 (2019)
10. Tayade, M.C., Wankhede, S.V., Bhamare, S.B., Sabale, B.B.: Role of image processing technology in healthcare sector: review. Int. J. Healthc. Biomed. Res. 2(3), 8–11 (2014)
11. Chen, I.Y., Szolovits, P., Ghassemi, M.: Can AI help reduce disparities in general medical and mental health care? AMA J. Ethics 21(2), 167–179 (2019)
12. Yang, C., Kerr, A., Stankovic, V., Stankovic, L., Rowe, P., Cheng, S.: Human upper limb motion analysis for post-stroke impairment assessment using video analytics. IEEE Access 4, 650–659 (2016)
13. Zhang, Q., Zhang, Q., Shi, W., Zhong, H.: Firework: data processing and sharing for hybrid cloud-edge analytics. IEEE Trans. Parallel Distrib. Syst. 29(9), 2004–2017 (2018)
14. Image Analytics Dataset Link. https://www.kaggle.com/paultimothymooney/chest-xray-pneumonia
15. Text Analytics Dataset Link. https://www.kaggle.com/kazanova/sentiment140
16. Barnouti, N.H.: Improve face recognition rate using different image pre-processing techniques. Am. J. Eng. Res. (AJER) 5(4), 46–53 (2016)
17. AAlAbdulsalam, A.K., Garvin, J.H., Redd, A., Carter, M.E., Sweeny, C., Meystre, S.M.: Automated extraction and classification of cancer stage mentions from unstructured text fields in a central cancer registry. In: AMIA Summits on Translational Science Proceedings, vol. 16 (2018)
18. Nguyen, G., Dlugolinsky, S., Bobák, M., Tran, V., García, Á.L., Heredia, I., Malík, P., Hluchý, L.: Machine learning and deep learning frameworks and libraries for large-scale data mining: a survey. Artif. Intell. Rev. 52(1), 77–124 (2019)
19. Shanmugamani, R.: Deep Learning for Computer Vision: Expert Techniques to Train Advanced Neural Networks Using TensorFlow and Keras. Packt Publishing Ltd. (2018)
20. Hsu, F.Y., Lee, H.M., Chang, T.H., Sung, Y.T.: Automated estimation of item difficulty for multiple-choice tests: an application of word embedding techniques. Inf. Process. Manag. 54(6), 969–984 (2018)

Security, Privacy and Visualization

Security and Privacy Issues in Health Care

B. L. Sandeep, Gouri Gavimath, and Siddesh G. M.

Abstract In today's world, because of technological advancement, it is extremely important to safeguard the data from the dark web and the cybercriminals. The healthcare data that is collected and analyzed online is in jeopardy. The task of the data handler is to ensure that the patient's information given to any healthcare organization is kept confidential so that their data is kept safe and secure. The information security and privacy are involved in the different phases like collection, usage, storage and transmission of the data especially with respect to Personal Health Information. With the advent of new technologies and because most of the devices are connected over the Internet and the data stored in cloud-based platforms, data could be compromised by the cybercriminals. It is about how well the data is protected and the confidentiality of the data is maintained. In this chapter, the challenges, threats, and concerns with respect to healthcare data and the solutions to the problems are looked at. Here we try and understand how these issues are handled by the various technology industries by looking at the several case studies in this area of healthcare and how the integrity of the data is maintained.

Keywords Health care · IoT · Medical records · Security · Privacy · Cloud computing

1 Introduction

Healthcare system plays a major role in a global world. From the early times of traditional treatment to rationalized treatment, healthcare sector has made its own impact and has achieved an important position due to the rapid growth of technology. The usage of technology has extended its hands to the global healthcare sector. The earlier healthcare system was using a manual record of patients and all the medical details of patients were maintained in the form of manual record books it was mostly

B. L. Sandeep (✉) · G. Gavimath · S. G. M.
Department of Information Science and Engineering, Ramaiah Institute of Technology, Bangalore, India

© The Author(s), under exclusive license to Springer Nature Singapore Pte Ltd. 2021   159
K. G. Srinivasa et al. (eds.), *Artificial Intelligence for Information Management: A Healthcare Perspective*, Studies in Big Data 88,
https://doi.org/10.1007/978-981-16-0415-7_8

the doctor centric. As the time changed and technology was introduced in health-care, manual form of storing records was replaced with digital forms of storage of records and now has become data centric [1]. Many digital record forms were created with different categories such as Personal Health Records (PHR), Electronic Health Records (EHR), Electronic Medical Records (EMR) or Electronic Health Data (EHD). These categories of records help in maintaining complete medical informa-tion of patients and these records can be accessed by the respective professionals who are handling the case, relatives, guardian, or patients themselves. By digitizing records, it helps in maintaining the transparency of the data between health profes-sionals and clients and can reduce manpower usage and physical storage space as well. These digital records contain computerized patients records in an orga-nized way which includes patients' medical histories, laboratory test reports, ECG reports, medication, demographics, and other medical-related details of the patients along with that it could also include the banking transactions made to cover the hospital expenses along with the bank account details. The advantages of digitizing the records in healthcare are more in comparison with manual storage. Digitally maintaining records helps in better clinical decision-making, reduce manual clinical error reporting and ensure patient safety. Because of the increasing technological advancement, approximately 90% of healthcare institutes have adopted e-healthcare services [2, 2].

At the present stage, the usage of e-healthcare services is tremendously growing. The use of EHD and EPR has helped in better management of healthcare system. EPR, Remote Patients monitoring, and many other integrated system concepts and approaches have made the most efficient impact in servicing global healthcare systems. Talking about the e-Healthcare, majority of healthcare organizations have created their own personalized web portals. This web portal helps patients to commu-nicate with doctors via the Internet and EPRs can be shared through websites and can easily accessed by login-id of respective patients or their caretakers. The Patient-Centered Access to Secure Systems Online (PCASSO) is one of the examples of healthcare websites, which is developed by the University of California, San Diego [3]. These websites will include a complete patient record history such as ECG, laboratory test reports, demographics and even patients' bill payment history can be maintained and accessible through these websites. Properly maintained patient clinical trial reports help the doctors to improvise the treatment method and help in providing better health care facilities. Many computational approaches such as Cloud Computing, AI concepts and data mining are being implemented on the data for understanding the patient's illness as part of e-healthcare services, which is providing a very good impact in remotely monitoring patients and healthcare groups. Hence modernizing the healthcare system has made healthy lifestyle easier and accessibility to medical professionals has increased.

However, now securing and maintaining the privacy of health information records is a major challenge. Maintaining the confidentiality of medical information and providing privacy and security is a major responsibility of every healthcare organi-zation. This chapter will discuss the major data security and privacy issues in health care, it gives us an overview of information flow in the health care system. This chapter also discusses the challenges identified in healthcare information security, different techniques to enhance data security and case studies on data security and privacy in health care to understand how the industries have managed to provides the required support for the current needs in maintaining the confidentiality of the patient's records.

2   Overview of Flow of Information in Healthcare Systems

Maintaining patient's health data, providing privacy and security to patient's health information is a major responsibility of every respective healthcare organizations and institutes. Providing confidentiality and transparency between doctors and patients or relatives or caretakers regarding the patient's health report is one of the ethical rules of medical professionals. In the era of modern healthcare system, health care information flow is in the form of digital records. They are categorized in different forms such as EPRs, PHRs, EMRs, EHD [4, 5]. People can opt to share the information with a certain set of known contacts. For the patients suffering from HIV and psychiatric illness, their health information (such as Personal Health Records—PHRs) cannot be shared with anyone except the respective person whom the patient wants to know and the government health survey department. Because these are sensitive information related to patients and may have a chance of causing discrimination in society. Hence securing the privacy of patient's health information is very vital in such cases.

Information flow in the healthcare system is a typical graphical flow with all privacy and security rules. Figure 1 shows a graphical overview of patient's information flow in the healthcare system. Here the information of the patient can be accessed by only a particular authorized resource body. In the past few decades, there is a vast revolution in the health system [6]. The Health Insurance Portability and Accountability Act 1996 (HIPAA) ensures that the patient's health-related information has been organized well. According to HIPAA rules and other National Health privacy and security Acts, only certain authorized groups can access the patient's records such as Health Bank groups, Extended Health Enterprise which includes subgroups such as pharmacists and insurance companies, which help in maintaining patient's health insurance records. Regional Health information organization which keeps a complete overview of health and disease reports of particular areas and complete health records from health enterprise groups is taken into consideration by government and other health department authorities under the public policy to control health disaster, disease control, provide national health information security and improve in better decision making in national health sector [7, 8]. In addition, many other health information related policies and legal stand have been created to improve the privacy and security in healthcare information flow.

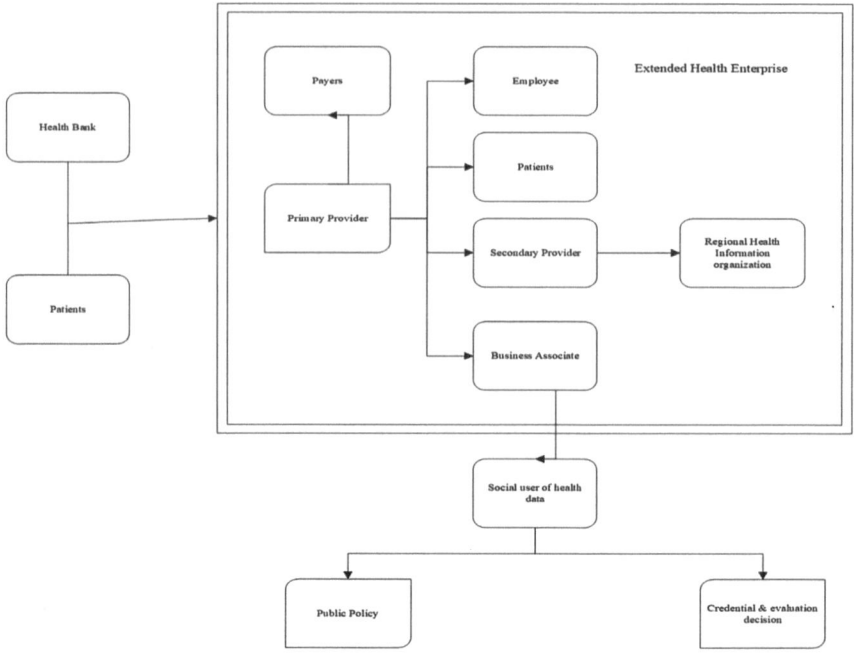

Fig. 1 An overview of patient information flow in the healthcare system

2.1 The Role of Information Security in Different Health Enterprises

Healthcare information security interlinks to different health domain enterprises such as healthcare consumers, providers, inter-organizational bodies and public policy. Figure 2 shows the role of Healthcare Information security in different Health domain enterprises. The review includes complete information systems, health informatics, policy, insurance, medicine and law. Research review has been made particularly on personal health records (PHRs) and Electronic health records (EHRs), that address security and privacy issues in healthcare record management system [9] and this has also helped in addressing IT drivers impacting medical security issues, medicine errors and mistakes caused due to corruption of health data.

The model will represent the role of healthcare data security in different health domains such as health consumers, healthcare providers, public policy sectors and other inter-organizational groups of healthcare system.

One of the major security issues with respect to the healthcare providers is, it impacts IT system due to medical errors, RFID deployment in medication, risk analysis and assessment, e-healthcare/telemedicine, and pervasive computing in health care. The information security issue in healthcare consumers is, it impacts personal health record (PHRs) management [10]. Clinical trial participation and personal

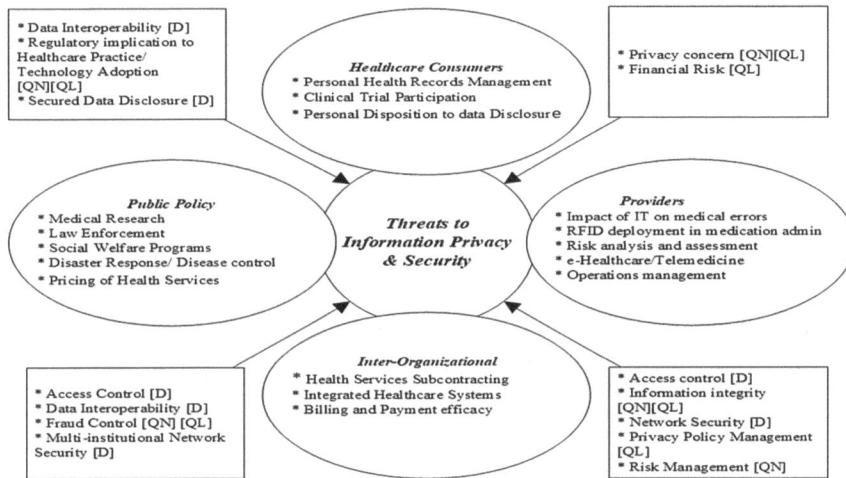

Fig. 2 The role of health care information security in different health enterprises

disposition to data disclosure. The information security issues in health care related to public policy are it impacts medical research, law enforcement, social welfare programs, disaster response/ disease control, pricing of health services. Finally, the information security issue in other inter-organizational groups is it impacts integrated healthcare systems, billing and payment efficacy and in providing subcontract in healthcare services. The review model will represent a thread of information security in mainly three research categories such as Design Research (D), Qualitative Research (QL), Quantitative Research (QR).

Design Research (D) mainly deals with developing algorithms, models, prototype, and provide a solution to information system problems. Design research deals with solving problems related to patient's privacy, patient data is disclosed only to authorized groups and deals with patient's data sharing in wireless networks and cloud platforms. Qualitative Research (QL) deals with explaining social healthcare facts. Here the social healthcare facts are examined by qualitative devices, and information's such as documents, data observation, reports, and healthcare informational details. Health Insurance Portability and Accountability Act (HIPAA) has made a measurable impact in Healthcare Information Research centers/Qualitative research centers. Quantitative Research (QN) deals with risk analysis and management, statistical analysis of patients, patient's data privacy, medical errors, fraud control.

3   Challenges Identified in HealthCare Information Security and Privacy

Safeguarding Healthcare Information flow and maintaining its privacy and security policy is a major challenge faced by every healthcare organization. As the e-health system is evolving, daily millions of health data flow all around the world in every health enterprise and an increase in the misuse of this health data and corruption of health data has been witnessed every day.

Adopting to e-healthcare system the information security plays an important role in a complete healthcare system. The e-healthcare system also increases the usage of electronic, telecommunication devices via the Internet in healthcare services. It has made an effective impact in treating remote patients and the main aim of the e-healthcare system is to enhance the efficiency and effectiveness in managing health care is to improve the quality of services. Hence the complete information flows in digital form, safeguarding this data is an important task [11]. By the comparative analysis of traditional healthcare system to e-healthcare system have made an effective impact in treating patients and maintaining proper health record of patients by using electronic devices leading to better decision-making. But compared to the benefits of e-healthcare, information security and privacy are a typical issue. Security threats such as virus or worm attacks in the software, data loss, hackers hacking healthcare information for self-benefits, confidentiality, and so on are challenges in the e-healthcare system. Some of the challenges identified in healthcare information security are discussed in the following subsections.

3.1   Threats to Information Privacy and Security

Talking about the healthcare systems, a lot of investigations are going on with regards to the privacy and security of its data. The threats to information security and privacy can broadly be identified and classified in two areas such as organizational threats and systemic threats.

Organizational Threats

Organizational threats are caused due to misusing authorized access of patient's data by any internal agents of the organization or by any external agents exploiting a vulnerability of the information system. These threats can occur in many forms such as an employee of a respective health organization having authorized access to data but misusing that data without any legitimate need or any outsider such as hackers (attackers) access the data by exploiting the vulnerability of healthcare information system for their economic or non-economic self-benefits. These organization threats can be explained clearly by characterizing them in some feature components such as motif, resource, accessibility and technical capabilities. The motif behind any of organization threats depends on attacker economic and non-economic benefits. Like attackers abusing the patient's data because of patient's economic background/for acquiring resource from patients or due to some non-economic benefits such as attackers involved with any relationship with patients. The organizational threats risk level is high depending on the attacker's/hacker's technical capabilities. The organizational threats risk level i s high due to some of the reasons like

- Accidentally disclosure of patient's data (Example: unintentionally healthcare organization sending patients health records to wrong mail address).
- Data breach by internal agents of organization (Example: insider member of healthcare organization using health data and transmitting to an outsider for their personal benefits or revenge.
- Data breach by external agents on healthcare organization agents with physical intrusion (Example: outsider with help of physical intrusion forcing insider member of healthcare organization for data access).
- Hacking of healthcare organization network system (Example: hacker may be a former member of healthcare organization trying to hack the network system due to some personal revenge).
- Curiosity (Example: any insider member of healthcare organization abusing access to investigate patients records without any legitimate need).

Systemic Threats

Systemic threats are being caused due to abuse of health data by any agents of health enterprise under the information flow chain of healthcare system. Every health enterprise shares some privacy and security rules with healthcare organizations and institutes to the safety of healthcare data. Whenever this healthcare enterprise denies these rules, it may lead to systemic threats.

3.2 Privacy Concern Among Patient's Health Records

Providing confidentiality for patient's health record is very important. Some of the patient's health records will be sensitive and if it is disclosed, it may result in discrimination in society. For example: if any patient suffering from human immunodeficiency virus infection (HIV) or any mental disorders. If their health records are disclosed publicly. These patients may be treated differently in society and this may cause trauma and become one of the reasons for patients' death. So, maintaining privacy in patient's health records is a challenge.

3.3 Healthcare Provider Viewpoint of Regulatory Compliance

Healthcare compliance such as HIPAA compliance has become a necessary part of business of health organizations. Patients' personal health records (PHRs) and medical history of any healthcare organization can be shared based on healthcare regulatory compliance. For example, if any researcher wants the medical history of a region to analyze the health status of that specific region. The respective health organization can share a medical history of that region based on HIPAA regulatory compliance and institute approval board (IAB). Maintaining health care for not been misused in the name of research is important. So, maintaining regulations in the viewpoint of a healthcare provider to protect healthcare data is a challenge.

3.4   Information Access Control in Healthcare System

The use of technology in healthcare enterprise has rapidly increased and daily millions of information flow in every sector of the healthcare enterprise. The data in the healthcare sector is very sensitive and the information flow is in the form of a largely distributed network system and maintaining its privacy and safeguarding it is very essential. So, role-based information access management systems and many other access control systems were implemented in every healthcare organization. The function of a role-based information access management system is to provide authority to only authorized people of an organization to access data. This helps in maintaining privacy and security in health data. But maintaining the information access control for unauthorized agents/hackers/attackers is a major challenge.

3.5   Data Interoperability and Information Security in the Healthcare System

Daily millions of information flow in healthcare enterprise and every healthcare enterprise stores the data in different formats. To improve the economic sector and research and development sector in the healthcare domain, interoperability of data is very important. Establishing interoperability in the healthcare domain helps to exchange the information and helps in saving a lot of amount in information flow chain system. Introducing interoperable electronic health records (EHRs) and maintaining information security is a challenge.

3.6   Information Integrity in Healthcare and Adverse Effects of Faulty Design

The major key concept for data security is maintaining data integrity. Data breach and hacking are the most frequently heard terms in issues of data security. There are many faulty system design models in the healthcare system. By improving data integrity and using it in faulty design helps in identifying faulty models. This helps in identifying errors caused human–machine interfaces. Hence maintaining information integrity in the healthcare system is a challenge.

3.7 Financial Risk in Healthcare System

When it comes to healthcare data, it includes healthcare financial data too, such as patients' bill payment records, hospital required equipment bills, financial data related to healthcare organization/institutes. Maintaining expenditure records is important to improve the economy of healthcare enterprises. The chances of misusing this data by internal agents or external agents of the healthcare system are more. Hence maintaining the financial data of the healthcare system is important. So, financial risk in the healthcare system is a challenge.

4 Security and Privacy Issues in Cloud Computing for Health Care and Its Solutions

Cloud computing is a platform that helps in delivering different services and resources over the Internet. These services and resources include tools and applications like data storage, servers, databases, networking and software. The major advantage of cloud computing platform is it is on-demand self-service which helps in the proper utilization of resources. Considering the healthcare domain, utilization of cloud computing platform has enormously increased in healthcare organizations/institutes [12, 13]. This section will explain cloud computing infrastructure, cloud computing in the healthcare sector, Possible risks acquiring in the cloud for healthcare applications, privacy and security control for the healthcare cloud.

4.1 Cloud Computing Infrastructure

Cloud computing platform will help the user to access resources and services whenever they need, and these resources, services are hosted by an outside party in "the cloud". Cloud computing will provide three types of services such as Software as a Service (SaaS), Platform as a Service (PaaS), and Infrastructure as a Service (IaaS) [14]

- Software as a service: This is a cloud service that provides us with many software applications deployed. Software applications are installed over the cloud and help us to use them whenever needed. For example, in healthcare sector, medical clinical assistant software are deployed in the cloud which helps interconnecting providers and consumers of healthcare and helps in maintaining healthcare data.

- Platform as a service: This is a cloud service that provides us many support tools deployed on the cloud. For example, an X-ray reports built on Microsoft Azure.
- Infrastructure as a service: This is a cloud service that provides us infrastructure facilities like networking, operating system applications. For example, transmitting patients' test reports to other departments in the organization is done with help of a cloud networking system.

Cloud computing users can use services over the internet whenever they need and cloud computing service providers will provide services such as storage, CPU, network system, and resources over the Internet with an outside party called cloud. The usage is in form of on-demand services called "pay as you use", which says user need to pay only for resource what he uses. Cloud computing infrastructure can be categorized into four types of clouds such as public cloud, private cloud, hybrid cloud, and community cloud [15]. This cloud helps in explaining the availability of the service depending upon ownerships.

- Public cloud: Cloud computing service offer public clouds which allow public to use resources by log-in to the respective cloud and paying only for resources used and these services providers are accountable for hosting and operations of resources. Some of the examples for public cloud is Elastic cloud provided by Amazon web services (AWS), Blue cloud provided by IBM.
- Private cloud: Cloud computing service offer private clouds which can be owned by organizations/institutes/company for their business use. Private cloud services can be accessed by only organizations which are owning them and the payment process depends on basis of bandwidth use or usage of resources. Private clouds can be accessed by only authorized peoples. Some examples for private cloud is Virtual Private Cloud provided by Amazon web services (AWS) and Smart cloud provided by IBM.
- Hybrid cloud: Cloud computing services offer hybrid clouds which are a combination of both public cloud and private cloud, which provide flexibility and scalability in deploying cloud services and helps in security control too. For example, most IT organizations use a hybrid cloud for interconnecting different clouds and accessing resources.
- Community cloud: Cloud computing services offer community clouds that allow sharing of resources among some community groups. For example, medical college and hospital come under healthcare community, these two-organization share cloud computing services.

4.2 Cloud Computing in Healthcare Sector

As technology is rapidly spanning in the healthcare sector, managing healthcare data have become easy with the use of electronic health records (EHRs), digital medical records (DMRs) and many new ways of storing data in digital form. Modernization in healthcare increased the use of new resources and services [16, 17]. Using cloud computing platforms in the healthcare system enhanced the information flow chain in the healthcare system. Using cloud infrastructure is also cost-effective in healthcare enterprise as it is "pay as you use" form.

4.3 Possible Risks Acquiring in Cloud for Healthcare Applications

Confidentiality of data is the main aim of the healthcare system. Using cloud platforms in health enterprise made information flow flexible. But maintaining high cloud security is very challenging. Many security and privacy issues are identified in cloud platform [18, 19]. Some of the possible risks acquired in the cloud for healthcare applications are as follows:

- Failure of cloud access tools/communication media: If there is any accidently failure of cloud access tools may result in huge human injury and economic harm.
- Flooding attacks by virus or malware programs are used by hackers.
- Distributed Denial of Service (DDoS).
- Bad IP Addresses.
- Change in cloud ownership.
- Technical failure or downtime period.
- Process interlocking.
- Access of data by unauthorized users.
- Cloud-based privacy and security.
- IP and port scanning.
- Policies and its changes.
- Legal, Ethical and Privacy lows.
- Different Geographical Regions or countries having different laws.

4.4 Privacy and Security Control for Healthcare Cloud

Considering security and privacy issue for the healthcare cloud, many security controls and privacy rules have been implemented in healthcare cloud infrastructure. Some of the key security and privacy controls/ access limitations for data security are used in the healthcare cloud for protecting data Safety [20, 21]. Figure 3 shows some of the key security and privacy controls used in healthcare cloud infrastructure.

- System monitoring: System monitoring can be used in order to maintain security and privacy in the healthcare cloud. System monitoring helps in controlling unauthorized access of data and it also helps in maintaining a record log for every

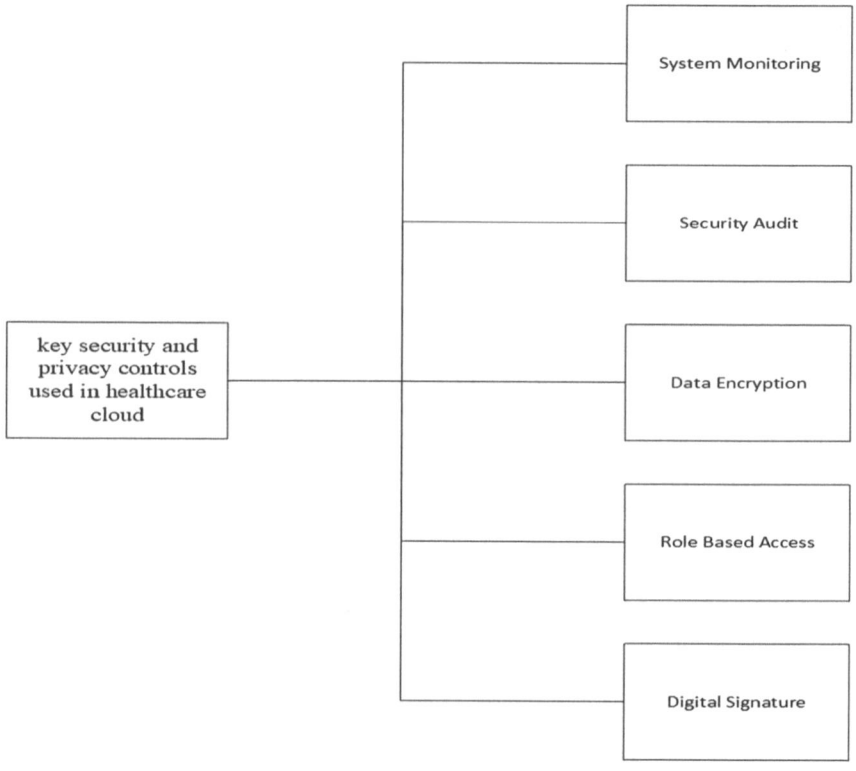

Fig. 3 Some of key security and privacy controls

activity, actions and events of a user while accessing cloud services. This helps in enhancing security checks.
- Security Audit: Regular security audits in an organization helps in enhancing the security system. Regular security training should be provided for employees of an organization. Protecting the data from a data breach is very important. So, improving auditing forms and upgrading security forms and admitting the importance of security in an organization is very helpful.
- It helps in protecting the data during transmitting from one cloud to another. It also helps in avoiding interception.
- Role-based access: Role-based access can help in securing the data from unauthorized people. Implementing role-based access in the hospital information system (HIS) will provide only access premises to authorized staff in organizations.
- Digital signature: Every document needs authentication for proving its legal. Using digital signature in electronic health records (EHRs) and patient's health records (PHRs) help patients and health enterprises to identify whether the records are authentic or not. Digital signature also helps in identifying shared information are from the right sources.

- Cloud users must have complete knowledge of cloud infrastructure and software.

5 Case Studies

Protecting healthcare data is important in every health organizations/institutes. Many companies have provided privacy and security guides to protect the data of healthcare organizations. Here are some of the case studies explaining about security and privacy provided by some companies (such as Deloitte, Cisco, Proof point) to protect the data of healthcare groups/organizations/institutes.

5.1 Case Study on Security and Privacy for Healthcare Providers by Deloitte

Deloitte is one among the leading consultancy companies, which largely provide security to healthcare enterprise. Himss D-A-CH Community collaborating with Deloitte started identifying security issues accruing in healthcare enterprises and provided a task force approach in whitepapers which helped in enhancing the security system in healthcare sectors [22].

Use of Modern Technologies in the Healthcare Sector

As IT extended its hands, modern approaches have been implied in the healthcare sector. Himss D-A-C-H community and Deloitte explained some IT trends in health care and their risks.

i. Cloud computing: Cloud computing technologies provide better service accessibility. Some risks identified in cloud computing technologies are as follows:

   - Meeting compliance challenges in a cloud,
   - Inadequate security administration,
   - Complicated legal situation,
   - Extends the corporate network boundary.

ii. Big data and healthcare analytics: Big data and healthcare analytics help in providing efficient clinical research and better outcomes, better quality in lowering costs. Some risks identified in big data and healthcare analytics are as follows:

   - Privacy issues,
   - Inaccurate data from data silos,
   - Difficult security administration,
   - Fast evolving technology.

iii. Telemedicine and e-Healthcare: Mobile health solutions help in providing remote care and remote patient monitoring. Some risks identified in telemedicine and e-healthcare are as follows:

- Advanced user identification required,
- Extends the corporate network boundary,
- Keeping compliance with industry security standards ensuring access monitoring.

iv. Ever increasing integration: Developing systems and platforms' integrating points. Some risks identified in integrating are as follows:

- Multiplying vulnerabilities,
- Limited visibility to who has the appropriate access,
- Health information exchanges,
- Heterogenic administration.

Existing IT Security Conditions in the Healthcare Sector

Himss D-A-CH community and Deloitte have found some of the existing IT security conditions in health care which helped them in providing taskforce approaches.

- Provide compliance with legal and regulatory rules.
- Ensure data protection with new medical devices and technologies.
- Protecting patient's data from cyber-attacks and prohibiting threats.

Taskforce approach provided by Himss D-A-CH community and Deloitte

Himss D-A-CH community and Deloitte helped in providing a taskforce approach, which helped in enhancing IT security for the healthcare sector. Figure 4 shows the taskforce approach by Himss D-A-CH community and Deloitte.

- Provide compliance with legal and regulatory rules.
- Ensure data protection with new medical devices and technologies.
- Protecting patient's data from cyber-attacks and prohibiting threats.

Taskforce Approach Provided by Himss D-A-CH Community and Deloitte

Himss D-A-CH community and Deloitte helped in providing a taskforce approach which helped in enhancing IT security for the healthcare sector. Figure 4 shows the taskforce approach by Himss D-A-CH community and Deloitte.

Taskforce approach provided by Himss D-A-CH community and Deloitte helped in identifying various issues faced in different perspectives in the healthcare sector and helped in providing solutions for it.

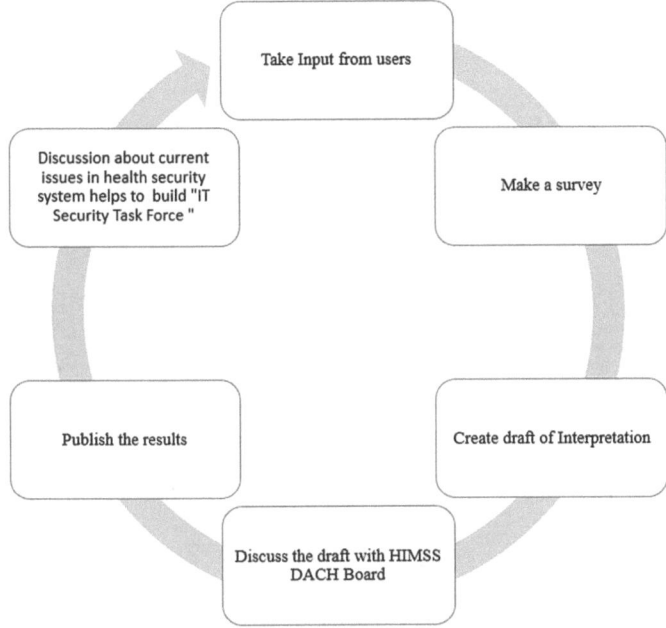

Fig. 4 Shows taskforce approach by HIMSS DACH C

5.2 *Case Study on Security and Privacy for Healthcare Providers by Cisco*

Cisco is one of the well-liked companies in providing networking applications. Considering the healthcare sector, Cisco explained about the importance of security in the healthcare network and how it is secured and managed [23].

Importance of Network Security in Healthcare

The use of modern technologies are tremendously increased in every sector, and it has extended to healthcare enterprise too. Now network-based applications have spread their roots deeply in the healthcare information system. Electronic medical records (EMRs), biomedical information, patient's billing details, medical administrative details, and many more information flows using modern network system. Daily millions of healthcare-related information moves in every healthcare enterprise network system. So, securing healthcare data and protecting the network from attackers is very important [24].

Government has started many policy and rules in order to secure healthcare information systems such as the U. S. government's health insurance portability and accountability act (HIPAA), which was established for policy requirements in protecting health information. But providing this policy and deploying a network firewall is not enough, in the proportion of securing a network system. The healthcare

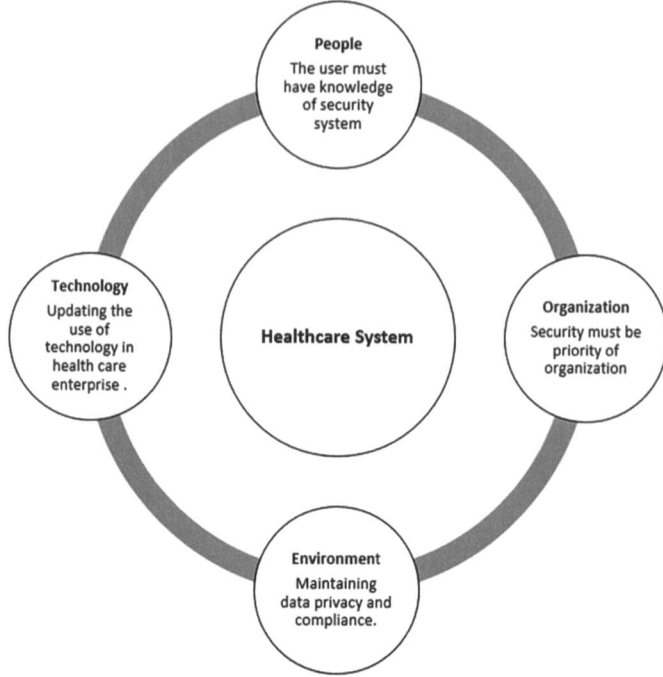

Fig. 5 Shows achieved results in different perspectives in the healthcare system in order to maintain health security

provider needs to enhance their potential with new approaches in order to protect the healthcare network. Most of the network attacks are not the same, they always vary from systems to systems and locations. Some of the network threats are as follows:

- Packet Sniffers,
- IP Spoofing,
- Defacing,
- Denial of Service (DoS),
- Spam,
- Viruses, Worms,
- HTTP Exploits,
- Application-Layer Attacks.

Poor Security Network

Agreeing on the importance of security, every organization has started maintaining its security system. But due to improper maintenances and poor security, network will result in some of the following problems such as

- Loss of patients and partner's confidence,
- Financial risks arise,
- Disruption of clinical and administrative processes.

So, maintaining a network security system in the health care is very essential.

Security Considered as Process

On the note of the importance of network security in health care by considering various network threats raised in the healthcare network system and poor maintenance of healthcare networking system. Cisco provides a security suite that is best in securing the information. Security must be considered as a process in every healthcare organization and not as a product-based point of solution.

Step 1: The initial step in the security process in a healthcare enterprise is to set up a secure network infrastructure with a proper security policy that defines all roles, responsibilities, acceptance use, and complete security system implementations.

Step 2: After setting up the policy, healthcare enterprises should closely observe the implementation of policy, and enterprises should provide some tests for examining network infrastructure. This helps in identifying vulnerabilities, including physical security and risk matrix.

Step 3: As implementation continues, healthcare enterprises must continuously evaluate each area of network infrastructure and help in identifying potential threats and provide appropriate security modules to prevent threats and protect security for healthcare data.

Threats Centric Security Model

Security network infrastructure will undergo continuous evolving and examining phase and changing network system, implementing with new devices is a regular process. Due to this, the complexity of the security system increase. So, Cisco introduced threats-centric security model for creating robust security solutions in the healthcare enterprise.

Threats-centric security model allows customers to provide protection before, during, and after an attack.

Before: Threats-centric security model will help to identify what is on the network, and activities the defense firewall and safeguard the network system.

During: Threats-centric model will always be inspecting what is on the network and looks the activities across and determine whether it is good or bad to the network system.

After: After any kind of attack in the network system, threats-centric model will examine and traverse the network behaviour and change the policy to secure the information.

Threats centric security models can be created by using three major categories such as

i.   Setting up the list of security policy,
ii.   Constantly monitoring and revising the organization's security policy,
iii. Implementing new security modules as indicated by organization's security
      policy and network needs.

Cisco also specified some of the elements which much be present is the security policy.

- Policy Statement,
- Scope,
- Roles and Responsibilities,
- Security Directives,
- Acceptable use policy (AUP),
- Incident Response Procedures,
- Document Control Factors.

Cisco also helps in providing most network security tools, which help healthcare providers to maintain their security system.

- Policy Access and Control Solutions,
- Next-Generation Firewalls,
- Next-Generation Intrusion Detection Systems,
- Advanced Malware Protection,
- Web Security,
- Email Security,
- Cisco Umbrella,
- Security Advisory, Managed and Implementation Services.

How Healthcare Provider Manages and Secures the Network

In today's world, operating virtually and access for mobility and access remotely is made easy. Healthcare providers need to secure their network and manage it by creating a security policy. Healthcare providers use some of the network security in order to secure their network systems.

- Deploying WLAN security,
- Satellite location (Tracking the network flow location using private WANs and public links),
- Deploying management tools in order to secure networks.

Benefits

- Access to information with trust,
- Helps in increasing productivity and reducing costs,
- Improved patient safety.

This case study helps in understanding the importance of network security healthcare enterprise, and identified common threats in the network system, what are the problem caused due to poor network security. Understanding Cisco security suite by explaining the security process in healthcare organizations, threats-centric security model and give details about the elements and tools included in cisco security policy and security system.

6 Conclusion

Healthcare data is confidential and sensitive. Maintaining its security is a major aim of healthcare enterprises. This chapter gives a brief introduction about the data security and privacy in healthcare by introducing storage of healthcare data in different categories of digital records. Also, it gives a complete overview of information flow in the healthcare system, and role of information security in different healthcare enterprises, various challenges identified in healthcare security and privacy system. It gives a brief explanation on security and privacy issue in cloud computing for the healthcare system and its solutions which helps in understanding cloud infrastructure, cloud computing in the healthcare environment, and understanding what are the possible risks identified in the healthcare sector under cloud platform and how it is controlled. The chapter ends by explaining two case studies. One case study explained the security and privacy for healthcare providers by Deloitte, which in turn explained about the modern technologies used in the healthcare sector and task force approaches explaining the security improvement provided by Deloitte and Himss D-A-CH community. The Cisco case study explains the network security provided by Cisco in the healthcare sector and explained how the healthcare provider secures the network system.

References

1. Hathaliya, J.J., Tanwar, S.: An exhaustive survey on security and privacy issues in Healthcare 4.0. Comput. Commun. **153**, 311–335 (2020). ISSN 0140-3664
2. Meingast, M., Roosta, T., Sastry, S.: Security and privacy issues with health care information technology. In: 2006 International Conference of the IEEE Engineering in Medicine and Biology Society. IEEE (2006)
3. Masys, D., Baker, D., Butros, A., Cowles, K.E.: Giving patients access to their medical records via the internet; the PCASSO experience. J. Am. Med. Inf. Assoc. Mar–Apr; **9**(2), 181–191 (2002)
4. ShekhaChenthara, K.A.: Hua Wang, Frank, "Security and Privacy-Preserving Challenges of e-Health Solutions in Cloud Computing." IEEE **7**, 74361–74382 (2019)
5. Dong, N., Jonker, H., Pang, J.: Challenges in ehealth: from enabling to enforcing privacy. In: Proceedings of International Symposium on Foundations of Health Informatics Engineering and Systems, pp. 195–206. Springer, Berlin, Germany (2011)
6. Appari, A., Johnson, E.: Information security and privacy in healthcare: current state of research. Int. J. Internet Enterp. Manag. **6**(4), 279–314 (2010)
7. Mercuri, R.T.: The HIPAA-potamus in health care data security. Commun. ACM 2004, **47**(7), 25–28 (2010)

8. Cate, F.H.: Principles for protecting privacy. Cato J. **22**(1), 33–57 (2017)
9. Zhang, R., Ling, L.: Security models and requirements for healthcare application clouds. In: IEEE 3rd International Conference on Cloud Computing, pp. 268–275 (2010)
10. Allard, T., Yin, S., Anciaux, N., et al.: Secure personal data servers. In: Proceedings of the VLDB Endowment, pp. 25–35 (2010)
11. Meingast, M., Roosta, T., Sastry, S.: Security and privacy issues with healthcare information technology. In: Ubiquitous Methodologies, pp. 5453–5458 (2006)
12. Daman, R., Manish, M.T., Mishra, S.: Security issues in cloud computing for healthcare. In: IEEE, International conference on computing for sustainable global development, pp. 1231–1236 (2016)
13. Methods of Minimizing Security Risks in Healthcare. https://healthtechmagazine.net/article/2020/03/3-methods-minimizing-security-risks-healthcare-perfcon (2020)
14. Wang,C.B., Xing, H.Y.: The application of cloud computing in education informatization, modern educational technology. In: Computer Science and Service System (CSSS), International Conference on IEEE, pp. 2673–2676 (2011)
15. Fusarol, V., Patil, P., Gafni, E., Tonellato, P.J.: Biomedical cloud computing with Amazon Web Services. PLOS Comput. Biol. **7**(8) (2011)
16. Kuo, A.M.-H.: Opportunities and challenges of cloud computing to improve healthcare services. J. Med. Internet Res. e67 (2011)
17. Wang, L., Alexander, C.A.: Medical applications and healthcare based on cloud computing. Int. J Cloud Comput. Serv. Sci. (IJ-CLOSER) **2**(4) (2014)
18. Takabi, H., James, B., Ahn, G.-J.: Security and privacy challenges in cloud computing environments. IEEE Secur. Priv. (2010)
19. Abouelmehdi, K., Beni-Hessane, A., Khaloufi, H.: Big healthcare data: preserving security and privacy. J. Big Data **5**, 1 (2018)
20. Wooten,R., et al.: Design and implementation of a secure healthcare social cloud system. In: 12th IEEE/ACM International Symposium in Cluster, Cloud and Grid Computing, pp. 805–810 (2012)
21. Xin, Z., Song-Qing, L.: Research on cloud computing data security model based on multidimension. IEEE (2012)
22. Benthin, F.: Cyber security for healthcare providers—approach to a whitepaper for the hospital management. In: World of Health IT (2016)
23. Cisco Healthcare Security. https://www.cisco.com/c/dam/en_us/solutions/industries/docs/healthcare/healthcare-security-white-paper.pdf (2014)
24. Kruse,C.S., Mileski, M., Vijaykumar, A.G., Viswanathan, S., Suskandla, U., Chidambraram, Y.: Impact of electronic health records on long-term care facilities: systematic review. JMIR Med. Inform. **5**(3), e35 (2017)

Healthcare Data Visualization

M. V. Manoj Kumar, B. S. Prashanth, Aditya Shastry, H. A. Sanjay, and H. R. Sneha

Abstract It is evident that a huge amount of data is currently being generated. Across the world, 2.5 quintillion bytes of data is being recorded currently. It i s almost equivalent to 0.5 Million TB or it is enough to occupy 10 Million Blue-ray disks. The amount of data is expected to surpass 44 trillion gigabytes at the end of 2020 (as compared to 4.4 trillion gigabytes during the end of 2013). The lion's share of the data being recorded in the information systems is basically related to healthcare activities. Extracting useful information/insights from a large quantity of data is very important. Visualizing data could yield wonderful results, and summaries hidden in data, especially, visualization could do a wonderful job in health care. Data visualization saves time and conveys information more meaningfully. It is a powerful way to summarize which assists all stakeholders. This chapter presents an attempt to summarize healthcare data through exploratory data analysis and process mining control-flow discovery techniques. Exploratory data analysis of healthcare data presents a way to explore healthcare data meaningfully, and process mining based control flow visualization presents the way to extract the causal relationships between the activities of the process. Process mining way of visualizing healthcare helps in identifying the discrepancies between planned and actual healthcare processes. Final sections of this chapter present Process Mining based control flow visualizations on real-time event log detailed in healthcare information systems.

M. V. Manoj Kumar (✉) · B. S. Prashanth · A. Shastry · H. A. Sanjay · H. R. Sneha
Department of Information Science and Engineering, Nitte Meenakshi Institute of Technology, Bengaluru 560064, India
e-mail: manojmv24@gmail.com

B. S. Prashanth
e-mail: prashanth.bshivanna@gmail.com

A. Shastry
e-mail: adityashastry.k@nmit.ac.in

H. A. Sanjay
e-mail: sanjay.ha@nmit.ac.in

K. G. Srinivasa et al. (eds.), *Artificial Intelligence for Information Management: A Healthcare Perspective*, Studies in Big Data 88,
https://doi.org/10.1007/978-981-16-0415-7_9

Keywords Data visualization · Electronic health data · Machine learning · Artificial neural network · Process mining

1 Introduction

Healthcare management as the name suggests is the overall management of the healthcare institution such as hospitals or a clinic. A healthcare manager is a person who monitors and manages all the activities involved in these facilities such as institute budget, managing the human and equipment resources coinciding with the facility mission and vision. A humongous amount of data is being generated daily by various medical facilities all over the world [1]. These data related to medical facilities can be used to draw abundant useful insights, using which the institution can prosper in terms of revenue, human relations, and technology in an effective manner. One of the horizons that the present study explores is to accumulate and organize these data in a proper structure and use this data to draw process models which will further help us to deduce an effective workflow for the medical personnel and various stakeholders involved in the medical facility.

There are two horizons from which exploring healthcare data in a meaningful way can be done, First is to interpret data using exploratory data analysis, and the other is to employ process mining techniques to discover the healthcare process models. Exploratory data analysis offers methods and techniques to dissect the data to obtain the key performance indicators, it acts as a tool that can dissect the data and gives a complete overview of it. On the other hand, process mining offers tools and techniques to extract the process model from the information recorded in the form of event log—typically in healthcare information systems. Availability of event logs is a starting point to apply process mining techniques. On the event logs, the range of techniques related to discovery, conformance and enhancement can be applied. The second section of this chapter discusses the process mining way of visualizing healthcare data.

Preliminary section of this chapter examines the various issues and challenges involved in medical data processing, characteristics of the medical data. The data coming from the various medical sources can be tuned for processing using Exploratory Data Analytics Techniques which is explored in detail in the coming sections of this chapter. A further section of the chapter explores the various topics related to health care management and data visualization. The final section of the chapter examines the application of process mining for healthcare process modelling and summarization.

2 Importance of Healthcare Management

Healthcare data management refers to the process of consolidating, storing, processing, and drawing out useful insights from the medical data from various sources which are available in many varieties. The abundant information available in the medical data can be used for summarization, patient diagnosis, treatment, and provides a structured way of healthcare management. Though on the outset the task seems simplistic, in action it involves us addressing many challenges due to the nature of the medical data itself. Healthcare data management is quite essential because of the following reasons:

- It helps to model various stakeholders such as patients, caretakers, consumers, and provides a way for guided interaction with the patients as well as the caretakers [2].
- It helps the hospital or medical institution to make important business decisions to improvise the relationship with the various stakeholders related to the medical institution.
- It also helps the institute or hospitals to analyze, monitor the physicians, doctors and patient activities and cross-check them against the institute vision and mission.
- To effectively use the healthcare system on a larger scale, we need to understand the health care data in a detailed manner. The following section explores the attributes of the healthcare data.

3 Critical Attributes of Healthcare Data

The four fundamental properties of the healthcare data [3] are

- **Non-Atomicity**—Medical datasets are non-atomic in nature, meaning that data is retrieved from multiple sources and these combined data are used to draw inferences. An example of this is a medical practitioner collects inference drawn from various sources such as X-ray, MRI, CT images and laboratory tests and patient history data to infer his diagnosis of the disease.
- **Cognition**—Healthcare data must be accessed with cognitive skills, rather than accessing it as bare data for inferences. Medical practitioners must have vast skills and knowledge base to have a better understanding of practices, medicine, and diagnosis methodology thereby they can draw specific clinical decisions [3].
- **Shareability**—Healthcare data should be published and shared online on medical platforms to get universally accepted by various doctors, clinicians all over the world. *Interprofessional Collaborations* [3] are vital for advanced diagnosis of the patients
- **Longitudinal**—Healthcare data should be observed and recorded longitudinally that is, a set of tests, medicines procedures conducted during patient treatment can be reviewed continuously to infer observable changes upon the method of treatment.

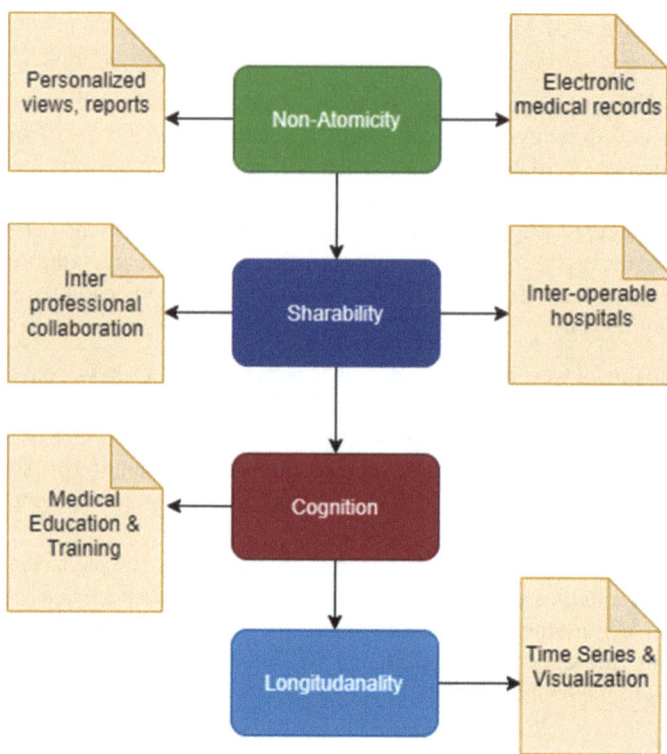

Fig. 1 Four characteristics of the Healthcare Data

Figure 1 shows the characteristics of the healthcare data.

4 Common Data Sources in Health Care

Following are some of the most common data sources found in any healthcare setup.

- **Electronic Medical Records (EMR)**—These categories of healthcare data recorded as a digital version of a patient's paper version of the report. It is used by medical professionals to keep track of a patient's condition, the upcoming treatment plan, etc. Electronic medical records normally stored digitally within the healthcare organization.
- **Electronic Health Records (EHR)**—It is a superset of digitized information related to a patient's complete health, it also includes treatment history of patients administered by other healthcare services, providers, laboratory reports, etc. HER basically moves with patients and is used by various providers as and when it is required.

- **Specific departmental data**—This data pertains to information collected by some internal departments of healthcare facilities. This data is not required by all departments, but critical for the functioning of some departments.
- **Administrative data**—It is gathered by Healthcare Management Systems, which take care of the complete healthcare setup's operation. It is a source of information for hospital top management. It also consists of data related to resource optimization/utilization (human/non-human)
- **Financial data**—It is proprietary data typically stored in financial information systems in large organizations.

4.1 Dashboard-Based Advanced Data Visualizations

Everyone likes to see the information briefly and in a simplified format. This led to the creation of dashboards. The dashboard is a part of GUI aimed at providing the bird's eye view of most important information for specific healthcare entities. Dashboards can even act as a driving force for immediate/long-term goals.

Individuals at various levels of the healthcare industry require information from different sources. A customized dashboard that shows critical patient and operational information will help healthcare professionals. It helps one to make informed decisions. Some of the key advantages of healthcare dashboards are

- Combining data from various sources—hence address the issues in care quality, hurdles in the decision process, informed decisions, critical reasoning.
- Helps in optimizing the process by turning the key parameters.
- Helps to monitor the healthcare process.
- Promotes transparency between various doctor and managerial levels.
- Promotes a collaborative environment among peers, specialists, and healthcare facility staff members.

4.2 Types of Healthcare Dashboards

To deliver superior service to patients, healthcare establishments need to offer several healthcare standards. Aligned to this, it is essential to optimize costs, maintain compliance with regulatory bodies, and reduce patient wait times. A tailor-made supervisory dashboard will help to address all these challenges.

Some of the dashboards currently used by healthcare providers are Clinical Dashboards, Healthcare Organization Dashboards, Patient Dashboards, Healthcare Provider Dashboards, and Quality Dashboards.

4.3 Population Health Analytics

The fundamental vision of healthcare professionals is to offer value-oriented superior care to patients. With population health analytics, one can identify patient populations, find out the care offered to these patients, based on this one can plan how to offer the best care to patients.

Customized population analytics facilitates quick and improved extraction of data from various data sources [4]. There are some models that offer the method to divide the patient population into low. Medium, high-risk tires. It can even help in foreseeing the risk score which allows one to assign patient-specific healthcare plans and get to know mass-oriented health trends. This can result in a range of dashboards, such as consolidated report medical history as shown in Fig. 2 (comprising medical diagnoses, emergency room visits, hospital stays, chronic care management, and medication).

5 Exploratory Data Analysis in Medical Dataset

In a lot of Machine Learning projects, before any algorithm is built for a dataset, Data Scientists perform two important steps, Data Pre-Processing, and Exploratory Data Analysis (EDA). It is famously quoted that data pre-processing and data exploration cover 80% of the project time and the rest 20% is dedicated for model building, validation, and deployment. While data pre-processing involves cleaning of data in terms of dealing with null values, manipulating categorical data, and analyzing and removing outliers if deemed necessary. Once this step is completed, next comes understanding the data via various statistical methods and graphs which allows us to get insights within the data, understand various patterns and relations of the features in the dataset,

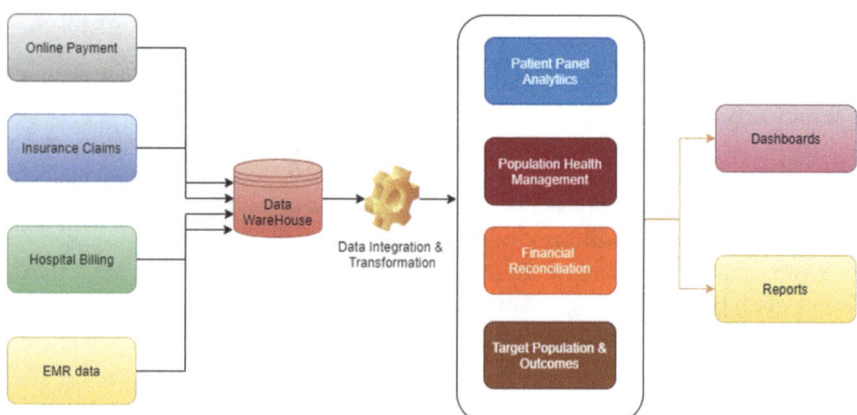

Fig. 2 Dashboard and reports

understand how the data is distributed, check for outliers, create hypotheses, etc. This step is known as Exploratory Data Analysis (EDA). This step is of paramount importance before applying any machine learning model, since understanding the features of the data, which can be univariate or multivariate, as well as understanding the correlations with the dependent feature (if dealing with supervised learning).

5.1 History of EDA

Before understanding the steps and processes under the umbrella of EDA, it is important to note the contributions made by some of the brilliant minds who are the driving force behind data exploration and analysis. One of the noted mathematicians named Karl Pearson proposed *Kurtosis coefficient* to measure the degree of flatness of frequency distribution in 1905. He also challenged the idea of either the data is normally distributed, or it should be transformed to normality. He suggested that the data should be represented as it is. In 1973, a Statistician named Francis Anscombe constructed *Anscombe's quartet* which suggested the importance of data to visualize it graphically before analyzing it. He also showed the effect of outliers on statistical properties. However, the main source of contribution and the term "Exploratory Data Analysis" came in 1977 by John W. Tukey, who is considered to be the *"Father of Exploratory Data Analysis"*. He introduced new plots and five-point boxplots with the help of computer-aided visualization, in his book titled Exploratory Data Analysis. He also implied that Confirmatory Data Analysis (CDA) can suffer from confirmation bias due to predetermined hypotheses, whereas Exploratory Data Analysis is more open-minded in discovering patterns within the data. Now we have understood the origin of EDA, in the next section let us understand the importance of the same, thus appreciating various techniques involved in this process and gaining a clear understanding of the same.

5.2 Need for EDA

In this section, let us discuss the necessity of EDA, thus equal weightage and motivation are channeled to this process while solving data-related problems.

- It helps you to spot missing values or erroneous values, which either can be an outlier or non-related values to that column.
- Understanding the structure and patterns within the data.
- Understanding and establishing the relationships within the variables in the dataset.
- Identifying the most important variables in the dataset.
- Creating and testing hypotheses related to a model.

As widely said, neglecting this step can lead to the following possibilities:

- Data can be skewed, has missing values and outliers, which can adversely affect the model performance.
- Generating incorrect assumptions and hypotheses.
- Wrong sets of variables can be extracted for the model.
- Incorrect understanding of the data can lead to biased models and thus reduce the performance of the model.

Now that we have understood the importance of EDA, let us understand certain basic terminologies, before analyzing various techniques involved in data exploration.

- **Dataset**—It is a collection of similar data which can be either in a form of tables, images, texts, graphs, etc.
- **Data frame**—It is a 2-dimensional data structure, i.e., it consists of 2 axes; rows and columns and it is in tabular format. It is generally used to store the dataset which is in Comma-Separated-Values (CSV) extension as a data structure for easy manipulation and operations on data.
- **Records**—These are the rows in a tabular dataset that contains information about a person or an entity and is unique to each other.
- **Attributes**—These are the columns in a tabular dataset that describe that person or an entity. The values in an attribute can be either categorical or numerical in nature. Attributes are of two types: Quantitative and Qualitative.

5.2.1 Qualitative Attributes

Qualitative attributes are of following types:

- **Nominal**—These are also known as categorical attributes which distinguish objects under the same type. Example: Brown, black and white are the three categories that fall under the umbrella of colors
- **Ordinal**—These variables contain the order or sequence between the objects. Example: Good, Better, Best.
- **Binary**—These are categories that have only two states or values.

  Example: Yes or No, 0 or 1.

5.2.2 Quantitative Attributes

Quantitative attributes are of the following types: Numeric, Discrete, and Continuous.

- **Numeric**—These are the attributes that contain either real or integer values. Numeric attributes are of two types: Interval and Ratio.

  - **Interval**—They are sequences of numbers or numerical values where the distance between them is standardized or equal. Example: Temperature.
  - **Ratio**—These are the numeric attributes with fixed zero-point.

- **Discrete**—These are the finite values that can be in the form of either numerical or categorical. They generally contain integer values. Example: Zip codes, counts etc.
- **Continuous**—These are the numerical values that have no finite states and can take float values as well. Example: Height of a person.
- **Independent attributes**—These are the input values from the dataset which are passed to any machine learning model. They are called independent attributes since they are assumed to have no direct relations between them.
- **Dependent attribute**—These are output or the predictor column in the dataset. They are known as dependent attributes since the value for that record is based on the values in the independent values of that record.

Now that we have understood the basic terminologies, let us know the basic steps involved in understanding and processing the dataset before diving into statistical analysis and EDA. For further explanations, the famous Pima-Indians diabetes dataset will be used to conduct and understand EDA.

Example: About the dataset: This dataset consists of 768 records and 9 attributes. The attributes are as follows:

- Pregnancies: Number of times pregnant.
- Glucose: Plasma glucose concentration.
- Blood Pressure: Diastolic blood pressure (mm Hg).
- Skin Thickness: Triceps skinfold thickness (mm).
- Insulin: 2-Hour serum insulin (mu U/ml).
- BMI: Body Mass Index (weight in kg/(height in m)^2).
- Diabetes Pedigree Function.
- Age: Age in years.
- Target: 1 (Patient has diabetes) or 0 (Patient does not have diabetes).

The dataset is stored in the form of a data frame thanks to Pandas library, which is written in Python programming language. Pandas library allows the developer to store and manipulate with data. Libraries can be imported in the following manner:

> import pandas as pd

This allows the developer to use the various functionalities under Pandas library. As keyword in Python stands for Alias, where a short form of any imported library is created to ease the use of calling the functions within that library in the future. After importing the library, the next step is to store the dataset in the form of a data frame. To do this, the following code segment is written:

> df = pd. read_csv("diabetes.csv")

The above line of code allows the user to store the dataset which is of the CSV extension into Pandas data frame. This data frame will be stored in the df variable. In the next step, let us look at the first five records of the dataset to get an idea about the dataset. To do this, we will be using the head (), which will allow the developers to

	Pregnancies	Glucose	Blood Pressure	Skin Thickness	Insulin	BMI	Diabetes Pedigree Function	Age	Outcome
0	6	148	72	35	0	36.6	0.627	50	1
1	1	85	66	29	0	26.6	0.351	31	0
2	8	183	64	0	0	23.3	0.672	32	1
3	1	89	66	23	94	28.1	0.167	21	0
4	0	137	40	35	168	43.1	2.288	33	1

Fig. 3 First five records in the dataset

view the first five records of the dataset. You can investigate any number of records in the dataset by passing that value within that function as follows,:

> **df. head()**

The result is as shown in Fig. 3.

Similarly, the last five records in the dataset can be observed using df.tail(). Now, let us look at the datatypes of the columns in the dataset. This will give the developers the idea to deal with the attributes while performing analysis. This is because certain data types such as String cannot be directly used for analysis. They need to be converted to numeric format before processing the data. To perform this step the code segment is as follows:

> **df. types()**

The result is as shown in Fig. 4.

In the next step, let us look at the statistical description of the dataset using describe (). This function allows you to analyze certain basic statistical analyses such as mean, standard deviation, percentile and displays the minimum and maximum values and count of each attribute.

> **df.describe()**

The result of this operation is as shown in Fig. 5.

Fig. 4 Datatypes of the columns in the dataset

Pregnancies	int64
Glucose	int64
Blood Pressure	int64
Skin Thickness	int64
Insulin	int64
BMI	float64
DiabetesPedigreeFunction	float64
Age	int64
Outcome	int64
dtype: object	

	count	mean	std	min	25%	50%	75%	max
Pregnancies	768	3.845052	3.369578	0	1	3	6	17
Glucose	768	120.89453	31.972618	0	99	117	170.25	199
Blood Pressure	768	69.105469	19.355807	0	62	72	80	122
Skin Thickness	768	20.536458	15.952218	0	0	23	32	99
Insulin	768	79.799479	115.244	0	0	30.5	127.25	846
BMI	768	31.992578	7.88416	0	27.3	32	36.6	67.1
DiabetesPedigreeFunction	768	0.471876	0.331329	0.078	0.24375	0.3725	0.6263	2.42
Age	768	33.240885	11.760232	21	24	29	41	81
Outcome	768	0.348958	0.476951	0	0	0	1	1

Fig. 5 Statistical description of the dataset

Let us look at each column and analyze them separately,

- Count: This column gives the count of non-null rows in a feature. For example, if there is one missing value in a record under any attribute, then one count will be subtracted from the total count. In this example, we have 768 records in the dataset and the total count of each attribute is 768. Hence, we have no missing value in the dataset. If there is any missing, then it should be dealt with by applying the appropriate technique.
- Mean: This column calculates and displays the mean of each attribute. Mean for the mean is given as follows: Where xi is the ith element of a set and n is the total number of elements. However, we need to remember that mean is not always the right metric to analyze the data, since they can be affected by outliers which often skews the data. Also, in this case, we can see that we do not have missing values, however certain attributes have 0 as a value in them. They must be taken care of by applying suitable statistical techniques such as median or other interpolation techniques.

$$Mean(\mu) = \frac{\sum_{i=0}^{n} x_i}{n}$$

- Standard deviation: Standard deviation allows us to understand the spread or dispersion of a set of values. They are generally compared to its distance with respect to mean. If they are close to the mean, those sets of values have a smaller standard deviation, whereas if they are farther away from the mean they have a larger standard deviation and these data points are spread over a wider range. Standard deviation is for a dataset X of size n given by

$$Standard\ Deviation(\sigma) = \frac{\sum_{i=0}^{n} x_i - \mu^2)}{n}$$

where xi is the *i*th element of the dataset and μ is the mean of all elements.

- Minimum—This column provides the least value present in an attribute for that dataset. The minimum value for any attribute may or may not be an outlier. It should be analyzed and dealt with if deemed necessary. 25, 50 and 75%—the values 25, 50 and 75% are known as percentiles. They are valuable in summarizing data distribution. They are also helpful in identifying the outliers in data. While 50% is the median value of the attribute, 25% is the median of data that lie between minimum value and median, whereas 75% is the median of data that lie between the median and maximum value. Percentile can also be viewed and analyzed using box plots which will be explained in the later sections.
- **Maximum**: This column provides the largest value present in an attribute for that dataset. The maximum value for any attribute may or may not be an outlier. It should be analyzed and dealt with if deemed necessary. Now that we have a basic understanding of the dataset, let us now conduct univariate and multivariate analysis using suitable graphs. Remember that analyzing attributes with continuous values are different from analyzing attributes with categorical values. We shall see different plots for each case using Seaborn and Matplotlib libraries which are written in python. Seaborn allows developers to plot statistical graphs and Matplotlib allows the developer to plot both static and interactive graphs. Let us also discuss the suitable techniques to deal with missing values and outliers in the upcoming sections.

5.2.3 Treating the Missing Values

In today's era, there is an abundance of data, collected from various sources, solving different problems across industries. In an ideal scenario, all the data would be caught seamlessly, and that data would be stored in a database, and that data is used for analysis. But this is not the case while solving real-world problems. The dataset often will be very messy, and it consumes a lot of time and effort in cleaning and understanding the data. Due to various reasons, certain values will not be recorded for an attribute and that missing value must be treated accordingly to obtain optimal performance after applying any machine learning algorithm.

In the considered example, we have seen that there are no missing values per se, since they are generally referred to as 'Not A Number' (NAN). But there are few records that contain 0 as its value. Of course, in some of the data problems, 0 might have some significance but for this dataset, it is not possible for attributes such as Blood Pressure, Glucose, BMI, and skin thickness to have the values 0. Thus, we either need to remove them or replace them based on the understanding of data. Mean and Median are used to find the missing values.

6   Healthcare Data Visualization with Process Mining

The basic techniques in process modelling using the bottom-up approach involves discovery, conformance checking, and enhancement.

The basic idea of process modelling is shown in Fig. 6. The information systems supporting and controlling various real-world processes record event log. With the availability of event log, different process modelling analysis techniques can be employed to analyze the observed behavior. Figure 7 describes the basic types of process model construction and related operations. Discovery, Conformance, and Enhancement [5].

6.1   Process Discovery

Process discovery methods are most useful to provide insights into what occurs. Discovery techniques produce control-flow, data, organizational, time, and case models. A plethora of methods exists in process mining to elicit the process model of various notations, the focus of the chapter is to discover the control-flow perspective. The control-flow perspective [6] depicts the causal relationships between the activities of the process. It discovers the visual process graph in terms of nodes and edges. It gives the ordering of the execution of activities. For example, Sect. 4 briefs modelling the process control flow perspective in more than 10+ different modelling formats such as Petri net, BPMN, EPN, etc.

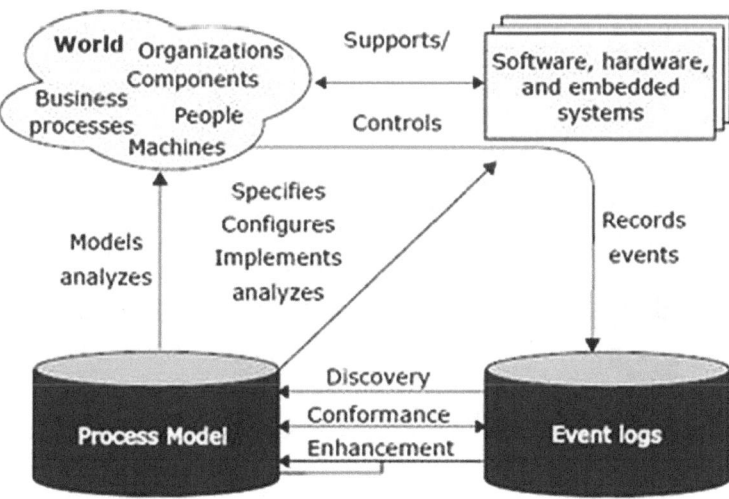

Fig. 6   Basic idea of process mining [31]

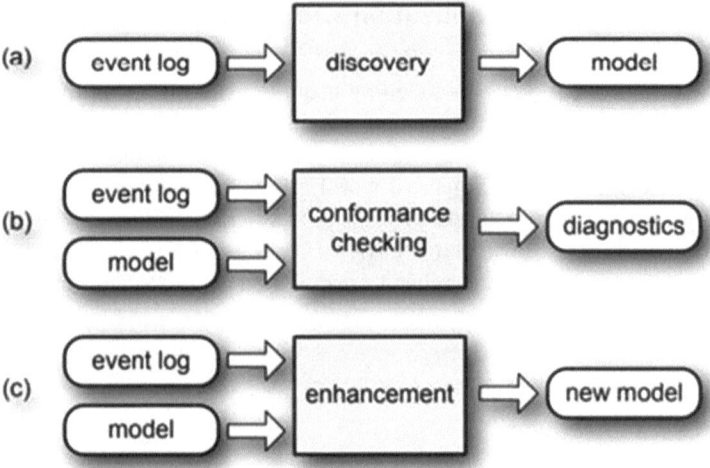

Fig. 7 Basic techniques in process model construction

7 Event Log

The starting point of process mining is the observed behavior of process executions, stored in event logs [7, 8]. An overview of recording the process execution data is shown in Fig. 8. We now formalize the various notations related to the event log,

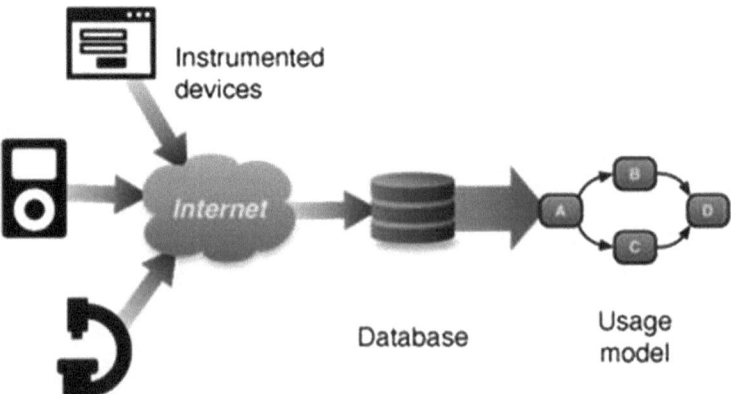

Fig. 8 Process of recording event log and model generation from recorded data

7.1 Event and Attribute

Since the event logs of information systems provide factual data about the underlying processes, they are a precious source of information [9, 10]. Figure 9 shows an example of an event log of the hospital patient admission process. This event log will be used for discussion and illustration in this chapter. Let E be the set of all event identifiers and AN be the set of all attributes. For an attribute, $s \in AN$ let X_x is a universal set (consists of a set of all possible values of x). Given E and an attribute $x \in AN$, $\#_x(e)$ is the value for all attributes x not defined in e and $\#_x$ [11, 12].

$$\#_{activity}(e) \in A$$

signifies the activity associated with the event e.

$$\#_{resource}(e) \in R$$

indicates the resource performing the event e.

$$\#_{time}(e) \in R$$

indicates the timestamp of event e.

$$\#_{trans}(e) \in TT$$

indicates the transaction type associated with the event e.

7.2 Case, Trace and Event log

$$\mathcal{L} = |\langle\, \text{Appointment, Admit patient, Check history, Decide, Begin treatment}\,\rangle, \langle\, \text{Appointment, Out patient, Check history, Decide, Discharge}\rangle, \langle\, \text{Appointment, Admit patient, Check history, Decide, Re-examine, Out patient, Check history, Decide, Discharge}\,\rangle, \langle\, \text{Appointment, Check history, Admit patient, Decide, Discharge}\rangle, \langle\, \text{Appointment, Out patient, Check history, Decide, Re-initiate, Admit patient, Check history, Decide, Begin treatment}\,\rangle, ..|$$

Event log on control perspective normally defined over a set of activity names. A sequence of activity is referred to as trace. A simple event log is defined as a

| Case id | Event id | Properties | | | | |
		Timestamp	Activity	Resource	Cost	...
	2342	10-10-2012:01.20	Appointment	Anne	200	...
	2343	11-10-2012:07.24	Admit patient	Jhon	100	...
xx12	2344	12-10-2012:08.24	Check history	Thomas	400	...
	2345	13-10-2012:12.24	Decide	Clar	50	...
	2346	13-10-2012:13.25	Begin treatment	Ram	10	...
	3347	14-10-2012:01.29	Appointment	Anne	200	...
	3348	14-10-2012:01.34	Out patient	Wil	20	...
xx13	3349	14-11-2012:16.34	Check history	Thomas	300	...
	3350	15-11-2012:08.22	Decide	Clar	50	...
	3351	15-11-2012:09.17	Discharge	Ram	100	...
	4352	22-11-2012:07.47	Appointment	Anne	200	...
	4353	23-11-2012:12.31	Admit patient	John	100	...
	4354	25-11-2012:19.41	Check history	Thomas	50	...
	4355	25-11-2012:18.14	Decide	Clar	50	...
xx14	4356	25-11-2012:19.37	Re-examine	Steven	100	...
	4357	26-11-2012:01.00	Out patient	Wil	20	...
	4358	28-11-2012:02.00	Check history	Thomas	100	...
	4359	29-11-2012:13.37	Decide	Clar	400	...
	4360	30-11-2012:02.20	Discharge	Ram	100	...
	5361	30-12-2013:02.20	Appointment	Anne	200	...
	5362	11-01-2013:02.20	Check history	Thomas	300	...
xx15	5363	12-01-2013:03.20	Admit patient	Jhon	20	...
	5364	12-01-2013:15.20	Decide	Clar	50	...
	5365	13-01-2013:17.20	Discharge	Ram	30	...
	6366	17-01-2013:22.20	Appointment	Anne	200	...
	6367	17-01-2013:23.17	Out patient	Wil	50	...
	6368	19-01-2013:01.20	Check history	Thomas	100	...
	6369	19-01-2013:04.20	Decide	Clar	20	...
xx16	6370	19-01-2013:15.20	Re-initiate	Steven	400	...
	6371	19-01-2013:22.20	Admit patient	Jhon	300	...
	6372	20-01-2013:05.20	Check history	Thomas	200	...
	6373	23-01-2013:07.20	Decide	Clar	300	...
	6374	24-01-2013:14.20	Begin treatment	Ram	200	...
...	...	...	...	...	...	...

Fig. 9 Event log of the hospital admission process

bag of traces [13, 14]. Projection using resource classifiers can be used in mining organizational models, social networks, etc. [15]. By choosing resource classifier, the sample event log results as

$$\mathcal{L} = [\langle \text{ Anne, Jhon, Thomas, Clar, Ram } \rangle, \langle \text{ Anne, Wil, Thomas, Clar, Ram} \rangle, \langle \text{ Anne,}$$
$$\text{John, Thomas, Clar, Steven, Wil, Thomas, Clar, Ram } \rangle, \langle \text{ Anne, Thomas, John,}$$
$$\text{Clar, Ram} \rangle, \langle \text{ Anne, Wil, Thomas, Clar, Steven, John, Thomas, Clar, Ram } \rangle, ..]$$

7.3   Structure of Event Log

To better understand the structure of an event log, a tree diagram of a hospital patient admission event log is given in Fig. 10. Using the tree structure, we can describe the structure of the event log as follows:

- **Case id** is used for distinctly identifying an instance of the process. For example, xx12, xx13, etc. represent the case ids in the hospital admission event log given in Fig. 9.
- **Event id** assigns a distinct identifier for every event related to a specific case. For example, event 2346 of case xx12 and event of 3347 of case xx13.
- **Activity** assigns a readable name for every event of a case. For example, event 2346 of case xx12 and event of 3347 of case xx13 points to an activity named Appointment. But activity Appointment will be carried out separately for both cases.
- **Resources** identify the individuals or machines who are assigned and responsible for executing a specific activity. For example, Ram is assigned as a resource for executing the activity Discharge related to all cases.
- **Timestamps** record the duration.
- The expenditure incurred while executing a specific activity is recorded in the **cost** field.
- **Data** objects related to the process are recorded in the data field. Typical data objects are messages, files, documents, guards, videos, voice, and conditions.

8   Control Perspective of Hospital Process Using Various Modelling Notations

The control flow notations connect activities (i.e., functions, tasks, transitions) in the process through constructs like condition, places, events, connectors, and gateways. Control flow perspective models, the causal relationship between different steps in the process execution [16]. Based on the transitions between activities, execution

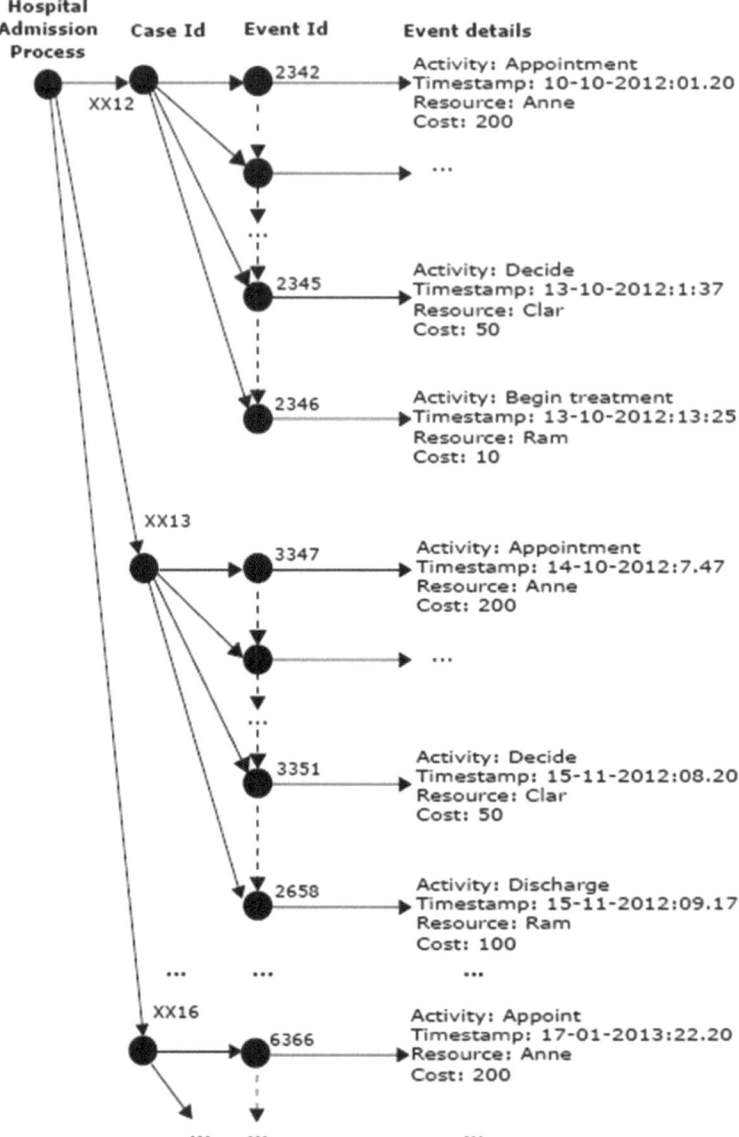

Fig. 10 Tree structure of process log

can be serial, concurrent, optional, and repeated. Process mining offers a plethora of techniques for discovering control-flow models out of event-log.

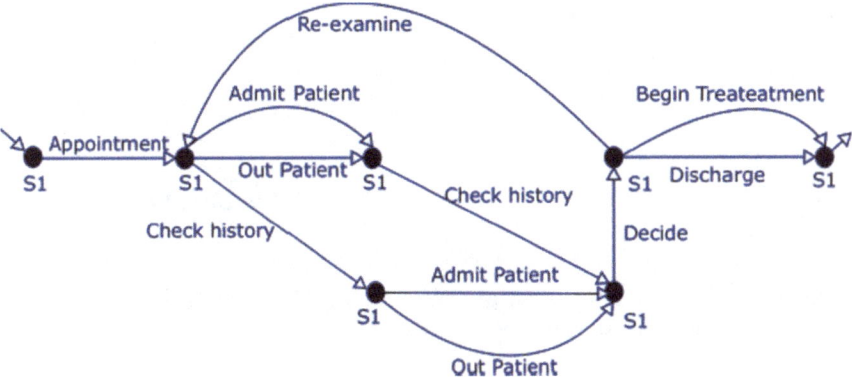

Fig. 11 Transition net

8.1 *Transition Systems*

Transition system is the most rudimentary control flow modelling notation. It consists of states and transitions. It is represented using triplet $TS = \{S, A, T\}$. Where S represents set of states T is set of Transitions, and A is set of Activities. A sample transition system is shown in Fig. 11.

8.2 *Petri Net*

α algorithm [17, 18] available in process mining can generate control flow of a process in the Petri net notation. Petri net model of the hospital admission process is

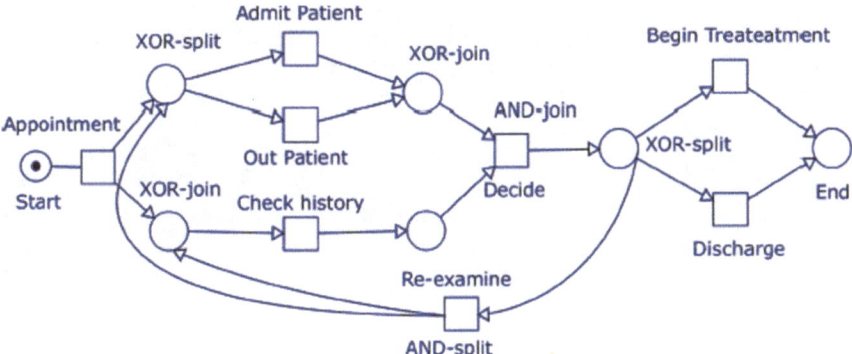

Fig. 12 Petri net

Fig. 13 Workflow nets

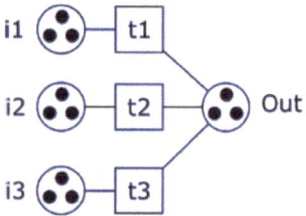

given in Fig. 12. A Petri net is a triplet $N = \{P, T, F\}$. Where, P is a set of places. T is a set of transitions such that $P \cap T = \phi$.

8.3 Workflow Nets

A workflow net is an extension of Petri nets with a specific start and end place [19–21]. A workflow net is represented with attributes as $N = \{P, T, F, A, L\}$, where N is workflow net, P is output place, F is final place. A sample workflow net is shown in Fig. 13.

8.4 Yet Another Workflow Language (YAWL)

YAWL is an amalgamation of the workflow system and modelling language. The development of YAWL was greatly driven by the workflow patterns initiative [22, 23]. Based on a regular investigation of the notations utilized by existing control flow notations. The following Fig. 14 shows a sample YAWL net.

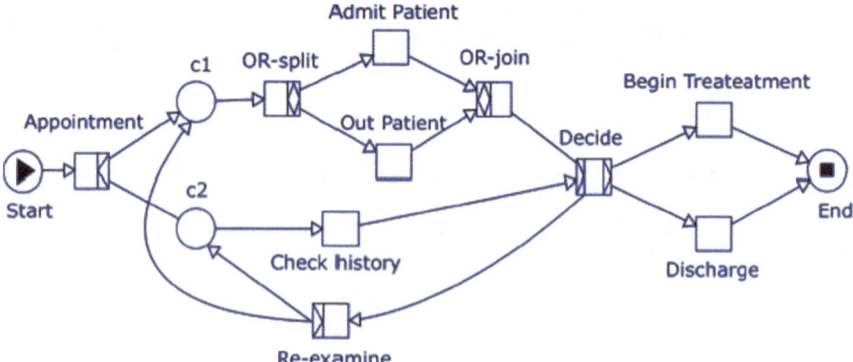

Fig. 14 Yet another workflow Language

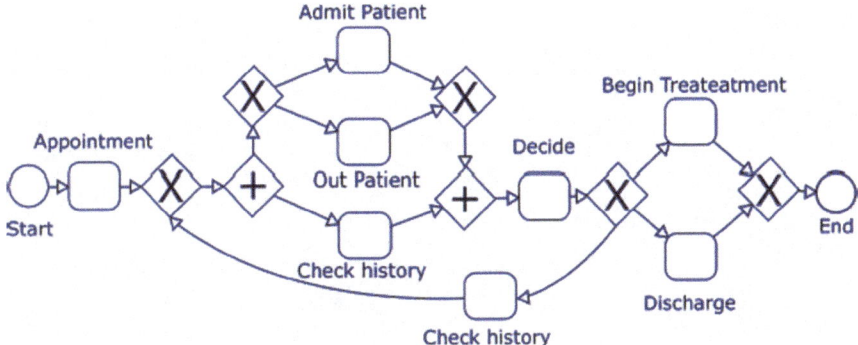

Fig. 15 Business process modelling notation

YAWL is based on the philosophy of facilitating a range of patterns without increasing the modelling language complexity.

8.5 Business Process Modelling Notation (BPMN)

In recent times, BPMN [24] has become a widely used notation to model operational processes. It preserves the concept of tasks from YAWL. BPMN model of the hospital admission process is shown in Fig. 15.

8.6 Event-Driven Process Chains (EPC)

EPCs [25, 26] fundamentally offers a subset of features from BPMN and YAWL with its own graphical notations. Activities in EPCs are called functions. Functions consist of one input and output arc. EPC of the hospital process is shown in Fig. 16.

8.7 Causal Nets

A causal net [27] is a graph where arcs signify causal dependencies and nodes signify activities. Each activity has a set of possible input and output bindings that guides routing logic in the causal net. Causal nets are highly suitable for control flow related tasks of process mining. Casual net representation of the hospital admission process is shown in Fig. 17.

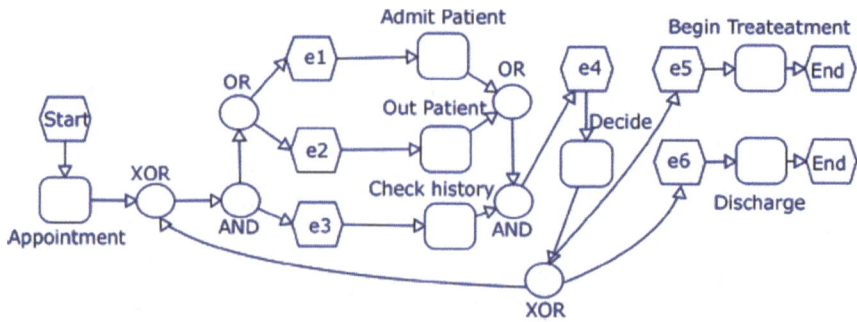

Fig. 16 Event-driven process chain

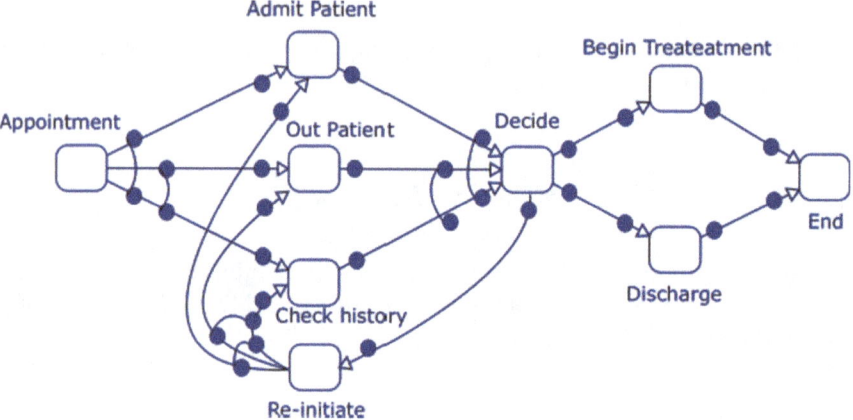

Fig. 17 Causal net

9 Predictive Modelling Control Flow of a Process Using Fuzzy Miner

This section presents a case study to illustrate the modelling of real-life health-care processes. We present a detailed analysis of the event log of hospital treatment process execution, and hospital billing process [28]. We have taken the data from 4TU.Center for Research Data [13]. The fuzzy miner will be used to predictively elucidate the control flow model of the process [29]. Using the fuzzy miner, the process is predictively reconstructed by vomiting the insignificant activities and paths in the process.

9.1 Hospital Process

The 'Hospital Billing' event log comprises events that are associated with the billing of medical facilities. Each trace of the event log accounts for the activities performed to bill a package of medical services. Typical activities found in the billing process have been depicted in Fig. 18, it shows the relative frequency of each of these significant activities. All activities in the process irrespective of execution frequency have been depicted in the table.

Figures 19 and 20 show the typical attributes and complexity of the dataset. There are 1 lakh cases, totaling 4,51,539 events over 18 different activities, other typical attributes of the event log are briefed in Figs. 19 and 20.

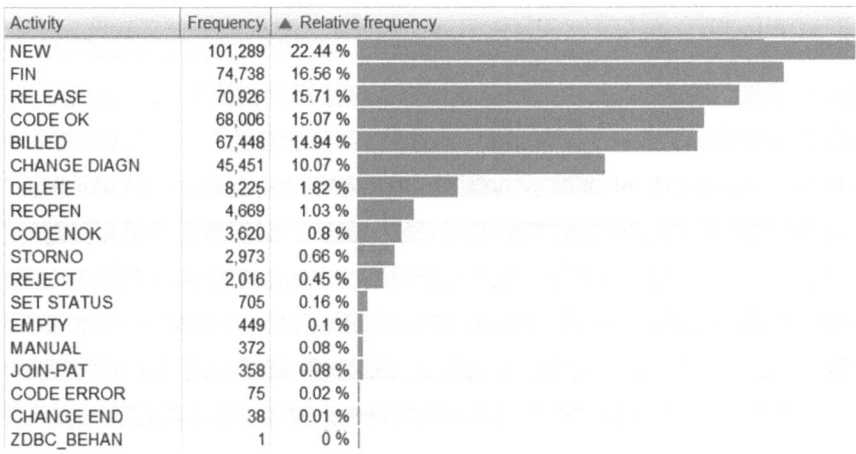

Activity	Frequency	▲ Relative frequency
NEW	101,289	22.44 %
FIN	74,738	16.56 %
RELEASE	70,926	15.71 %
CODE OK	68,006	15.07 %
BILLED	67,448	14.94 %
CHANGE DIAGN	45,451	10.07 %
DELETE	8,225	1.82 %
REOPEN	4,669	1.03 %
CODE NOK	3,620	0.8 %
STORNO	2,973	0.66 %
REJECT	2,016	0.45 %
SET STATUS	705	0.16 %
EMPTY	449	0.1 %
MANUAL	372	0.08 %
JOIN-PAT	358	0.08 %
CODE ERROR	75	0.02 %
CHANGE END	38	0.01 %
ZDBC_BEHAN	1	0 %

Fig. 18 Activities in the process and relative frequency

Fig. 19 Overview of the hospital billing process

Events	451,359
Cases	100,000
Activities	18
Median case duration	14.6 wks
Mean case duration	18.2 wks
Start	13.12.2012 14:43:18
End	19.01.2016 13:28:56

Activities	18
Minimal frequency	1
Median frequency	3,296
Mean frequency	25,075.5
Maximal frequency	101,289
Frequency std. deviation	35,074.67

Fig. 20 Overview of activity classes in the hospital billing process

A predictive model of the hospital billing process with 100% paths and 100% activities are given in Fig. 21, the control flow model resembles a spaghetti structure and cumbersome. It cannot be comprehended, neither used for any sort of analysis. Further, it is predictively simplified by decreasing the number of activities and paths in it. For predictively generating the simple control flow models, the activities and paths

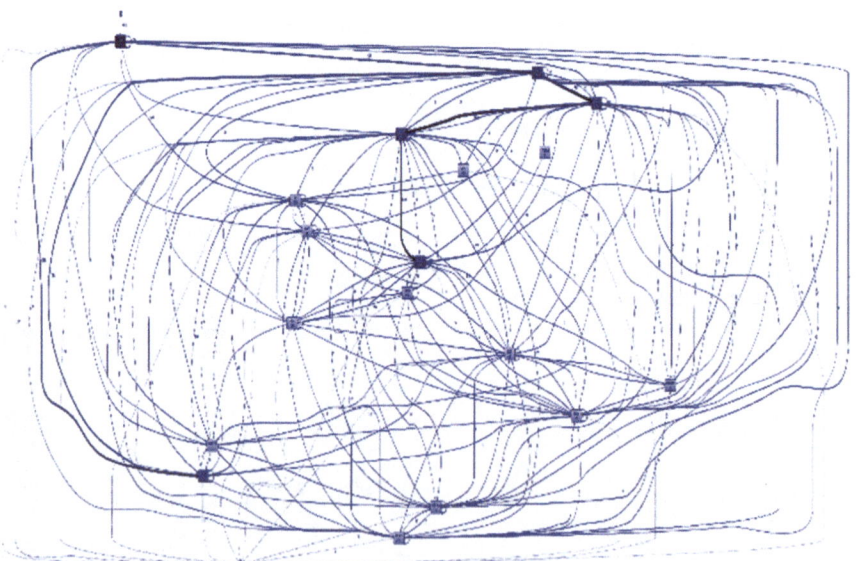

Fig. 21 100% activity and 100% Paths in the process[1]

---

[1]Fuzzy net is used to construct the process mode.

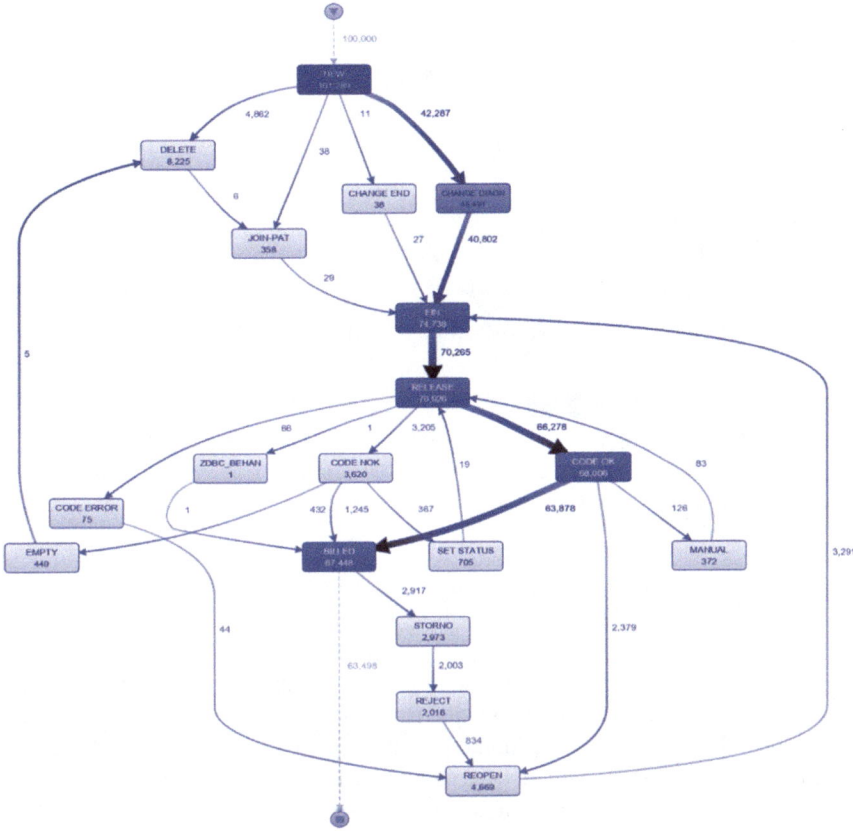

Fig. 22 100% activity with significant paths

are filtered out at some threshold value decided by the domain expert. A simplified control flow model of the hospital billing process is shown in Fig. 22. This model considers all the 18 activities and most significant paths out of several insignificant ones. The model is much cleaner and simple compared to the one given in Fig. 21, which considers all activities and paths in the process. The predictive model shown in the figure can be easily comprehended and can guide to identify the discrepancies in planned and executed processes.

Another predictive model of the hospital billing process which considers all significant activities (out of 18) and all paths is shown in Fig. 23. The much-simplified predictive version of the control flow of the hospital billing process is shown in Fig. 24. This control flow model considers both significant activities and paths. All path activities in the process which are insignificant are ommitted, the rest of the activities/paths which are significant are considered. Predictive control flow model given in Fig. 24 is the simplest control flow model that one can produce, and it could be used to guide the information system process.

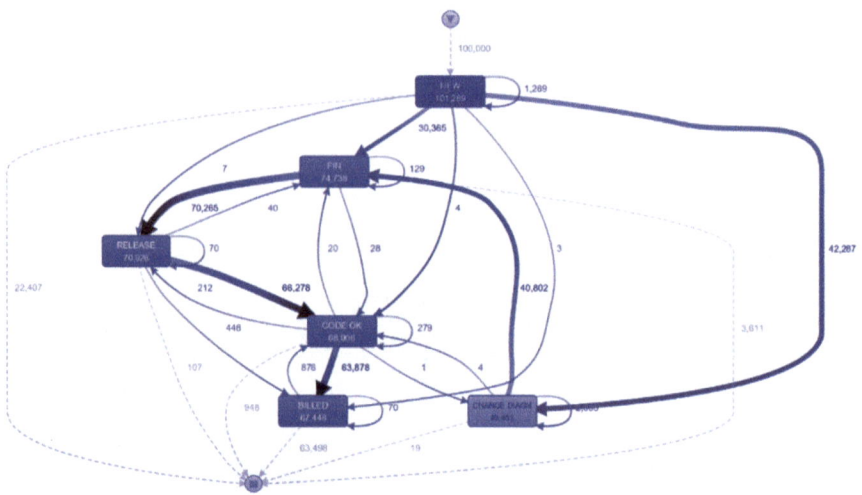

Fig. 23 Significant activities and 100% paths

9.2 Hospital Treatment Process

This section briefs the predictive modelling of the hospital treatment process—the event log of the process has been obtained from 4TU center for research data [11]—link for download is given in the footnote section. Figure 25 shows some of the most significant activities and the relative frequencies, due to the sheer number of activities in the process, we have only considered the activities which have been executed 1% of the total number of total activity executions.

The event log information has been given in Figs. 26 and 27. The hospital treatment process comprises 1.5 Lakh+ events over 625 activities making 1143 distinct cases. When compared to the hospital billing process, which had 18 activities, 625 activities signify a large process. The predictive control flow model of the hospital process is given in Fig. 28. It uses 100% of all activities and paths in the event log. The generated model is not comprehensive, and it cannot be used to guide the future execution of the same process—due to its spaghettiness. A much simpler version of the process could be produced by chopping out the insignificant activities and paths from the event log. The same threshold criteria are used here to predictively generate the simplified control flow models from the original control flow model. As usual, the threshold limit is set by domain experts.

The simplified predictive model considering all activities and significant paths are given in Fig. 29. Figure 30 shows the predictive control flow model constructed by considering only significant activities and all paths.

A much simplified predictive model of the hospital process is shown in Fig. 31. It considers both significant activities and paths. All insignificant paths and activities are removed while constructing the predictive control flow model.

Fig. 24 Significant activities
and paths

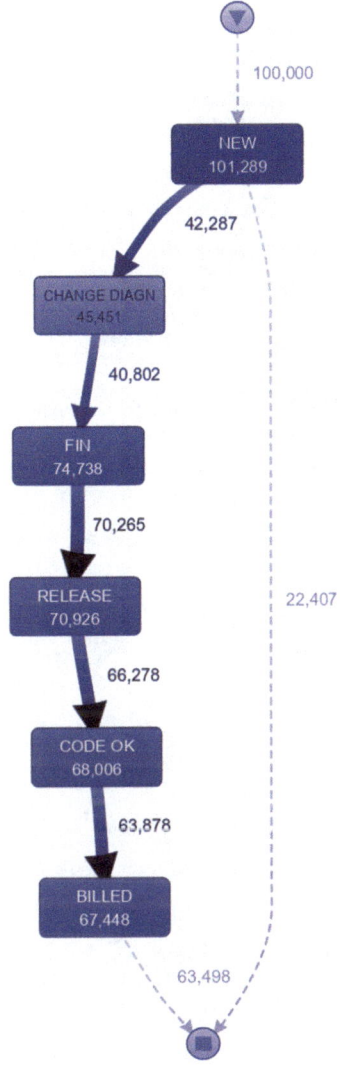

10 Open Challenges and Future Research Directions in Healthcare Data Visualization

This chapter presented a sincere attempt to illustrate the uses of exploratory data analysis and process mining for meaningfully visualizing and analyzing the healthcare data. There are several perspectives from which the visualization of the healthcare data can still be improved, for this, there are numerous challenges to be addressed. Following are a few of the challenges that can be considered for further exploration.

Activity	Frequency	Relative frequency
aanname laboratoriumonderzoek	15,353	10.22 %
ligdagen - alle spec.beh.kinderg.-reval.	10,897	7.25 %
190205 klasse 3b a205	9,351	6.22 %
ordertarief	9,008	5.99 %
190101 bovenreg.toesl. a101	6,241	4.15 %
vervolgconsult poliklinisch	5,239	3.49 %
kalium potentiometrisch	4,328	2.88 %
natrium vlamfotometrisch	4,304	2.86 %
hemoglobine foto-elektrisch	4,275	2.84 %
creatinine	3,955	2.63 %
leukocyten tellen elektronisch	2,968	1.97 %
trombocyten tellen - elektronisch	2,724	1.81 %
differentiele telling automatisch	2,370	1.58 %
administratief tarief - eerste pol	2,171	1.44 %
190021 klinische opname a002	2,118	1.41 %
calcium	2,042	1.36 %
glucose	1,950	1.3 %
kruisproef volledig -drie methoden-	1,705	1.13 %
haemoglobine foto-electrisch - spoed	1,676	1.12 %

Fig. 25 Significant activities in the process that forms the control-flow perspective

Fig. 26 Overview of the hospital treatment process

Events	150,291
Cases	1,143
Activities	624
Median case duration	47.6 wks
Mean case duration	12.7 mths
Start	03.01.2005 04:30:00
End	20.03.2008 04:30:00

Fig. 27 Overview of activity classes in the hospital process

Activities	624
Minimal frequency	1
Median frequency	4
Mean frequency	240.85
Maximal frequency	15,353
Frequency std. deviation	1,074.53

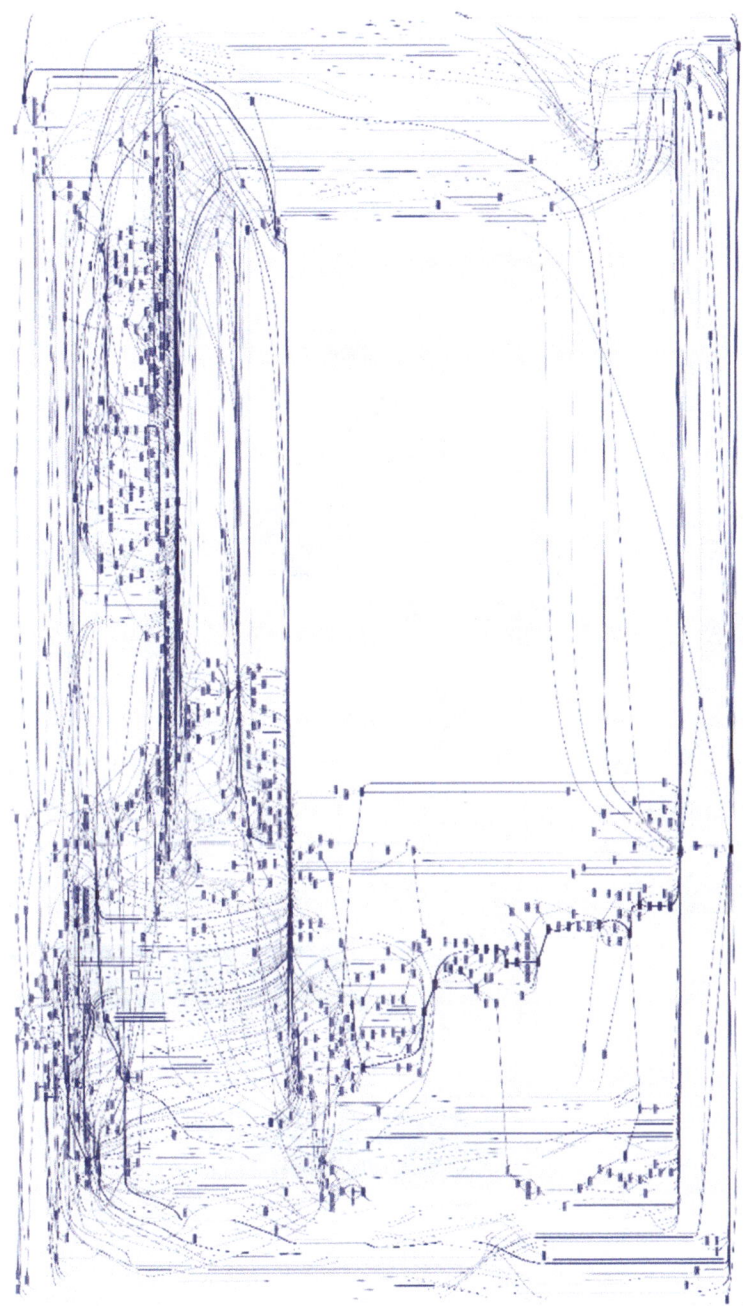

Fig. 28 100% activity and 100% paths

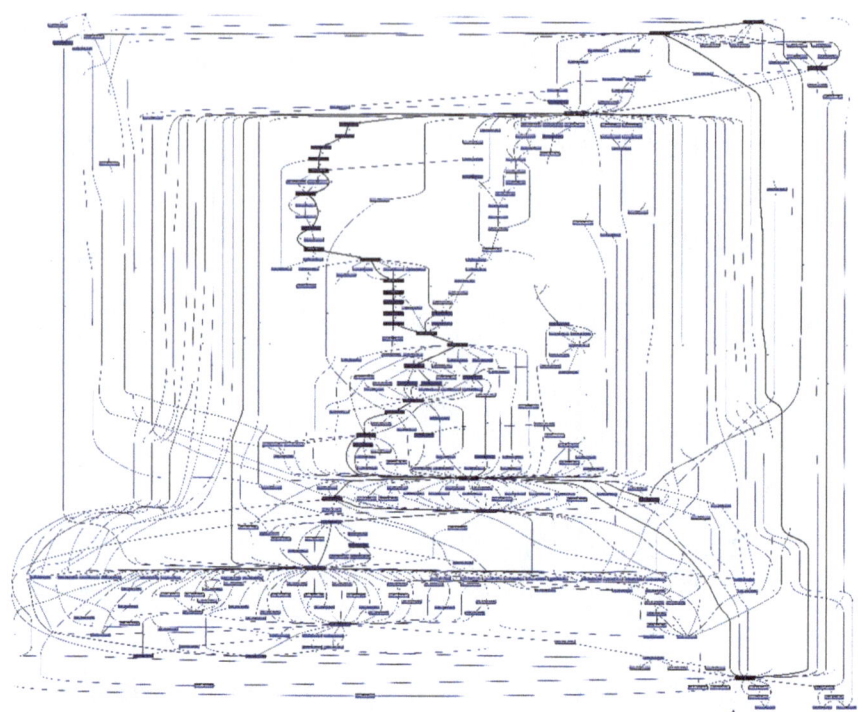

Fig. 29 100% activity with significant paths

Fig. 30 Significant activities 100% paths

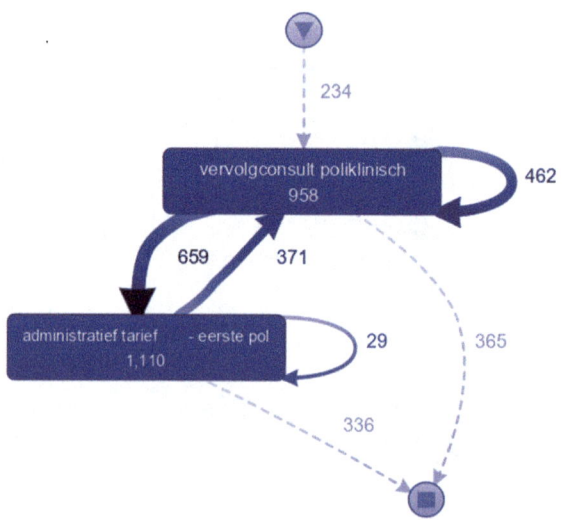

Fig. 31 Significant activity
and paths

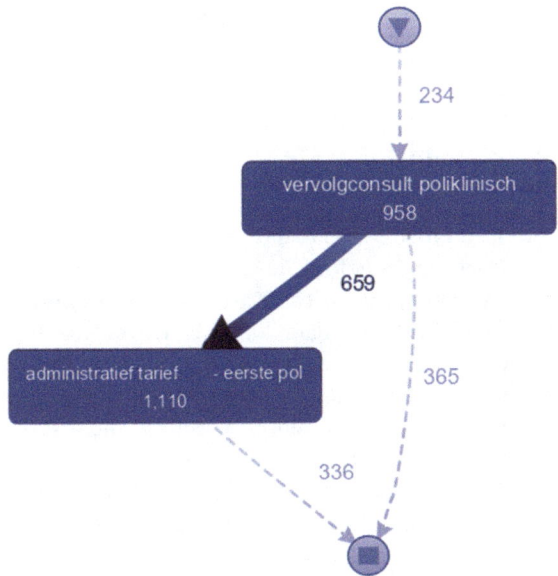

- **Collating the information from multiple sources**—Health care consisting of various parallel operating departments. Real-time collation of data and extracting the information and visualizing it is a challenge to be explored.
- **Concept drift**—Healthcare data tend to change depending on ever-changing disease parameters. Over the period, the model constructed based on the historical data becomes obsolete. It is required to update the constructed model to illustrate the contemporary healthcare process. The process of ever-evolving systems is termed concept drift. It is an inherent problem in any research discipline which deals with data. Concept drift in healthcare data is a promising research direction that requires further exploration.
- **Real time recommendations**—The very essence of visualization in health care is making informed decisions at various levels of the system. It is utmost necessary to derive real-time recommendations through visualizing healthcare data. The recommendation in healthcare based on data visualization is an area that is not explored to the detail it demands. Through further investigations, it may yield a promising result
- **Collaboration**—It is highly necessary to combine the patient data from multiple organizations, to arrive at a visualization that can be specifically used for reasoning and decision-making.
- **Pattern recognition and Pattern Matching**—Healthcare visualization is an easy aid for pattern recognition and matching. Depending on the problem context and domain it is necessary to develop a system that can cater to visualize data that highlights patterns in data.

The list presented here is a minuscule of opportunities to be further explored, healthcare data visualization is a promising field to explore further.

11 Conclusion

Currently, Process-Aware Information Systems [30] which are supporting healthcare operations are generating huge amounts of data. It is required to extract meaningful insights from this data. There are several ways in which tabular data can be summarized. Visualization of data is an effective method that can summarize the entire data, provides insights, helps to make reasoned/informed decisions, helps to understand the key parameters, etc. This chapter presented an attempt to summarize the healthcare data from two different perspectives, the first sections of the chapter discussed how exploratory data analysis can be applied to extract the key parameters of the healthcare dataset. It has also presented an approach for summarizing the entire dataset. The second part of the chapter entirely concentrates on extracting the meaningful control flow models from the event logs recorded in information systems. Process discovery techniques from process mining are used to extract the control flow models. The chapter also presents various process modeling notations. Control flow models extracted from the real-life event logs recorded in hospital information systems are presented.

References

1. Adriansyah, A., van Dongen, B.F., van der Aalst, W.M.: Towards robust conformance checking. In: International Conference on Business Process Management, pp. 122–133. Springer, Berlin, Heidelberg (2010)
2. Mani Sekhar, S.R., Siddesh, G.M., Kumar, S., Manvi, S.: Introduction to bioinformatics. In: Statistical Modelling and Machine Learning Principles for Bioinformatics Techniques, Tools, and Applications. Algorithms for Intelligent Systems book series (AIS). Springer (2020). https://doi.org/10.1007/978-981-15-2445-5_1
3. Four Fundamental Properties of HealthCare Data. (n.d.): Retrieved July 17, 2020, from https://www.linkedin.com/pulse/four-fundamental-properties-health-care-data-dimitrios-zikos
4. Reichert, M., Weber, B.: Enabling flexibility in process-aware information systems: challenges, methods, technologies. Springer Science & Business Media (2012)
5. Xia, J.: Automatic determination of graph simplification parameter values for fuzzy miner. Eindhoven University of Technology, Netherlands (2010)
6. Van Der Aalst, W., Adriansyah, A., Van Dongen, B.: Causal nets: a modelling language tailored towards process discovery. In: International Conference on Concurrency Theory, pp. 28–42. Springer, Berlin, Heidelberg (2011)
7. Mans, R.S., Schonenberg, M.H., Song, M., van der Aalst, W.M., Bakker, P.J.: Application of process mining in healthcare–a case study in a Dutch hospital. In: International Joint Conference on Biomedical Engineering Systems and Technologies, pp. 425–438. Springer, Berlin, Heidelberg (2008)
8. Mans, R.S., Van der Aalst, W.M., Vanwersch, R.J.: Process Mining in Healthcare: Evaluating and Exploiting Operational Healthcare Processes, pp. 17–26. Springer, Cham (2015)

9. Van Der Aalst, W.M., Reijers, H.A., Weijters, A.J., van Dongen, B.F., De Medeiros, A.A., Song, M., Verbeek, H.M.W.: Business process mining: An industrial application. Inf. Syst. **32**(5), 713–732 (2007)

10. Rojas, E., Munoz-Gama, J., Sepúlveda, M., Capurro, D.: Process mining in healthcare: a literature review. J. Biomed. Inform. **61**, 224–236 (2016)

11. Zhao, W., Zhao, X.: Process mining from the organizational perspective. In: Foundations of Intelligent Systems, pp. 701–708. Springer, Berlin, Heidelberg (2014)

12. Mans, R.S., van der Aalst, W.M., Vanwersch, R.J., Moleman, A.J.: Process mining in healthcare: data challenges when answering frequently posed questions. In: Process Support and Knowledge Representation in Health Care, pp. 140–153. Springer, Berlin, Heidelberg (2012)

13. Sarshar, K., Loos, P.: Comparing the control-flow of epc and petri net from the end-user perspective. In: International Conference on Business Process Management, pp. 434–439. Springer, Berlin, Heidelberg (2005)

14. Günther, C.W., Van Der Aalst, W.M.: Fuzzy mining–adaptive process simplification based on multi-perspective metrics. In: International Conference on Business Process Management, pp. 328–343. Springer, Berlin, Heidelberg (2007)

15. Gupta, S.: Workflow and process mining in healthcare. Master's thesis, Technische Universiteit Eindhoven (2007)

16. Weijters, A.J.M.M., van Der Aalst, W.M., De Medeiros, A.A.: Process mining with the heuristic miner-algorithm. Technische Universiteit Eindhoven, Tech. Rep. WP **166**, 1–34 (2006)

17. De Medeiros, A.A., Van Dongen, B.F., Van der Aalst, W.M., Weijters, A.J.M.M.: Process mining: Extending the α-algorithm to mine short loops (2004)

18. Valmari, A.: The state explosion problem. In: Advanced Course on Petri Nets (1996)

19. Van Der Aalst, W.M., Ter Hofstede, A.H.: YAWL: yet another workflow language. Inf. Syst. **30**(4), 245–275 (2005)

20. Van der Aalst, W., Weijters, T., Maruster, L.: Workflow mining: discovering process models from event logs. IEEE Trans. Knowl. Data Eng. **16**(9), 1128–1142 (2004)

21. Delft, T.: 4TU. Center of Research Data (2010)

22. Van Eck, M.L., Lu, X., Leemans, S.J., van der Aalst, W.M.: A process mining project methodology. In: International Conference on Advanced Information Systems Engineering, pp. 297–313. Springer, Cham (2015)

23. Van der Aalst, W.M.: The application of Petri nets to workflow management. J. Circ. Syst. Comput. **8**(01), 21–66 (1998)

24. Weijters, A.J., Van der Aalst, W.M.: Rediscovering workflow models from event-based data using the little thumb. Integ. Comput.-Aided Eng. **10**(2), 151–162 (2003)

25. Lawrence, P., Bouzeghoub, M., Fabret, F., Matulovic-broqué, M.: Workflow handbook. In: Proceedings of International Workshop on Design and Management of Data Warehouses (DMDW'99) (1997)

26. White, S.A.: Introduction to BPMN. IBM Coop.**2**(0), 0 (2004)

27. Scheer, A.W., Thomas, O., Adam, O.: Process modeling using event-driven process chains. In: Process-Aware Information Systems, p. 119 (2005)

28. Rebuge, Á., Ferreira, D.R.: Business process analysis in healthcare environments: a methodology based on process mining. Inf. Syst. **37**(2), 99–116 (2012)

29. Jansen-Vullers, M.H., van der Aalst, W.M., Rosemann, M.: Mining configurable enterprise information systems. Data Knowl. Eng. **56**(3), 195–244 (2006)

30. Dumas, M., Van der Aalst, W.M., Ter Hofstede, A.H.: Process-aware information systems: bridging people and software through process technology. Wiley (2005)

31. Belle, A., Thiagarajan, R., Soroushmehr, S.M., Navidi, F., Beard, D.A., Najarian, K.: Big data analytics in healthcare. BioMed Res. Int. (2015)

Data Science Tools and Techniques for Healthcare Applications

Srinidhi Hiriyannaiah, Siddesh G. M., Divya, R. Aravind Shreyas, Dheeraj Bhat, V. Gaurav, Kushagra Mishra, and K. G. Srinivasa

Abstract Data analytics in healthcare applications play an important role as it gives insights into various aspects. In the present digital world, many gadgets are used for health monitoring. The data from these devices need to be collected in a careful manner as the privacy of the data also needs to be ensured. Machine learning methods such as clustering, random forests can be used for the analysis of various healthcare records. The patterns and trends in data become much more useful to predict and analyze data specifically in the sphere of healthcare. The aim of this chapter is to provide the different data science-oriented tools and methods for healthcare analytics. A case study on the usage of different tools and techniques is also presented at the end of the chapter that provides the complete life-cycle of the analytics phase for healthcare applications.

S. Hiriyannaiah (✉) · S. G. M. · Divya · R. Aravind Shreyas · D. Bhat · V. Gaurav
Ramaiah Institute of Technology, Bengaluru, India
e-mail: srinidhi.hiriyannaiah@gmail.com

S. G. M.
e-mail: siddeshgm@gmail.com

Divya
e-mail: divyasanjeevni@gmail.com

R. Aravind Shreyas
e-mail: aravindshreyasramesh@gmail.com

D. Bhat
e-mail: bhatdheeraj19@gmail.com

V. Gaurav
e-mail: gaurav.vinay2020@gmail.com

K. Mishra
Member of Technical Staff at Nutanix, San Jose, USA
e-mail: kmishra@ncsu.edu

K. G. Srinivasa
National Institute of Technical Teachers Training & Research, Chandigarh, India
e-mail: kgsrinivasa@gmail.com

K. G. Srinivasa et al. (eds.), *Artificial Intelligence for Information Management: A Healthcare Perspective*, Studies in Big Data 88,
https://doi.org/10.1007/978-981-16-0415-7_10

1 Introduction

The steep rise in dependency on technology in healthcare is, in turn, driving the need to be able to both, obtain data, and use the data generated in a systematic manner. This paves the way for Data Analytics and Data Engineering to come into play. Statistics show that skin cancer affects one in every five Americans by the age of 70 [1]. Today, there exists a possibility of being able to detect certain types of skin cancers with just a mobile application, with a relatively high degree of accuracy [2].

It is also possible for surgeons to perform surgeries that were previously almost impossible, thanks to great strides in image processing and computer vision (both of which require data to function and show results) [3]. These are just a few in a plethora of examples. It does not end with just diagnoses of diseases. In a fitness conscious world of smartwatches today that gives the user an idea of step count, heart rate, calories burnt and so on and so forth, abstracted behind the scenes, is a mammoth collection of data which is being structured, clustered and analyzed by an algorithm before it appears as a neat integer on your device.

Data Science also plays a key role in being able to monitor and manage a world being plagued by a virus [4]. When you have millions of people being affected, data can be key in monitoring and identifying persons of interest and will go a long way in reducing the strain on the healthcare system and in curbing the virus.

Where there is technology, there exists data. Now that we understand technology is more or less an integral component of a given healthcare system, it follows that knowing to structure and utilize this data is of utmost importance. As you proceed through the chapter, you will have a clear understanding of the tools and software used to study data and different techniques used to be able to make sense of large collections of data. With real-world examples, you will be guided through applications of Data Science in healthcare.

2 Machine Learning Techniques for Healthcare Applications

2.1 Clustering

Clustering is an *unsupervised* Machine Learning routine in which a given set of data is "clustered" or grouped into subsets in which any element in a given subset shares some common characteristic with other elements in the subset [5]. In Layman's terms, the process by which a huge chunk of data is segregated into groups of data according to some property/properties is termed as clustering.

According to the most popular classification, there exist two types of Clustering, namely:

i. **Hard Clustering**: It is a type of Clustering in which a given data point is assigned one definite cluster.
ii. **Soft Clustering**: It is a type of Clustering in which any given data point is assigned a probability of being in every cluster.

Another popular classification of Clustering is as follows:

i. **Partitional Clustering**: Clustering occurs in such a way that the dataset is considered as a set which is to be clustered into subsets in which each element of a given cluster is similar to each other, different from elements in other clusters
ii. **Hierarchical Clustering**: Clustering occurs in a nested manner, that appear to be in the form of trees
iii. **Density-based Clustering**: Clustering occurs in areas of the graph where there exist a high density of data points.

2.1.1 Example of Usage of Clustering

The Dataset considered is a public dataset that comprises thirteen key parameters that are used to determine the heart health of individuals. These factors are a group of numerical and categorical data collected from different types of patients. Among these, there are five numerical parameters, which are age, resting blood pressure, cholesterol level, ST depression induced by exercise relative to rest, slope of the peak exercise ST segment, maximum heart rate achieved. Each individual is mapped to a value called target, which is an integer that ranges from 0 to 4 that indicates the chance of having a heart disease, 0 being the least and 4 being the most [6].

First, we import the necessary libraries. These include *numpy, seaborn, pandas* and *sklearn*. Then, we read our file that consists of the public data set. Python implementation for reading from a CSV file and storing the data in a *pandas' DataFrame* object is as follows:

```
df = pd.read_csv(path)
```

In order to visualize the dataset in a way that is relatively easy to analyze and to perform K-means clustering, it is highly recommended to choose numerical data rather than categorical data. In this example, we have selectively chosen numerical data from the dataset and dropped all the categorical factors from the *DataFrame df*.

Since all the five numerical factors have to be considered in order to get accurate results and owing to our inability to understand a 5-dimensional graph, we need to reduce the dimensionality of the data set to either 2D or 3D. For this, there exists a class called *PCA* in the *sklearn.decomposition* module that does all the math for the user and converts the data into a dimensionality of the user's choice. The code to combine all factors so that our data can easily be plotted on a graph is as follows:

```
pca = PCA(n_components = 2)
cols = df.columns
df['x'] = pca.fit_transform(df[cols[:6]])[:,0]
df['y'] = pca.fit_transform(df[cols[:6]])[:, 1]
data = df[['x', 'y']]
```

Here "*n_components* = 2" indicates that we desire a two-dimensional graph. Now we organize our data into clusters after combining all the factors and plot it out. To apply the K-Means algorithm, we have imported called *KMeans* from the *sklearn* library to perform the clustering for us.

```
clusters= KMeans(n_clusters= 6)
df["clusters"]=clusters.fit_predict(df[df.columns[7:9]])
seaborn.lmplot(x='x', y='y', hue='clusters', fit_reg=
False, data= df)
```

The above code snippet produces the output as shown in Fig. 1.

In Fig. 1, observe that there exists 6 clusters in this particular example. One can pick the number of clusters according to the dataset and desired results. In this example, 6 clusters are chosen as results can be analyzed relatively easily.

NOTE: In the above graph, the x and y axis do not point to one single quantity each, rather, they represent a combination of factors.

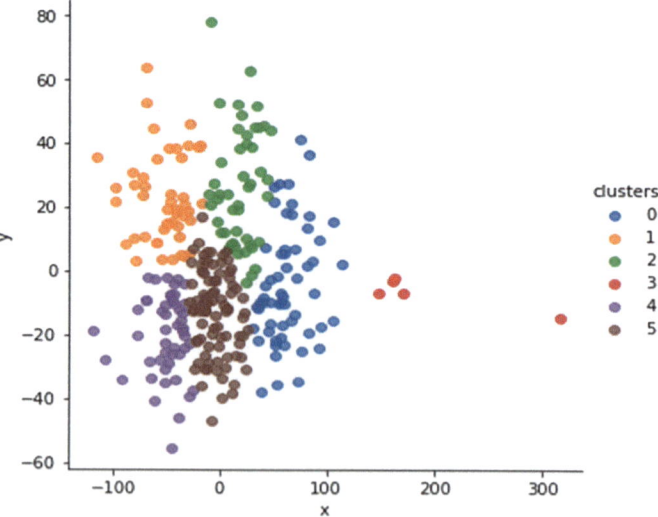

Fig. 1 K-means clustering for heart disease dataset

On analysis of clusters, it was found that the values from cluster 4 had the least average of target values, then came cluster 5, 0, 3, 2, and 1, respectively. We can observe that higher the centre of the cluster, higher the chance of having heart disease.

2.2 Decision Trees

Decision Tree is a supervised ML technique which involves a tree in which the parent node represents a statement, the branches represent a conditional operation on that statement (ex: True/False) and the child nodes represent the outcome. It is a useful method to represent an algorithm that comprises of many conditionals.

Each node usually contains a value called "Gini Value" or the "Gini Index" which represents the impurity of an outcome. The node with the lowest Gini value (highest accuracy) is chosen as the root node. Calculation of Gini value for a node in a yes/no decision tree is as follows:

$$\text{Gini Value} = 1 - \left[P(\text{yes})\right]^2 - [P(\text{no})]^2, \text{ where P(x) represents probability of x.} \tag{1}$$

There are many other quantities, however, that represent the impurity or accuracy of an outcome that can be used in Decision Trees. Entropy is one such popularly used quantity.

Let us understand this concept with a real-life example.

2.2.1 Example of Usage of Decision Trees

The dataset considered for this example is a public dataset that contains key factors that determine if a woman is prone to diabetes or not [7]. We will call it as the Diabetes Dataset. In this example, the main factors take in the number of pregnancies the patient has experienced, their glucose level, blood pressure, skin thickness, insulin levels, their diabetes pedigree function and age.

The libraries that are required for decision trees include *pandas, sklearn, matplotlib* and *pydotplus*. From *sklearn*, we import *DecisionTreeClassifier*. Again, the first step is to read the file. Then, we input the factors (columns) as one variable and we partition the data into testing and training data. Python implementation for the same is as follows:

```
diabetes_dataset = pd.read_csv(path)
Xdata = ['Pregnancies', 'Glucose', 'BloodPressure',
'SkinThickness', 'Insulin', 'DiabetesPedigreeFunction',
'Age']
X = diabetes_dataset[Xdata]
Y = diabetes_dataset['Outcome']
X_train, X_test, Y_train, Y_test = train_test_split(X,
Y, test_size = 0.15)
```

Now, by means of *DecisionTreeClassifier* class, we create a decision tree of desired height with the following code:

```
decisionTree= DecisionTreeClassifier(criterion=
"gini",max_depth= 3)
decisionTree= decisionTree.fit(X_train, Y_train)
```

Note that *criterion* = " *gini*" indicates that we are using *gini* indices as a base reference for our decision tree and *max_depth* = *3*indicates that the desired result is a decision tree of height. After this, we output the resultant decision tree using the code that follows:

```
data= tree.export_graphviz(dtree, filled= True,
out_file= None, feature_names= Xdata, rounded= True)
graph = pydotplus.graph_from_dot_data(data)
graph.write_png('mydecisiontree.png')
img= pltimg.imread('mydecisiontree.png')
imgplot = plt.imshow(img,cmap="rainbow")
plt.show()
```

The above code produces the output as shown in Fig. 2.

Looking at the tree as shown in Fig. 2, we can infer that the most important factor initially for a person to be diagnosed with diabetes would be higher glucose levels in your blood. As you move down the tree, we observe that other lesser important factors also weigh in being diagnosed with diabetes. In the tree, blue nodes would represent a higher probability of being diagnosed with diabetes and the brown ones would mean that you would be less susceptible to be diagnosed with diabetes.

2.3 Random Forests

Random forests are a collective learning approach for regression, classification, and other machine learnable tasks that work by creating various decisions at the training

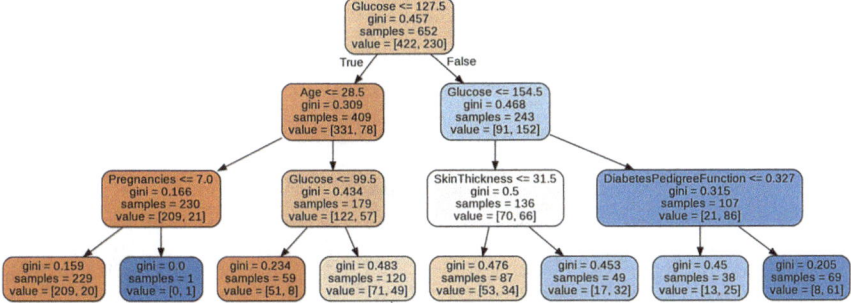

Fig. 2 Decision tree obtained in the analysis of the diabetes dataset

stage and return the class which is the mode of all classes predicted in case of a classification task or mean prediction of the individual trees in case of a regression task [8].

While predicting for testing data set, a Random Forest gets prediction results from every possible decision tree and voting is performed on the results based on the prediction from each decision tree, the output value is the most voted prediction. Random forests provide a more efficient result by not overfitting even a large dataset making it more accurate than decision trees.

2.3.1   Example of Usage of Random Forests

We consider the same dataset we used for Decision trees that is the Diabetes Dataset for this example too. The libraries required to be imported for decision trees include *pandas, sklearn, matplotlib* and *pydotplus*. From *sklearn.ensemble*, we import *RandomForestClassifier*.

Again, the initial steps are to read the file, assign the list of factors to a variable for later use, and split the data into testing and training data (in the ratio 1:9) as done in Sect. 2.2.1.

Now, using the *RandomForestClassifier* class, we create a random forest with each tree of desired height.

```
randomForest = RandomForestClassifier(n_estimators=500,
bootstrap= True,max_depth=3)
   randomForest.fit(X_train, Y_train)
```

Now we output the resultant decision tree using the code that follows:

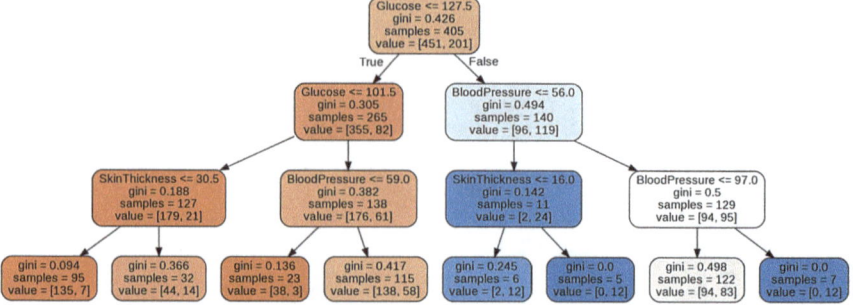

Fig. 3 Random forest obtained in the analysis of the diabetes dataset

```
data= tree.export_graphviz(randomForest.estimators_[0],
filled= True ,out_file=None,
feature_names=Xdata,rounded=True)
  graph= pydotplus.graph_from_dot_data(data)
  graph.write_png('rf.png')
  img=pltimg.imread('rf.png')
  imgplot = plt.imshow(img,cmap="rainbow")
  plt.show()
```

The above code produces the output as shown in Fig. 3.

By looking at the tree as shown in Fig. 3, we can infer that glucose was still the most important factor in being diagnosed with diabetes, as we move further down the tree, we see other factors weigh in. The nodes in blue represent a higher probability of being diagnosed with diabetes and the brown nodes a lesser chance.

The important difference to notice would be that a single decision tree gives an accuracy of 74.13% while random forests give an accuracy of 85.34% on the same training and testing data as demonstrated in the code below:

```
accuracy_dtree = decisionTree.score(X_test, Y_test)
accuracy_rf = randomForest.score(X_test, Y_test)
print("Accuracy of Decision Tree = ", accuracy_dtree,
"\n Accuracy of Random Forest = ", accuracy_rf)
```

The above code gives the output as shown below:

```
Accuracy of Decision Tree = 0.7413793103448276
Accuracy of Random Forest = 0.853448275862069
```

3 Cloud-Based Tools

3.1 Microsoft Azure

Microsoft Azure is a cloud-based computing package conceived by the engineers and researchers of Microsoft for creating, testing, deploying and managing applications and services. It provides support for all modern cloud computing paradigms like infrastructure as a service (IaaS), platform as a service (PaaS) and software as a service (SaaS), and provides many different programming languages, tools and frameworks [9].

Azure is a rich feature-packed cloud-based software solution with wide ranging use cases and applications, but w e shall dive deep into one of its services which aids as a data science and machine learning tool, Azure Notebooks—A playground for analytics and machine learning.

3.1.1 Azure Notebooks

Getting to grips with machine learning and data science can be tricky. It is hard to visualize data at scale, and harder still to understand how analytics can drive machine learning. This is where Microsoft Azure Notebooks come in. As the company states it, Azure Notebooks is a free service enabling anyone and everyone to develop and run code on their web browser using Jupyter formerly known as IPython.

A Jupyter Notebook is an open-source web application that enables you to develop and share documents which consist of live code, equations, graphical visualizations and text. It is extensively used for data cleaning and transformation of datasets, complex numerical simulation, statistical modelling, data visualization using various informative graphs and machine learning tasks.

3.1.2 Support and Pricing

Azure Notebooks currently has support for Python 2, Python 3, F#, R and their widespread packages. All your code and data is persisted. The only requirement is a modern web browser with a good internet connection. This means you can just login with your Microsoft account and get going since no installation/setup is necessary.

Azure Notebook is a free service, but there is a limitation. Each project is limited to 1 GB data and 4 GB memory. Users who require a bit more muscle can go through a verification process and enhance their service.

3.1.3 Key Features and Use Cases

Azure Notebooks assist you to get going quickly on prototyping, data science, academic research, or gain knowledge of Python. Because it allows for flexible coding, execution and has robust sharing capabilities, it can be used for numerous varied scenarios.

- **Access your Code from Anywhere**: There is no need to carry a USB stick or download your code from an online storage service. Azure Notebooks allow you to keep all your projects online securely. It also provides seamless integration with version control softwares like GitHub.
- **Easily Share Code**: Azure Notebooks is a great way to share code and collaborate with other people. Each project has a unique link which will allow others to view your code or clone it into their own copy of your project, and start playing and editing notebooks online.
- **Run the Code on Different Compute**: Azure Notebooks allow you to work with small and large data sets dynamically and help you run your code optimally. You can start off with the free compute option to work with smaller data sets and when more data needs to be crunched you can then switch to a powerful virtual machine. Azure will ensure that the same project environment is mounted to the target virtual machine and used there seamlessly with no data loss.

3.1.4 Drawbacks

While Azure Notebooks is a great tool, there are few disadvantages. A few of them are as follows:

- Limited network access
- Can access data only from verified sources like Azure resources, GitHub, Kaggle, OneDrive and a few more
- GPU Access is not included in Free Compute options for Azure Notebooks at this point of time.

3.1.5 Azure as a Data Science Tool for Healthcare

Azure provides plenty of tools which helps in elevating healthcare through enterprise level scalable services and analytics backed by AI, ML and APIs. Few well known tools are Synapse, Healthcare Assistant and Azure API for FHIR.

3.1.6 Azure Data Science Virtual Machines and Tools

Azure Data Science Virtual Machines (DSVMs) contain a variety of tools and libraries for ML and are available in many widely used languages like R, Python and Julia [10].

Few machine learning tools and libraries are as follows:

- **Azure Machine Learning SDK for Python**: It is a cloud-based service which can be used to develop and deploy ML models.
- **H20**: It is an open-source AI platform that promotes in-memory, distributed, fast and scalable machine learning.
- **LightGBM**: It is a high-performance gradient-boosting framework based on decision tree algorithms. It is extensively used for classification, ranking and several other ML tasks.
- **Vowpal Wabbit**: It is an open-source, out-of-core learning system library which is extremely fast.

Few other relevant tools and libraries are Weka, XGBoost, Apache Drill.

3.2 Google Colab

Colaboratory is a Google research project developed to support the propagation of ML education and research [11]. It is a Jupyter notebook environment that does not require any setup as it completely runs on the cloud. It is a free notebook environment with dynamic collaboration capabilities. Colab supports several prevalent machine learning libraries which can be imported into the notebooks effortlessly. Google Colab is Jupyter Notebook + Cloud + Google Drive. Introduction of Google Colab has simplified the understanding and development of robust and durable ML applications.

3.2.1 Support and Pricing

Google Colab currently supports Python 3.6, but not R or Scala yet. Much like Azure notebooks, the only requirement for working on Colab is a modern web browser with a good internet connection.

Google Colab is a completely free service but there is a limit to your size and sessions. Customers who want more reliable access and enhanced resources may be attracted to use Colab Pro, a subscription-based version with added benefits of faster GPUs, extra memory and extended uninterrupted sessions.

3.2.2 What Is the Difference Between Colab and Jupyter?

Jupyter is an open-source project on which Colab is established. Colab lets you use and share Jupyter notebooks with others without any hassle of downloading, installing, or running anything.

3.2.3 Key Features

The best feature that differentiates Colab from other free cloud services is that Colab offers GPU and is entirely free. You can perform the following operations on Google Colab.

- One can create, upload and share notebooks in a hassle free manner
- Notebooks can be saved on Google Drive and Github.
- Notebooks can be imported from Google Drive and Github.
- External datasets can be imported from websites such as Kaggle.
- One can write and execute code in Python.
- Libraries such as PyTorch, TensorFlow, Keras, OpenCV can be imported easily.

3.2.4 GPU? What Does that Do?

A graphics processing unit (GPU) is a computer component that is designed to rapidly generate images or data in a frame buffer. Let us draw a comparison. Architecturally, the CPU comprises of small number of cores with plenty of cache memory that can store a small number of software threads at any instance of time. In comparison, a GPU consists of a high number of cores (un hundreds) that can carry a large number of threads simultaneously. It basically means a GPU can perform high intensity tasks at an extremely fast rate. GPUs perform much more work for every unit of energy than CPUs which renders them more powerful and efficient.

Purchasing a good GPU for data science and machine learning is often very costly and this is where Colab helps us. The GPUs that are available in Colab are usually the Nvidia K80s, T4s, P4s and P100s. Colab lets us use one of these GPUs for free and lets the user focus on the important things while it takes care of the cost, compute and maintenance.

3.2.5 Drawbacks

While Google Colab provides many amazing features, there are few disadvantages:

- All Colab notebooks must be stored in Google Drive
- Long-running background computations may be stopped—session based
- Certain libraries which are not preinstalled with python by default have to be installed during every single session.
- Google Drive Storage is used with the developer's current session, hence if the developer has downloaded a file to use later, the developer would be required to save it before quitting the session.
- Problems could arise when working with large datasets as the dataset has to be uploaded to Google drive which has a storage cap of 15 GB on its free tier.

3.3 NVIDIA RAPIDS

RAPIDS is a set of software libraries that allows data scientists to run end-to-end data science and analytics pipelines completely on the GPUs. It makes use of NVIDIA's own API, CUDA(Compute Unified Device Architecture), to expose parallelism on GPU and high-bandwidth memory speed through Python interfaces which are very user friendly [12].

It is a useful tool to perform tasks in analytics and data science and has the DataFrame API which enables various machine learning algorithms to run at ease. Another building block that forms the foundation of RAPIDS along with the DataFrame API and its ML libraries is Graph Analytics Libraries or "cuGRAPH" which is simply a set of graph analytics libraries just like matplotlib or seaborn.

3.3.1 Advantages and Key Features

- **Open Source**: Free to be customized and interoperable. Provides a highly collaborative user experience.
- **Ease of Integration**: Can be integrated with your Python code with minimal changes
- **Low cost in terms of training time**: Low training time, in turn, boasts increased productivity. RAPIDS also has a relatively interactive data science experience.
- **High Accuracy**: Faster iteration and quick deployment of the necessary modules and models.

4 Example of a Healthcare-Care Application Using Azure

4.1 Dataset and Scenario

To show a practical example of data analytics in healthcare, we are going to use a dataset that is the UCI ML Breast Cancer Wisconsin (Diagnostic) datasets [13]. It is a real-valued multivariate data collected in 1995, by Dr. William H. Wolberg, W. Nick Street, Olvi L. Mangasarian. The target of the dataset is one of the two classes of tumor, that signifies if a patient has breast cancer or not. It has the class of tumor and 30 numeric, predictive attributes.

Features of the dataset describe properties of a cell nuclei present in the image of a fine needle aspirate (FNA) of breast mass. These features are area, perimeter, radius, which is the mean of distances from centre to points on the perimeter, texture, which is the standard deviation of grey-scale values, smoothness, which are local variation in radius lengths, symmetry, compactness, which is calculated by using the formula "perimeter^2/area-1.0", fractal dimension, which is "coastline approximation"-1, concavity, which denotes the severity of concave portions of the contour, and concave points, which is the number of concave portions of the contour. Each of the ten attributes is available in three categories which are mean, standard error, and "worst" or largest (mean of the three worst/largest values) [14].

The two classes of the data are WDBC-Malignant, WDBC-Benign. Benign tumors are not harmful and pose no danger towards cancer. Malignant tumors can be life-threatening as they can become cancerous and cause serious problems. The dataset that we are going to use has 212 data points of malignant class and 357 data points of benign class.

4.2 Step-by-Step Analysis of Healthcare Data

The initial steps of data analysis are defining the questions carefully, setting clear measurement priorities according to the questions, followed by the collection of data based on the previously set priorities.

In the dataset being used for this example, the question is clear: Given the 30 attribute values for a new case of breast tumour, which class will the tumour belong to? In other words, if the values for all the features are known for the tumour, will it be classified as a cancerous tumour or a non-cancerous one?

The measurement priorities and collection of data based on the question have already been set by the owners and collectors of the data. Now the next steps include understanding the data and determining the algorithm that will be used for further predictions.

We will load our dataset from *sklearn's* module *datasets.*

```
from sklearn.datasets import load_breast_cancer
breastCancer = load_breast_cancer()
factorsData = breastCancer.data
targetClass = breastCancer.target
```

From the above code, all the values for features are in the variable *factorsData* and the tumour class values for the same is in *targetClass*. On checking the shape of the features, we find it to be (569, 30), meaning there are 30 characteristics (or columns) to the dataset and 569 data points (or rows). On checking the same for classes, we find the shape to be (569,), which means that there is one column representing the target class for each row in the features ndarray. The values of target are of type float, 0.0 for Benign and 1.0 for Malignant. None of the data points or class values have any field as empty (or NaN) so we can assume our dataset to be complete and ready for further analysis.

For further analysis, we want to visualize the data points and see if there is any relationship among those of the same class. Since we have 30 features and we can only visualize on 2D or 3D space, we will again make use of *PCA* as we did in Sect. 2.1.1 to reduce the dimensionality of the data as per our convenience. For this, we need to have one *DataFrame* that will have all the values of the features and the target for each case in a single row. So the next steps include: reshaping *targetClass* into an array of shape (569, 1), concatenating it with the *factorsData* along the vertical axis, followed by storing them in a *DataFrame* with appropriate column labels for further convenient analysis.

```
import numpy
import pandas
targetClassesArray = numpy.reshape(targetClass,(569,1))
completeDatasetArray = numpy.concatenate([factorsData,
targetClassesArray], axis = 1)
breastCancerDataFrame = pandas.DataFrame(
completeDatasetArray, columns = numpy.append(breastCancer
.feature_names, 'class'))
```

From the code snippet, we now have the complete data in a *DataFrame* called *breastCancerDataFrame* of shape (569, 31). After this, we also need to standardize the data. It is a suggested practice to feed in normalized data to any machine learning algorithm to avoid inoperable errors. To apply normalization, we need to import the *StandardScaler* module from the *sklearn* library [15]. When *StandardScaler* is applied, each feature of the data has to be normally distributed to ensure that after normalization, the mean of the new data is close to zero and the standard deviation is close to one. Note that, we must only normalize the 30 features of the *DataFrame* and not the last column, that is the class. Further steps include: normalizing the first 30 columns of the *breastCancerDataFrame*, rename the features to the string denoting feature number, followed by storing it in a *DataFrame*.

```
from sklearn.preprocessing import StandardScaler
factorsValues = breastCancerDataFrame.loc[:, breastCanc
er.feature_names].values
factorsValues = StandardScaler().fit_transform(factorsV
alues)
normalizedFeatureNames = ['Feature '+str(i) for i in ra
nge(factorsValues.shape[1])]
normalisedDataset = pandas.DataFrame(factorsValues,colu
mns=normalizedFeatureNames)
```

After running the above code, we are ready to use *PCA* and reduce the dimensionality to 2D. Further steps are: importing *PCA*, followed by reducing their dimensionality to two principal components [16].

	Principal Component 1	Principal Component 2	Tumour Type
564	6.439315	-3.576817	Benign
565	3.793382	-3.584048	Benign
566	1.256179	-1.902297	Benign
567	10.374794	1.672010	Benign
568	-5.475243	-0.670637	Malignant

Fig. 4 Example rows of the DataFrame

```
from sklearn.decomposition import PCA
pcaObject = PCA(n_components=2)
principalComponents = pcaObject.fit_transform(factorsVa
lues)
principalComponents = numpy.concatenate([principalCompo
nents, targetClassesArray], axis = 1)
principalComponentsDataFrame = pandas.DataFrame(data =
principalComponents, columns = ['Principal Component 1',
'Principal Component 2', 'Tumour Type'])
principalComponentsDataFrame['Tumour Type'].replace(0,
'Benign',inplace=True)
principalComponentsDataFrame['Tumour Type'].replace(1,
'Malignant',inplace=True)
principalComponentsDataFrame.tail()
```

The above code produces the output as shown in Fig. 4.

We can see that the *DataFrame principalComponentsDataFrame* is ready for visualization. Further steps are: plotting the two components against each other on a scatter plot with the hue of class using *seaborn* library.

```
import seaborn as sns
sns.lmplot(x = 'Principal Component 1', y= 'Principal C
omponent 2', hue='Tumour Type', fit_reg=False, data=princ
ipalComponentsDataFrame, height=8)
```

The above code produces the output as shown in Fig. 5.

From the graph in Fig. 5, it can be observed that all the data points belonging to the same class are together in the form of clusters, in our case, benign and malignant. In the situation that there exists another person who's tumour type is to be predicted, the new data point has to belong to one of the two clusters. To classify which cluster it will belong to, one of the optimal approaches can be KNN (K-Nearest Neighbours), especially because our dataset is not relatively large.

KNN is a supervised ML algorithm that can be applied for both classification and regression-based tasks. Imagine a new data point in the above graph between

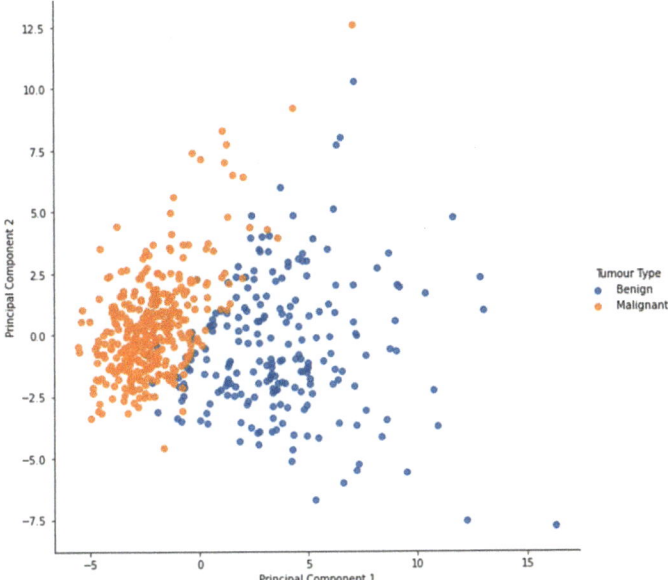

Fig. 5 Visualization of data points belonging to benign and malignant classes of breast cancer dataset

the orange and blue clusters, how will we classify if the new data point belongs to someone who's tumour is benign or malignant? We calculate the distances using a standard measure from a given metric system from the point to 'k' number of nearest neighbours around the new data point and determine which cluster the data point should be a part of. The data point is assigned to the cluster in which the maximum number of its k neighbours belong to. A classic example of classification.

To apply KNN, we make use of *sklearn's KNeighborsClassifier* class [17]. Before feeding into the model, we need to split the data into testing and training sets (in a ratio of 1:9) so that the model is trained with the training dataset and later the testing accuracy of the model is observed by testing it on the test dataset. This is done using the *model_selection* module of *sklearn* library. Further steps are: importing the class for use, preparing X and Y arrays out of the features and class arrays, respectively, dividing the dataset into training and testing datasets.

```
from sklearn.model_selection import train_test_split
X = numpy.array(factorsData)
Y = numpy.array(targetClass)
trainingX, testingX, trainingY, testingY= train_test_sp
lit(X, Y, test_size = 0.1)
```

Now, we are ready to choose the number of neighbours and feed the data into the algorithm. We consider the number of neighbours to be 4, reasons for which will be discussed in the next section. Further steps are: importing the required class, training the model on the training set and then checking the accuracy of the model by testing it on the testing set.

```
from sklearn.neighbors import KNeighborsClassifier
knnObject = KNeighborsClassifier(n_neighbors=4)
knnObject.fit(trainingX, trainingY)
accuracy = knnObject.score(testingX, testingY)
print(accuracy)
```

The above code produces the following output:

```
0.9649122807017544
```

4.3 Results and Discussion

To produce accurate results through this algorithm, it is critical that we choose an optimal 'k' value. How is this value chosen? Simple, just check which value of k produces most accurate results over a set range of values as shown below.

```
for i in range(1,15):
    knnObject = KNeighborsClassifier(n_neighbors=i)
    knnObject.fit(trainingX, trainingY)
    accuracy = knnObject.score(testingX, testingY)
    print(str(i) + " = " + str(accuracy))
```

The above code produces the following output:

```
 1  =  0.9122807017543859
 2  =  0.9649122807017544
 3  =  0.9298245614035088
 4  =  0.9473684210526315
 5  =  0.9649122807017544
 6  =  0.9473684210526315
 7  =  0.9473684210526315
 8  =  0.9649122807017544
 9  =  0.9298245614035088
10  =  0.9473684210526315
11  =  0.9298245614035088
12  =  0.9298245614035088
13  =  0.8947368421052632
14  =  0.9122807017543859
15  =  0.9122807017543859
```

From the above output, it is clear that $k = 2$, 5 and 8 produces the same high accuracy. You can choose any number as k value, keeping in mind that it should not be a multiple of the number of classes. For the same reason, we have chosen the number of neighbours to be 5.

Thus, with $k = 5$, we have developed a model that is trained to classify women who have a high chance of getting diabetes and those who do not. Out of every 100 predictions made in the data set, about 97 of them are right. This makes it quite an impressive, reliable model.

It does not end with only diabetes, diagnosing cancer patients, classifying types of cancer, and identifying Alzheimer's genes can all be done, maybe not up to this high level o f accuracy but in a fairly accurate manner.

There have been some discussions on improving this algorithm, however, because of its inability to handle relatively larger datasets. Most K-NN models use either Euclidean or Manhattan distance as the standard distance metric. These metrics are simple, robust and perform well in a wide range of situations and circumstances. However, research shows that when the distance between data points is measured using a metric called "cosine similarity" in our KNN algorithm (which obviously requires modification to the traditional algorithm), it outperforms the traditionally imported "Scikit-Learn" model in terms of both, speed and accuracy [18].

There are several papers published which discuss several other ways to modify the traditional KNN algorithm to make it more amiable to relatively larger datasets. But one thing is clear and that is the fact that KNN is an algorithm that can easily be understood, implemented and explained. With a dataset that gives enough information for it to be classified, this technique of classification can produce impressive results.

4.4 Conclusion

Data Science for healthcare applications plays an important role in the current scenario of the world. In this chapter, the different kinds of data science tools for healthcare were explored with their advantages. The machine learning methods that are useful for the analysis of the healthcare data are also explored in this chapter. The last section presented a case study on healthcare data analytics. The KNN algorithm was used for the analysis that shows the different types of clusters in a typical healthcare application. Healthcare analytics provide support for the patients through various interpretations of the data.

References

1. Hogarty, D.T., Su, J.C., Phan, K., Attia, M., Hossny, M., Nahavandi, S., Yazdabadi, A.: Artificial intelligence in dermatology—where we are and the way to the future: a review. Am. J. Clin. Dermatol. 21(1), 41–47 (2020) (SkinVision Service)
2. Tong, S.T., Sopory, P.: Does integral affect influence intentions to use artificial intelligence for skin cancer screening? A test of the affect heuristic. Psychol. Health 34(7), 828–849 (2019)
3. Nelson, C.A., Pérez-Chada, L.M., Creadore, A., Li, S.J., Lo, K., Manjaly, P., Menon, A.V.: Patient perspectives on the use of artificial intelligence for skin cancer screening: a qualitative study. JAMA Dermatol. 156(5), 501–512 (2020)
4. Chegini, M., Bernard, J., Berger, P., Sourin, A., Andrews, K., Schreck, T.: Interactive labelling of a multivariate dataset for supervised machine learning using linked visualisations, clustering, and active learning. Vis. Inform. 3(1), 9–17 (2019)
5. Huang, L., Shea, A.L., Qian, H., Masurkar, A., Deng, H., Liu, D.: Patient clustering improves efficiency of federated machine learning to predict mortality and hospital stay time using distributed electronic medical records. J. Biomed. Inform. 99, 103291 (2019)
6. Heart Disease UCI: https://www.kaggle.com/ronitf/heart-disease-uci
7. Pima Indians Diabetes Database: https://www.kaggle.com/uciml/pima-indians-diabetes-database
8. Athey, S., Tibshirani, J., Wager, S.: Generalized random forests. Ann. Stat. 47(2), 1148–1178 (2019)
9. Copeland, M., Soh, J., Puca, A., Manning, M., Gollob, D.: Microsoft azure and cloud computing. In: Microsoft Azure, pp. 3–26. Apress, Berkeley, CA (2015)
10. Qian, L., Luo, Z., Du, Y., Guo, L.: Cloud computing: an overview. In: IEEE International Conference on Cloud Computing, pp. 626–631. Springer, Berlin, Heidelberg, Dec 2009
11. Carneiro, T., Da Nóbrega, R.V.M., Nepomuceno, T., Bian, G.B., De Albuquerque, V.H.C., Reboucas Filho, P.P.: Performance analysis of Google colaboratory as a tool for accelerating deep learning applications. IEEE Access 6, 61677–61685 (2018)
12. Jiang, B., Canny, J.: Interactive machine learning via a GPU-accelerated toolkit. In: Proceedings of the 22nd International Conference on Intelligent User Interfaces, pp. 535–546, Mar 2017
13. UCI ML Breast Cancer Wisconsin (Diagnostic) Dataset: https://archive.ics.uci.edu/ml/datasets/Breast+Cancer+Wisconsin+(Diagnostic)
14. Garreta, R., Moncecchi, G.: Learning Scikit-Learn: Machine Learning in Python. Packt Publishing Ltd. (2013)
15. Buitinck, L., Louppe, G., Blondel, M., Pedregosa, F., Mueller, A., Grisel, O., Niculae, V., Prettenhofer, P., Gramfort, A., Grobler, J., Layton, R.: API design for machine learning software: experiences from the scikit-learn project. arXiv:1309.0238 (2013)

16. Garcia-Larsen, V., Morton, V., Norat, T., Moreira, A., Potts, J.F., Reeves, T., Bakolis, I.: Dietary patterns derived from principal component analysis (PCA) and risk of colorectal cancer: a systematic review and meta-analysis. Eur. J. Clin. Nutr. **73**(3), 366–386 (2019)
17. Heyburn, R., Bond, R., Black, M., Mulvenna, M., Wallace, J., Rankin, D., Cleland, B.: Machine learning using synthetic and real data: similarity of evaluation metrics for different healthcare datasets and for different algorithms. In: Proceedings of the 13th International FLINS Conference (FLINS2018), Aug 2018
18. Subasi, A., Radhwan, M., Kurdi, R., Khateeb, K.: IoT based mobile healthcare system for human activity recognition. In: 2018 15th Learning and Technology Conference (L&T), pp. 29–34. IEEE, Feb 2018

Applications in Health Data Analytics

Management of Dementia Through Self-help and Assistive Technologies

Poulami Majumder

Abstract Dementia is often referred to as a cluster of symptoms that is largely associated with neural diseases that include declined memory and reduced ability of a person's daily activities. Plenty of research has been carried out toward the treatment and management of dementia. Some of the supportive medicines can treat this condition to a given extent but cannot cure it permanently. In this chapter, we present new ways of managing dementia by involving self-help, behavioral practices, and affective assistive technologies. We propose a scenario of the mentioned self-help that could be achieved by the patients and their caregivers themselves. We show how assistive technologies can support the patients and their family members to counter the societal restrictions of dementia while involving assistive instruments and tools such as mobile, smart device, and smart sensors. We discuss the effectiveness of such technologies and their impacts on self-help measures. Further, we present various benefits and limitations related to assistive technologies. We conclude the chapter by prescribing some techniques to manage dementia through new practices and technologies.

Keywords Dementia · Neural disease · Self-help · Assistive technology

1 Introduction

Dementia can be considered as the most viable factor to such memory losses [1, 2]. Dementia is a syndrome where a cluster of symptoms are involved such as progressive loss of memory along with daily activities, irregular thinking, and behavioral impairment [3]. It is mostly found in old people though it is not a normal part of aging. Neurodegeneration or damaged brain nerve cells are majorly responsible for dementia. These damaged cells cannot communicate to the surrounding normal cells which affects memory, thinking, behavior, and motor action [4, 5]. There are several

P. Majumder (✉)
Department of Biotechnology, Maulana Abul Kalam Azad University of Technology, Kolkata, India
e-mail: plm89.majumder@gmail.com

© The Author(s), under exclusive license to Springer Nature Singapore Pte Ltd. 2021 237
K. G. Srinivasa et al. (eds.), *Artificial Intelligence for Information Management: A Healthcare Perspective*, Studies in Big Data 88,
https://doi.org/10.1007/978-981-16-0415-7_11

causes that can be related to dementia, for example, progressive brain cell death, brain tumor, stroke, cerebrovascular disease, head injury through brain cell death, or neurodegeneration [6–9]. The early signs of dementia include mood change, short-term memory, trouble in finding the right words, confusion, repetition in work, trouble in task completion [10]. The general symptoms of dementia are memory problems, remembering recent events, lack of concentration.

There are four stages of dementia, e.g., (i) mild cognitive impairment, (ii) mild dementia, (iii) moderate dementia, and (iv) severe dementia [11]. Mild cognitive impairment is characterized by general forgetfulness. In the case of mild dementia, the cognitive impairment occurs in their daily life occasionally. Moderate dementia creates more confusion in daily life, like facing problem in getting dressed, hair combing, significant changes in personality, sleep apnea. Severe dementia is the last stage of dementia that causes loss of ability to communicate, facing trouble in completing simple task, moaning or yelling, imbalance during walk, uncontrolled bowel and bladder function [12–16]. The major types of dementia are as follows [17]:

a. Alzheimer's Disease (AD),
b. Dementia with Lewy Bodies (DLB),
c. Frontotemporal Dementia (FTD),
d. Parkinson's Disease Dementia (PD),
e. Huntington's Disease (HD).

Alzheimer's disease is one of the most discussed diseases in recent times. The other above-mentioned types of dementia are also a matter of concern. In recent times, the use of technologies is very much appreciated in the field of diagnosis and mostly in management. Artificial intelligence has been used in the diagnosis of Alzheimer's disease by analyzing blood samples. It can also diagnose the stage of the disease accurately by monitoring the progress of neurodegeneration. These kinds of technologies are including GPS (global positioning system) tracking systems, assistive robots, and smart homes full of smart technologies such as smart devices, safety aids, remote controlling systems, etc. [5, 18–27].

The major aim of this chapter is to discuss the management of dementia patients through assistive technologies and self-help including behavioral practices. In this chapter, there are three major sections that have been discussed. Section 2 described the various problems in dementia faced by both patients and caregivers. Section 3 focused on dementia management through self-help and use of assistive technology. Section 4 discussed the various consequences regarding the benefits and limitations of assistive technologies.

2 Problems in Dementia

2.1 Problems Faced by the Dementia Patients

The general challenges faced by patients with dementia are as follows [28–32].

a. General loss of memory means dementia patients are unable to remember recent events, relatives, even the name of their own. Even they cannot remember their own life events, dates, etc.
b. They lose the ability of cognitive thinking. They cannot acquire or assemble the activities through knowledge.
c. Mood swing has become their daily problem.
d. Disorientation in daily tasks such as keeping things such as spectacle, mobile, torch, etc.
e. An individual with dementia cannot hold a continuous conversation for a long time due to lack of concentration.
f. Disbalanced while walking.
g. Facing difficulty in food or water swallowing.
h. They cannot remember individuals, particular places, exact times such as whether it is day or night.
i. They are unable to perform any regular activities such as personal care.

2.2 Problems Faced by the Caregivers

Caregivers of dementia patients are none other than family members, nurses, and medical professionals. Each dementia patient suffers differently based on their mental behavior and physical activities. In accordance of such differences, the caregivers also experience a variety of challenges. The basic duties of a caregiver include help in walking, cooking, and medical assistance [33, 34]. In principle, caregivers should be physically fit, intellectually prepared, and emotionally strong [35]. Most of the dementia patients suffer from loneliness while companionship is very important to them. Caregivers can help them emotionally through continuous interaction [36]. There are such unique challenges the caregivers face to a different level during their duties. Following problems are generally faced by them [37–40].

a. Emotion: Rigorous emotional ups and downs can be seen in dementia patients. Caregivers must cope up with such variation of moods otherwise they may land into a range of difficulties in their duty.
b. Education: Caregivers should be aware of a dementia patient's cognitive activity. A proper education and training scheme should be developed and imposed upon them to support dementia patients in a better way.
c. Adaptation: Adaptability issue of caregivers sometimes comes into the questionable mode as they need to adapt themselves to the sudden changes in the

patient's behavior. Sometimes it becomes worse which may cause problems toward the caregiver's adaptability.

d. Self-care: To take proper care for the patients, the caregivers often forget to take care of themselves. It is common that the caregivers are losing their patience in order to deal with the ill behaviors, hurtful sayings, and sudden mood swings. In this adverse situation, proper care is needed for their own physique as well as their mind but the caregivers get a hard time for self-care during this difficult job.

3 Management of Dementia

Henceforth, facing the challenges of dementia is difficult for both patients and care-givers. Caregivers should be prepared in all of the situations associated with dementia patient care and for that, they must be strong in all aspects regarding physical, emotional, and intellectual health [40]. Dementia patients are also needed care at its level which can be taken by themselves. To manage this disease there are notable assistances that are existing such as medicine, assistive technologies, and self-help. There are a lot of medicines in the market which are prescribed for the patients to lower the advancement of the symptoms or manage the disease. But the daily challenges can be managed better through self-help and assistive technologies as well.

3.1 Self-help

An individual with dementia is facing both good day and bad day as well. The self-help of dementia patients has been a neglected area in practice and research [32]. At the early onset of dementia, the patients are able to help or manage themselves from the difficult condition of dementia. The help of family members is also considered as self-help. Self-help can manage the cognitive impairment of patients [33]. There are several tasks that are advised by the doctors and or caregivers that may help the patient to fight against their condition at an early stage of dementia. Some following tasks the patients may try as self-help for better results [34–39, 41]:

Patients should list all their daily problems that they face in their daily activities. During check-ups, they can present that list to the doctor and can find strategic solutions to those problems. The summarized key points also may help the patient to assess themselves on their own and help themselves from those impairments.

a. Sometimes, it is common that the patients are unable to identify their particular health issues. They may disregard the implications of ill-health. Sometimes their decision regarding any activities is dismissive. They may get help from family members and doctors to identify their illness. In accordance with the impact of the ill-health the patient should stop such activities like driving a car, playing bowls, etc.

b. Some home-based assistance like nursing, home help can be the support of the patient through their regular monitoring and assurance which may build up the self-confidence of patients. There are some home works like making flowcharts, checklist, decision tables may be done by the patients and actually help themselves in future.

c. Time to time appointments with a psychologist may be beneficial for patients to support and monitor their own health.

d. The use of medical devices which help to monitor the allied disease condition such as diabetes, blood pressure, speech pathology, occupational therapy, physiotherapy, sleep apnea, respiratory distress, etc. The direct observation of diseases through the use of medical devices help them to manage the disease to some extent.

e. Patients are mostly unable to express their symptoms or feelings and even cannot be able to seek appropriate help to describe their problems. This is caused due to reduction of their expressive languages. The limitation of language skills makes them argumentative and frustrated. So, if clinicians or caregivers manage the situation by teaching them with particular comprehensive and receptive words or languages the situation can be managed in a better way.

f. The regulation of intact response in addition to emotional control is needed to behave properly in social circumstances. Family members or friends can encourage the patients to attend the clinic with a supportive individual of his/her choice. The aggressive or extremely emotional behaviors can be written point-wise by the patient or the family members which may be useful for the patient and the clinicians also.

g. It is general to be impulsive as the patients execute impaired activities. This kind of behavior is getting more fluctuated as they failed to adhere to the prescribed management. The wall calendar listing appointments with doctors or others may help themselves to adhere to the health monitoring and societal connection.

h. Additional supports can be obtained from the community nursing. Electronic diaries with automated and or customized reminders (e.g., tablet, phone), medicine dose administration aid (blister packs) are helpful in dementia management. Though the most important part in the self-help mode is motivation which must remain in family members and caregivers who are also able to motivate dementia patients.

i. It is advised by doctors and researchers that the practice of some cognitive activities such as Sudoku, crosswords, chess, etc., may develop cognitive impairment and can manage the disease condition to some extent.

3.2   Assistive Technologies

In recent times there are several aids and/or technologies that act as assistance for the dementia patients, the caregivers, and family members as well. The situations around dementia patient can be frustrating and exhausting for both the loved ones living with the patient and caregivers. As it is discussed earlier that the self-help is quite helpful for both dementia patient and the caregivers, family members to manage the cognitive domain. In addition to this, assistive technologies are also catching the attention of the digital world. The new technologies help the situation in different ways such as health monitoring, medication management, personal care through robot, in-home cameras, sensor-based tracking of patients, etc. [40]. These technologies are assistive towards managing the anxiety, aggression, and different situations of the patients. This kind of "assistive technology" supports autonomy, independence and can manage potential safety risks around the home and help to reduce the stress of both the patient and family members/caregivers [42]. Ray et al. described different wearable GPS tracking devices which are different kinds of assistive technologies (Fig. 1) [43].

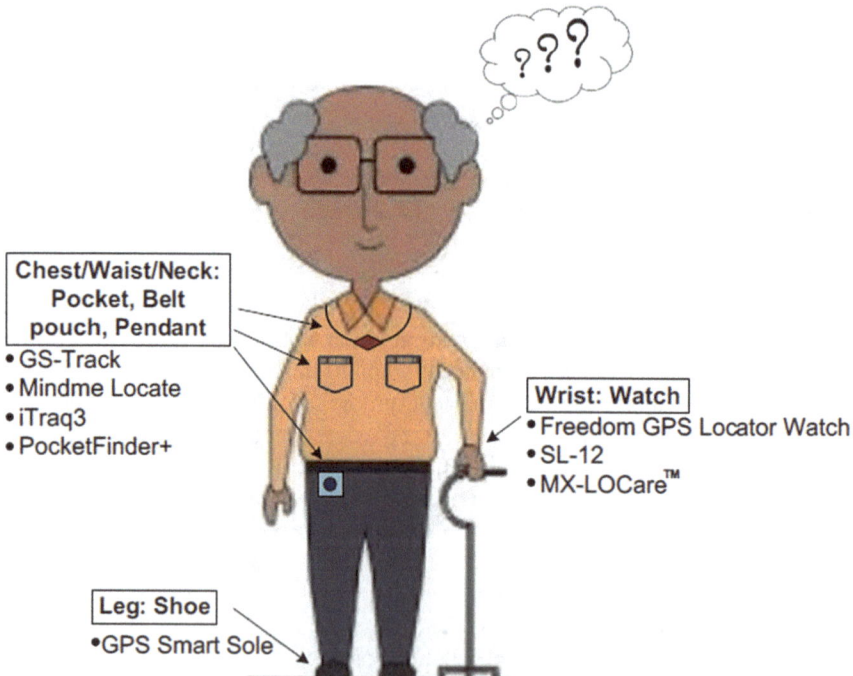

Fig. 1 The placement of GPS-enabled wearable tracking devices on patient's body. GSTrack, Mindme Locate, PocketFinder+, and iTraq3 and can be placed either in Pendant/Pocket/Bag/Keyfob/Belt pouch [43]

Here is a list of different possible technological innovations for both the patient and family members/caregivers [44–50].

a. Tracking: Dementia patients are prone to wander so it is very difficult to track them if they are getting lost. It is necessary to track their movement in a sophisticated and easier way. Wearable sensors and Internet of Things are combined together and make a smart system that can easily track the patient's exact position. There are several smart products available in the market which can easily track the current position of the patient. Those wearable sensor-based tracking devices are available as different wearing parts such as waist belt, pendant, chest pocket or pouch, GPS locator wristwatch, smart shoes with GPS sole, etc. These smart wearable GPS locators easily monitor the patient's every step and their location.

b. Fall Detection: Automated fall alert technology is very helpful for dementia patients. It is useful for patients with an advanced stage of dementia. At this stage, the cognitive impairment is getting worse and patients get disoriented and imbalanced while standing or walking that results in falling. This kind of alert system is generally combined with software and sensor, the sensor is getting attached to the patient's body through socks or shoes. If they fall the sensor attached to their body parts is giving a signal to the smart device through software in no time.

c. Communication: Staying connected with the loved one or the trusted one, the dementia patient needs hassle-free communication. The communication is getting tough and difficult with the progression of the dementia stage. Another popular app is Talking Mats that allows dementia patient to communicate their own feelings by selecting pictures, emojis, and symbols. The preprogrammed adapted telephones can be dialed numbers frequently and easier to watch the numbers by its large buttons. Video chat services such as Skype are another useful way to keep in touch with patients' loved ones who are distant geographically.

d. Robotic Care: With the progression of robotic science and technology home care robots are being made specifically designed for dementia patient's care. This kind of robots helps to reduce the burden of the caregivers. The personal home care robots are generally designed to do daily housework like cleaning, help to remind the medications and dose. These kinds of robots are needed to be more improved for their swifter actions. Though the robots cannot replace the human presence but can make the work of caregivers easier at some point.

e. Alerting Clock: This kind of clocks is specifically designed for dementia patients which is helpful to ease anxiety by reducing the confusion between day and night time. This is also helpful for the caregivers to set a routine for the patients. There are several alerting clocks are available such as Day Clock, DayClox, Alzheimer's Dementia Day Clock, Day/Night Clock, Thousand Clock Widgets, etc. Alzheimer's Dementia Day Clock and Thousand Clock Widgets are apps that display the clock in the phone as a screensaver and it can be set desirably. Some clocks are analog and digital which help the patients to distinguish between day and night time.

f. Home Monitoring: This technology is especially for the loved ones who are located distantly from the patient. Home monitoring devices manage the switch of electric lights to be on and off in accordance with the changed thermostats and can also alert and increase the safety measures by sending alarms through a smartphone. It is very encouraging for the long distance caregivers who can monitor the home and do safety measures for the patients remotely. In-home cameras are also other helpful aids through which the safety of the patient can be monitored distantly.

g. Picture phone: It is very difficult to remember the phone number for the dementia patient. Picture phone is being used by them as it shows pictures of their caregiver, family member. Whenever they need their loved ones, they just need to click on the picture displayed on the picture phone and make call them easily.

h. Pervasive biomedical informatics (PBI): As an emerging research domain, the PBI must be sought for managing the dementia patients [51]. With the inclusion of the pervasive computing, biomedical engineering and machine-learning-centric informatics, PBI could certainly improve the existing scenario of dementia tracking as well as care and management.

4 Consequences of Assistive Technology

There are consequences of assistive technologies in dementia management and those include benefits along with some limitations.

4.1 Benefits

The followings are the benefits of assistive technology [52, 53]:

a. Assist a dementia person to communicate through phone.
b. Help to distinguish between day and night time.
c. Automatic switch on and off electric appliances during and after use.
d. Safety measures by the chemical or thermal sensors for smoke, heat or toxic gas.
e. Long-distance monitoring.
f. Falls alert/safety at night.
g. Medication reminders.
h. Tracking the patients who are roaming around cluelessly.

4.2 Limitations

Assistive technology is useful in recent times though does have some limitations [53].

a. Sometimes the patient or family members have their different needs, preferences which cannot be fulfilled by the technology.
b. Sometimes sensors or electric appliances are not working properly due to some technological limitations.
c. False alarms may create confusion in both patients and caregivers.
d. Repeated alarm or reminding recorded messages sometimes irked the patient and family members as well.
e. During monitoring, tracking, or safety measures the assistive technologies sometimes invade privacy and may affect the freedom of individuals.
f. Technologies can do only alert the risk or threat but unable to strengthen the patient mentally.
g. Ethical issue is a major drawback in using of assistive technologies as the use of smart devices or systems are not properly obey the user's consent process.
h. Nowadays, assistive technology is very useful but can never be a replacement for human support and interaction.

5 Conclusion

In this chapter, the management of dementia through self-help and assistive technologies have been discussed. Self-help through continuous practices may improve the cognitive impairment of dementia patients though it is still a topic of debate. Assistive technologies are also helpful and getting popular also day by day. It is easy to list down the management processes but very difficult to adapt them by the dementia patients and caregivers. Sometimes the dementia patients are unable to do the practices related to self-help while assistive technologies have also their own limitations as discussed earlier. Myriad researches are carried out toward the management of dementia and there are various novel ideas and processes are being pointed out for better outcomes. However, the exact procedures of management can only be decided and adapted by the patients and their caregivers only.

References

1. Aalten, P., Van Valen, E., Clare, L., Kenny, G., Verhey, F.: Awareness in dementia: a review of clinical correlates. Aging Ment. Health **9**(5), 414–422 (2005)
2. Alzheimer's Disease and Dementia. Dementia Types: Signs, Symptoms, and Diagnosis. https://www.alz.org/dementia/types-of-dementia.asp (2019)
3. Dementia—Symptoms, Causes, Diagnosis, Treatments. https://www.alz.org/alzheimers-dementia/what-is-dementia (2019)

4. Duong, S., Patel, T., Chang, F.: Dementia: what pharmacists need to know. Can. Pharm. J./Revue Des Pharmaciens Du Canada **150**(2), 118–129 (2017)
5. Smith, S.K., Mountain, G.A.: New forms of information and communication technology (ICT) and the potential to facilitate social and leisure activity for people living with dementia. Int. J. Comput. Healthc. **1**(4), 332–345 (2012)
6. Garand, L., Buckwalter, K.C., Hall, G.R.: The biological basis of behavioral symptoms in dementia. Issues Ment. Health Nurs. **21**(1), 91–107 (2000)
7. Lantos, P.L., Cairns, N.J.: The neuropathology of Alzheimer's disease. In: Dementia, pp. 185–207. Springer, Boston, MA (1994)
8. Forman, M.S., Farmer, J., Johnson, J.K., Clark, C.M., Arnold, S.E., Branch Coslett, H., Chatterjee, A., et al.: Frontotemporal dementia: clinicopathological correlations. Ann. Neurol.: Off. J. Am. Neurol. Assoc. Child Neurol. Soc. **59**(6), 952–962 (2006)
9. Blacker, D., Lovestone, S.: Genetics and dementia nosology. J. Geriatr. Psychiatry Neurol. **19**(3), 186–191 (2006)
10. What is dementia? Alzheimer's Association. https://www.alz.org/alzheimers-dementia/what-is-dementia. Accessed 18 Jan 2020
11. Larson, E.B.: Risk factors for cognitive decline and dementia. https://www.uptodate.com/contents/search. Accessed 22 Jan 2020
12. AAN guideline summary for clinicians: detection, diagnosis and management of dementia. American Academy of Neurology. https://www.aan.com/Guidelines/Home/ByTopic?topicId=15. Accessed 1 Feb 2020
13. Cunningham, E.L., McGuinness, B., Herron, B., Passmore, A.P.: Dementia. Ulst. Med. J. **84**(2), 79–87 (2015)
14. McKeith, I.G., Dickson, D.W., Lowe, J., Emre, M., O'brien, J.T., Feldman, H., Cummings, J., et al.: Diagnosis and management of dementia with Lewy bodies: third report of the DLB Consortium. Neurology **65**(12), 1863–1872 (2005)
15. Petersen, R.C., Morris, J.C.: Mild cognitive impairment as a clinical entity and treatment target. Arch. Neurol. **62**(7), 1160–1163 (2005)
16. Todd, S., Barr, S., Roberts, M., Peter Passmore, A.: Survival in dementia and predictors of mortality: a review. Int. J. Geriatr. Psychiatry **28**(11), 1109–1124 (2013)
17. Prince, M., Bryce, R., Albanese, E., Wimo, A., Ribeiro, W., Ferri, C.P.: The global prevalence of dementia: a systematic review and metaanalysis. Alzheimer's Dement. **9**(1), 63–75 (2013)
18. Mani Sekhar, S.R., Siddesh, G.M., Manvi, S.S.: Introduction to bioinformatics. In: Statistical Modelling and Machine Learning Principles for Bioinformatics Techniques, Tools, and Applications. Algorithms for Intelligent Systems book series (AIS). Springer, Mar 2020
19. Mani Sekhar, S.R., Siddesh, G.M., Tiwari, A., Anand, A.: Submitted a chapter on "Bioinspired techniques for data security in IoT". In: For the book Internet of Things (IoT): Concept and Applications, S.M.A.R.T. Environments. Springer
20. Kiranmai, V.P., Siddesh, G.M., Mani Sekhar, S.R.: Supervised techniques in proteomics. In: Statistical Modelling and Machine Learning Principles for Bioinformatics Techniques, Tools, and Applications. Algorithms for Intelligent Systems book series (AIS). Springer, Mar 2020
21. Mani Sekhar, S.R., Siddesh, G.M.: A chapter on "Introduction and implementation of machine learning algorithms in R". In: For the book title Sentiment Analysis and Knowledge Discovery in Contemporary Business. IGI Global, Aug 2018. https://www.igi-global.com/book/sentiment-analysis-knowledge-discovery-contemporary/185750. ISBN13: 9781522549994
22. Patil, S.B., Mani Sekhar, S.R., Siddesh, G.M., Manvi, S.S.: A method for predicting essential proteins using gene expression. In: IEEE Conference, SmartTechCon2017, Oct 2017
23. Mani Sekhar, S.R., Siddesh, G.M., Manvi, S.S., Srinivasa, K.G.: Optimized focused web crawler with natural language processing based relevance measure in bioinformatics web sources. Cybern. Inf. Technol. **19**(2) (2019). Print ISSN: 1311-9702; Online ISSN: 1314-4081. https://doi.org/10.2478/cait-2019-0021
24. Mani Sekhar, S.R., Siddesh, G.M., Manvi, S.S., Srinivasa, K.G.: Identification of essential proteins in yeast using mean weighted average and recursive feature elimination. Recent Pat. Comput. Sci. **12**(1) (2019). https://doi.org/10.2174/2213275911666180918155521

25. Mani Sekhar, S.R., Tewari, S., Rahman, H., Siddesh, G.M.: A chapter on "Data collection in fog data analytics". In: Book Title: Fog Data Analytics for IoT Applications: Next Generation Process Model with State-of-the-Art Technologies. Studies in Big Data. Springer (2020)
26. Mani Sekhar, S.R., Siddesh, G.M., Tiwari, A., Khator, A., Singh, R.: Identification and analysis of nitrogen dioxide concentration for air quality prediction using seasonal autoregression integrated with moving average. Aerosol Sci. Eng. 4(2), 137–146 (2020) (Springer). ISSN: 2510-375X. https://doi.org/10.1007/s41810-020-00061-7
27. Mani Sekhar, S.R., Siddesh, G.M., Kalra, S., Anand, S.: A study of use cases for smart contracts using Blockchain technology. Int. J. Inf. Syst. Soc. Change 10(2), (2019)
28. Boustani, M., Schubert, C., Sennour, Y.: The challenge of supporting care for dementia in primary care. Clin. Interv. Aging 2(4), 631 (2007)
29. Haupt, M., Kurz, A., Jänner, M.: A 2-year follow-up of behavioural and psychological symptoms in Alzheimer's disease. Dement. Geriatr. Cogn. Disord. 11(3), 147–152 (2000)
30. McDaniel Jr., R.R., Jordan, M.E., Fleeman, B.F.: Surprise, surprise, surprise! A complexity science view of the unexpected. Health Care Manag. Rev. 28(3), 266–278 (2003)
31. Dementia: how to overcome common challenges. https://www.netdoctor.co.uk/healthy-living/a28347/living-with-dementia-challenges/. Accessed 20 Jan 2020.
32. Schubert, C.C., Boustani, M., Callahan, C.M., Perkins, A.J., Carney, C.P., Fox, C., Unverzagt, F., Hui, S., Hendrie, H.C.: Comorbidity profile of dementia patients in primary care: are they sicker? J. Am. Geriatr. Soc. 54(1), 104–109 (2006)
33. Boustani, M., Peterson, B., Harris, R., Lux, L.J., Krasnov, C., Sutton, S.F., Hanson, L., Lohr, K.N.: Screening for dementia (2003)
34. Guerriero Austrom, M., Damush, T.M., Hartwell, C.W., Perkins, T., Unverzagt, F., Boustani, M., Hendrie, H.C., Callahan, C.M.: Development and implementation of nonpharmacologic protocols for the management of patients with Alzheimer's disease and their families in a multiracial primary care setting. The Gerontologist 44(4), 548–553 (2004)
35. Tan, Z.S., Jennings, L., Reuben, D.: Coordinated care management for dementia in a large academic health system. Health Aff. 33(4), 619–625 (2014)
36. Callahan, C.M., Boustani, M.A., Unverzagt, F.W., Austrom, M.G., Damush, T.M., Perkins, A.J., Fultz, B.A., Hui, S.L., Counsell, S.R., Hendrie, H.C.: Effectiveness of collaborative care for older adults with Alzheimer disease in primary care: a randomized controlled trial. JAMA 295(18), 2148–2157 (2006)
37. Brodaty, H., Donkin, M.: Family caregivers of people with dementia. Dialogues Clin. Neurosci. 11(2), 217 (2009)
38. Sörensen, S., Conwell, Y.: Issues in dementia caregiving: effects on mental and physical health, intervention strategies, and research needs. Am. J. Geriatr. Psychiatry 19(6), 491–496 (2011)
39. Unique Challenges Faced by Alzheimer's & Dementia Caregivers. https://www.caringseniorservice.com/blog/challenges-alzheimers-dementia-caregivers. Accessed 28 Jan 2020
40. Arvanitakis, Z., Shah, R.C., Bennett, D.A.: Diagnosis and management of dementia. JAMA 322(16), 1589–1599 (2019)
41. Challenges facing primary carers of people with dementia: opportunities for research. https://www.alzheimers.org.uk/sites/default/files/2018-05/Challengesfacingprimarycarers.pdf. Accessed 25 Jan 2020
42. De Vreese, L.P., Neri, M., Fioravanti, M., Belloi, L., Zanetti, O.: Memory rehabilitation in Alzheimer's disease: a review of progress. Int. J. Geriatr. Psychiatry 16(8), 794–809 (2001)
43. Fillit, H., Knopman, D., Cummings, J., Appel, F.: Opportunities for improving managed care for individuals with dementia: part 1—the issues. Am. J. Manag. Care 5(3), 309–315 (1999)
44. Ray, P.P., Dash, D., De, D.: A systematic review and implementation of IoT-based pervasive sensor-enabled tracking system for dementia patients. J. Med. Syst. 43(9), 287 (2019)
45. Bennett, B., McDonald, F., Beattie, E., Carney, T., Freckelton, I., White, B., Willmott, L.: Assistive technologies for people with dementia: ethical considerations. Bull. World Health Organ. 95(11), 749 (2017)
46. Technological Innovations for Caregivers and Those Living with Dementia. https://www.alzheimers.net/9-22-14-technology-for-dementia/. Accessed 31 Jan 2020

47. The Future Role of Robots and Humans in Caretaking. https://hitconsultant.net/2018/08/06/robots-humans-caretaking/#.Xjr2ZGgzbIV. Accessed 01 Feb 2020
48. How technology can help. https://www.alzheimers.org.uk/get-support/staying-independent/how-technology-can-help. Accessed 02 Feb 2020
49. Inoue, T.: Assistive Technology and Robotic Technology for Dementia Care. https://www.who.int/mental_health/neurology/dementia/NSA_National_Rehabilitation_Center_for_Persons_with_Disabilities.pdf. Accessed 02 Feb 2020
50. Evans, J., Brown, M., Coughlan, T., Lawson, G., Craven, M.P.: A systematic review of dementia focused assistive technology. In: International Conference on Human-Computer Interaction, pp. 406–417. Springer, Cham (2015)
51. Ray, P.P., Majumder, P.: An introduction to pervasive biomedical informatics. CSI Commun. Mag. Comput. Soc. India **62** (2019)
52. Sriram, V., Jenkinson, C., Peters, M.: Informal carers' experience of assistive technology use in dementia care at home: a systematic review. BMC Geriatr. **19**(1), 160 (2019)
53. The benefits and limitations of assistive technology. https://www.atdementia.org.uk/editorial.asp?page_id=45 (2007). Accessed 02 Feb 2020

Classification and Prediction of Leukemia Using Gene Expression Profile

Pothuraju Rajarajeswari, G. Navya Krishna, G. Sai Pooja, V. Yamini Radha, and B. Naga Sri Ram

Abstract Cancer is one of the leading and major causes of death nowadays. While developing the approaches for healing the cancer is key, the role of correct classification is always encouraged. In the proposed system, we are going to classify Leukemia into Acute Lymphocytic Leukemia (ALL) and Acute Myeloid Leukemia (AML) and also going to predict who is at cancer risk by monitoring gene expressions. Leukemia is a blood or bone marrow type of cancer which can be treated with aggressive chemotherapy, bone marrow, or stem cell transplant therapy in major cases. But many of the Leukemic patients may not need chemotherapy if found in the initial stages. While chemotherapy is known to be effective, but it may not be the best option for every cancer patient. The main motivation is to help society to reduce the cost of treatment for cancer as many people cannot afford the cost of chemotherapy. It is also better to predict the type and intensity of cancer at early stages through gene expression monitoring. To solve this problem, we chose the domain of Bioinformatics, which is an interdisciplinary field mainly involving molecular biology, genetics, statistics, and computer science.

Keywords Bioinformatics · Cancer · Gene monitoring · Genetics · Leukemia

1 Introduction

In the current century, enormous factors contribute to causing cancer. So, cancer classification needs not depend only on the doctor's decision. Intelligent algorithms concerning doctor's help are inevitable. Most of the algorithms failed to classify data with better accuracy. Leukemia consists of four types (Acute Myeloid Leukemia (AML), Chronic Myeloid Leukemia (CML), Acute Lymphocytic Leukemia (ALL), Chronic Lymphocytic Leukemia (CCL). Here, in this proposed system, we are mainly concentrating on ALL and AML. These are the two important types for the cancer

P. Rajarajeswari (✉) · G. Navya Krishna · G. Sai Pooja · V. Yamini Radha · B. Naga Sri Ram
Department of CSE, Koneru Lakshmaiah Education Foundation, Guntur, Andhra Pradesh, India
e-mail: rajilikhitha@gmail.com

© The Author(s), under exclusive license to Springer Nature Singapore Pte Ltd. 2021   249
K. G. Srinivasa et al. (eds.), *Artificial Intelligence for Information Management: A Healthcare Perspective*, Studies in Big Data 88,
https://doi.org/10.1007/978-981-16-0415-7_12

classification of Leukemia prognosis that are: AML is mainly observed in childhood. ALL are also observed in both childhood and young adults. According to the condition of cancer, affected person may be prevented or may not be from cancer. Chemotherapy is one of the main and genesis types of treatment for cancer patients. Chemotherapy dwindles cancer or slows down its growth of cancer in the tissues and it reduces the chances of the cancer repetition again. But chemotherapy is mainly having side effects during the treatment. Some people can fit the therapy due to their body resistance power. That treatment cost very high common; people can't afford the cost. If cancer is identified in the initial stage itself then some precautions of using tablets and taking treatments in the hospital can be done. ALL and AML prognosis can be identified by the gene. It is mainly helpful for the function of the genes in the body. Here nowadays for the forecast of cancer, machine learning is used as machine learning gives the optimistic output for any classification of the data. The gene levels are observed at a time to time during tests performed in the hospital so that the changes can be observed one after one test. In this thesis, we are taking the top 10 gene-level patients for the main chances will be there for cancer to the patients. They can be predicted by these gene expression values. In this proposed system, cancer is predicted and classified using gene expression which is a supervised classification problem using the Random Forest method for classification based on GENE expression. The rest of the paper is as follows. Section 2 discussed research methodology of the literature survey, Sect. 3 follows the proposed system explanation, and Sect. 4 for the result and discussion and follows the conclusion.

2   Research Methodology

It is possible to predict cancer in the initial stages through a computer and gene monitoring by various methodologies. Hence, this issue had become much easier to solve via gene expression monitoring combining the machine learning techniques.

2.1   Techniques

Chu et al. [1] introduced a technique of FNN (Fuzzy Neural Networks) in the year 2004. Nahar et al. [2] introduced SVM Classifications based on associations scheme by adding the future scope that can be extended to a large scale of microarray datasets to provide a unique solution for SVM kernel selection in the year 2007. Wang et al. [3] introduced the supervised machine learning method to accurately classify cancer in the year 2007 with the future scope of consideration of cooperation between genes is for accurate predictions. The review presented by Rui Xu, Georgios in the year 2007 through a paper semi-supervised Ellipsoid ARTMAP [4] that classifies and verifies through a model called semi-supervised ellipsoid ARTMAP having a future scope of having more advanced feature selection approaches are required to find information of genes that are more efficient in prediction. Yukinwa et al. [5] proposed that the investigated algorithms are good for pathological diagnosis of cancer in near future by the methodology of weight tuning method, various classification algorithms, optimal coding problem. Luo et al. 2009 proposed classification based on SVM" [6] that uses the SVM (Support Vector Machine) for the classification system.

Bilen et al. [7] by the methodology of ANN (Artificial Neural Networks) and Genetic algorithm classified microarray data [8]. In the year 2016, Pablo Guillen and Jerry Ebalunode proposed an algorithm based deep learning based on a multi-layer perceptron for cancer classification based on microarray gene expression data. Tasci et al. [9] state that further research of all other selected genes relation with Leukemia may have great importance for the diagnosis and treatment and prognosis phases of cancer by using the methodology SVM (Support Vector Machine), Relief algorithm, correlation [9].

Benjamin Simeon, Soon Yeon Ji proposed an algorithm on Wavelet-based thresholding [8, 10], Cloud computing used for "Cloud-scale Genomic signals processing for robust large scale cancer Genomic Microarray data analysis" in the year 2017 which also had a computationally expensive limitation [11]. In the year 2018, Kavitha and Nair Harishankar developed a "PSO based feature selection of gene for cancer classification" using SVM (Support Vector Machine), recursive feature extraction, particle swarm optimization [12] which show that error rates are very high when the number of features involved is very high/low [13].

The paper "Effective cancer classification using Multidimensional Mutual Information ELM" [14], presented by Qun-Xing, Yuan fan, and Yan-Lin He introduced ELM (Extreme Learning Machine), multi-dimensional mutual information (MMI), feature selection which is an unstable algorithm, in the year 2018 [15].

As per the analysis made with various existing methods, an algorithm that takes less time, maintains high accuracy, for easy identification, the visualization should also work with large data sets [16–18]. According to my survey, the Random Forest (RF) algorithm is the one that satisfies all the conditions by omitting the limitations which are in the above-related techniques and papers [19, 20]. The advantage of random forest over the neural network technique [8] is that tree ensemble models like random forest are very interpretable and in fields like bioinformatics. So using random forest helps us to easily identify the type of cancer through correct accuracy and precision [21].

Random Forest method [RF] which is an ensemble tree technique, is mainly used for classification purposes which can be deployed very easily through learning novices of relative Machine Learning techniques to obtain reasonably good results that runs efficiently on large data sets. It is a good technique and provides effective methods for estimating missing data. The main advantage of the tree ensemble method is that the generated forests can be used for the future on various data for predicting the results.

3 Theory and Experimentation

To implement the proposed solution of classification of leukemia into ALL and AML, we simulate the operations using Random Forest (RF) with the help of the R language.

3.1 Proposed Solution

Random Forest (RF) is trained on the given gene expression data set so that it can predict whether the given cancer type is ALL or AML, where our goal is to predict which class the input image belongs to. By training a Random Forest (RF) on gene expression data set on cancer predicts the type, whether it is ALL or AML.

Random Forests (RF) are used in Bioinformatics area also with the combination of feature selection, representation, and finally through visualization. RF, feature extraction, and classification occur naturally within a single framework. This is a major advantage when compared to other techniques, while they need a lot of computations only for the pre-processing step and also show low expertise [4] and which are also difficult to interpret and much slower than RF.

3.2 Architecture of RF

For our experiment, we have used different R libraries like Tidyverse, Caret, Reshape2, and Amelia for pre-processing, implementing, and training the learning model. As it is a widely used Machine Learning classifier, it naturally leads to find the measure of the dissimilarity among the observations. The classification of the output class is done on voting or averaging several trees that are ensemble in the RF (Fig. 1). Each tree will be formed based on several parameters like GINI, VALUES, and SAMPLES. RF continues until there is a large difference in the classifier or accuracy. Once two or more iterations are having the same values as the result, then automatically splitting of the tress will be stopped.

3.3 Dataset Generation

We collected a dataset from a article, "Class Prediction by Gene Expression Monitoring" [16] which was published in the year 1999 by Golub et al. It was shown that how new cases of cancer can be classified through DNA microarray or gene expression profile through a general approach. This data was used to classify patients with AML and acute lymphoblastic leukemia (ALL) (Fig. 2). Two datasets containing

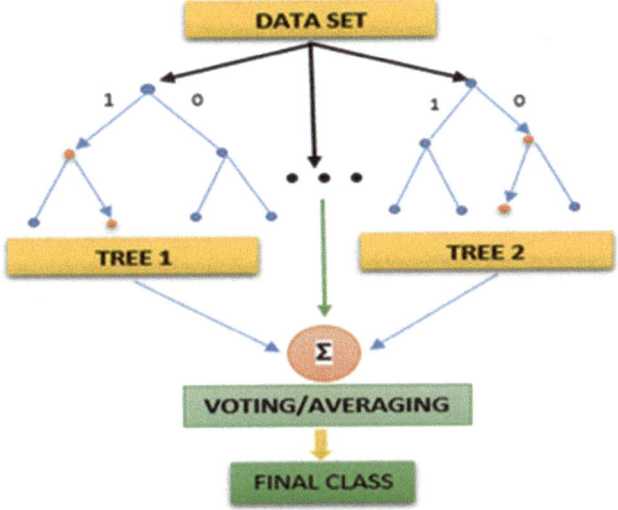

Fig. 1 Random forest process

the "initial" (training with 38 samples) and "independent" (test with 34 samples) samples were used for the proposed model. These datasets contain practical measurements that correspond to Bone Marrow (ALL) and Peripheral Blood (AML), which consists of gene accession number, gene description, and experiments of patients corresponding to the particular gene. These practical values are the intensity values that were rescaled and used such that intensities corresponding to each patient's practical measurements will be equivalent. These datasets are thus great for classification purposes and we converted++ the data set to .CSV (comma-separated value) files and used them for the proposed model to do the task of classification.

3.4 Methodology

Data set of gene expression which consists of gene accession number, gene description, and experiments of patients corresponding to a particular gene is taken first (Fig. 3). Now from this data set, we are going to select the features which are necessary for classification purpose.

Gene.Description	Gene.Accession.Number	X1	call	X2	call.1	X3	call.2	X4	call.3	...	X29	call.33	X30	call.'
AFFX-BioB-5_at (endogenous control)	AFFX-BioB-5_at	-214	A	-139	A	-76	A	-135	A	...	15	A	-318	A
AFFX-BioB-M_at (endogenous control)	AFFX-BioB-M_at	-153	A	-73	A	-49	A	-114	A	...	-114	A	-192	A
AFFX-BioB-3_at (endogenous control)	AFFX-BioB-3_at	-58	A	-1	A	-307	A	265	A	...	2	A	-95	A
AFFX-BioC-5_at (endogenous control)	AFFX-BioC-5_at	88	A	283	A	309	A	12	A	...	193	A	312	A
AFFX-BioC-3_at (endogenous control)	AFFX-BioC-3_at	-295	A	-264	A	-376	A	-419	A	...	-51	A	-139	A
AFFX-BioDn-5_at (endogenous control)	AFFX-BioDn-5_at	-558	A	-400	A	-650	A	-585	A	...	-155	A	-344	A
AFFX-BioDn-3_at (endogenous control)	AFFX-BioDn-3_at	199	A	-330	A	33	A	158	A	...	29	A	324	A

Fig. 2 Training data set sample

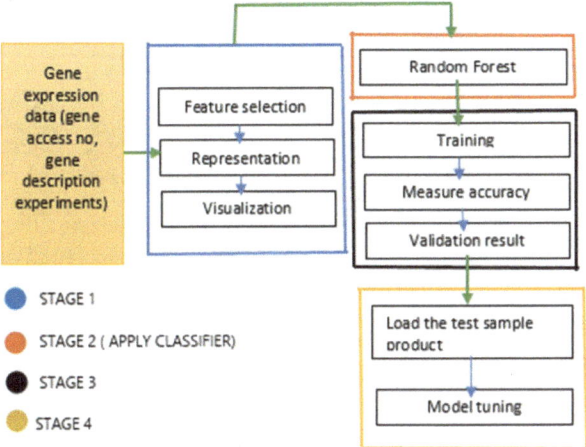

Fig. 3 Block diagram of the proposed model

3.5 Stage 1

3.5.1 Pre-processing Stage

In the pre-processing stage, we first select the features and then reshape the data. For reshaping the data we use a library called reshape2, which has a package that "melt" data sets from wide to long formats. Doing this may have a clear understanding of what the data set depicts.

Now we replace everything that starts with "X" as come other name and "num" as our experiment number.

After re-shaping and replacing the data set, we then see if there are missing values in our data. Then finally we process with training the data.

3.5.2 Representation

Now, we load the actual data which contains no missing values. We now took the provided actual data and made a subset and bind it to the training set using the mutate function (Fig. 4).

3.5.3 Visualization

In this part, we will visualize the top 10 gene expression levels since the data set is huge. For this, we use gene accession number on one axis and count in another axis which makes a plot on gene levels for each accession number. We choose the R language mainly for visualization purposes (Fig. 5).

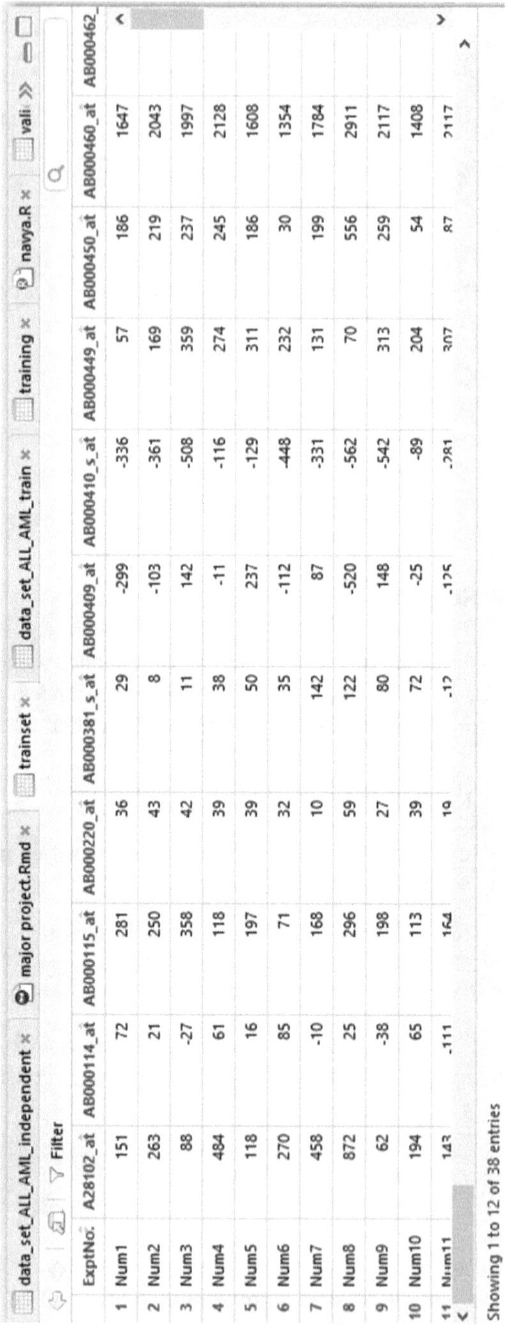

ExptNo.	A28102_at	AB000114_at	AB000115_at	AB000220_at	AB000381_s_at	AB000409_at	AB000410_s_at	AB000449_at	AB000450_at	AB000460_at	AB000462_
1 Num1	151	72	281	36	29	-299	-336	57	186	1647	
2 Num2	263	21	250	43	8	-103	-361	169	219	2043	
3 Num3	88	-27	358	42	11	142	-508	359	237	1997	
4 Num4	484	61	118	39	38	-11	-116	274	245	2128	
5 Num5	118	16	197	39	50	237	-129	311	186	1608	
6 Num6	270	85	71	32	35	-112	-448	232	30	1354	
7 Num7	458	-10	168	10	142	87	-331	131	199	1784	
8 Num8	872	25	296	59	122	-520	-562	70	556	2911	
9 Num9	62	-38	198	27	80	148	-542	313	259	2117	
10 Num10	194	65	113	39	72	-25	-89	204	54	1408	
11 Num11	143	-111	164	19	-12	-125	-281	207	87	2117	

Showing 1 to 12 of 38 entries

Fig. 4 Training set data after replacing and re-shaping

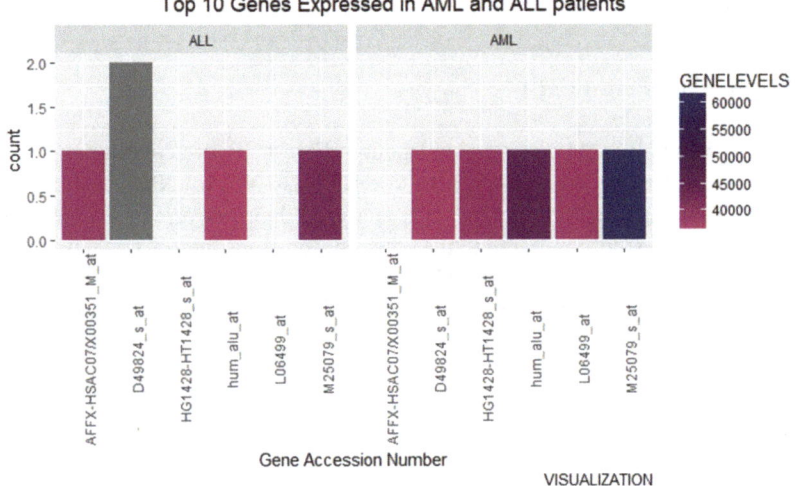

Fig. 5 Top 10 genes expressed in ALL and AML patients

From Fig. 6, we can conclude that the most distinguishing feature should be expression levels of M25079s_ though there is some overlap in gene expression between patients of both cancer types.

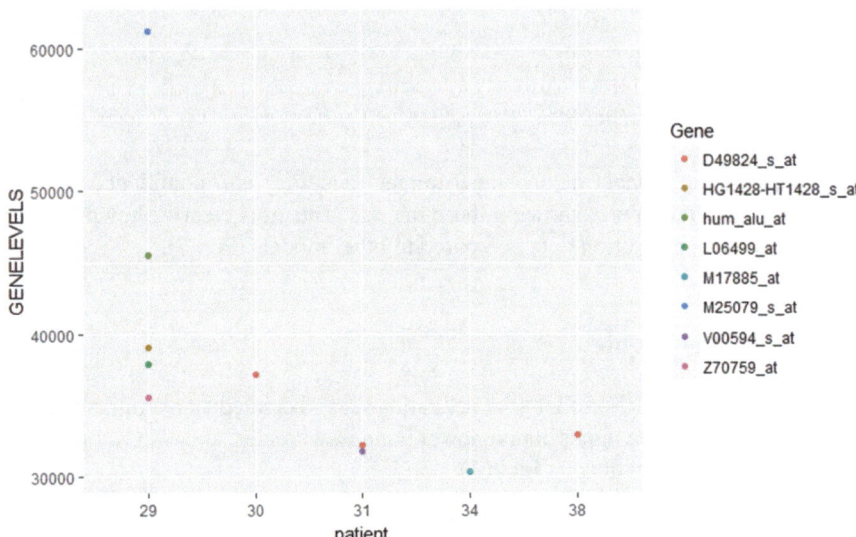

Fig. 6 Patient 29 shows several genes of which the most common gene is M25079s_At

3.6 Stage 2

3.6.1   Random Forest (RF)

In stage 2, we apply a classifier called Random Forest. Before concluding to apply RF, we also worked on other algorithms like KNN (K-Nearest Neighbours), GBM, and SVM (Support Vector Machine) and analyzed their performance to show that RF shows better results compared to the other chosen algorithms. Thus it proves that RF is the gold standard method to solve all the bioinformatics problems related to Genetics or Genomics. Here we took 5 trees initially where the interaction depth is 3.

3.7 Stage 3

3.7.1   Training

At first, we have to partition the data into training and validation sets. Load the train set and perform training in which 85% of the data will go into training and 15% of the data to the validation set. To split the data, we use the caret library for classification and regression tasks. Set up metrics and control in which we will use accuracy as our main metric. Now, set up the models SVM, KNN, GBM, and RF to train + the data.

3.7.2   Measure Accuracy

We compared the models of and measurement accuracy and confidence of each model. We also have a plot showing these metrics. Thus it is clearly shown that RF performs well on prediction data compared to other models (Fig. 7).

3.7.3   Validation Result

We now predicted the RF model with validation set and created an overall confusion matrix which shows the upper bound, lower bound accuracies, and also Kappa value which lists out the confidence (Table 1).

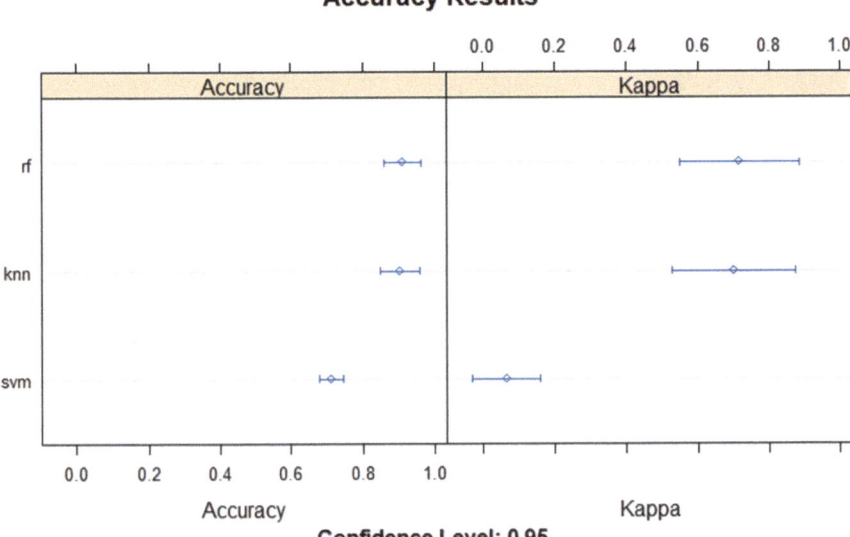

Fig. 7 Comparison of RF, KNN, and SVM

Table 1 Confusion matrix of accuracy levels

Accuracy	0.8000000
Kappa	0.0000000
Accuracy lower	0.283582063881911
Accuracy upper	0.994949236620532
Accuracy null	0.8000000

3.8 Stage 4

3.8.1 Load the Test Sample

Test sample is loaded to predict the cancer type. The data which we load is the independent data. After loading, we process our data which looks exactly like training data by changing column headings. Again for predicting the cancer type we have to check missing values first then after applying the model RF. To check the accuracies after prediction, we again have to create a confusion matrix (Table 2).

3.8.2 Model Tuning

We will now try to improve the accuracy of our GBM. To do this, we should first tune the model parameters like the number of trees, interaction depth, and shrinkage.

Table 2 Confusion matrix accuracy after prediction

Accuracy	1.0000000
Kappa	1.0000000
Accuracy lower	0.4781762
Accuracy upper	1.0000000
Accuracy null	0.8000000

Let the # of trees be 150 and maintaining the constant interaction depth, shrinkage be 0.001. Now train the model and measure the accuracies several times.

After seeing several times at the tuning model, there is no real change in the training accuracy. Thus there is no mere advantage of GBM model tuning.

4 Results

When we compare the existing experimental model with the actual data, our model does a pretty good job. We have compared our predictions to the actual test results.

When we observe the difference between the actual and predicted results (Figs. 8 and 9) there is a minute difference which can also be observed in the graph plot for visualization and estimation of accuracies.

In Fig. 10, we plotted a graph between actual (red) and predicted (green) data. But to plot a graph, we need accurate integers whereas our data set contains the cancer class in characters like ALL and AML. This may not be an accurate data type to plot a graph. Therefore, we have set a new output class named "out" which is an integer data type. To get this output class, we made cancer type ALL as 1 and AML as 0 (Figs. 8 and 9).

	patient <int>	cancer <chr>	out <dbl>
25	25	ALL	1
26	26	ALL	1
27	27	ALL	1
28	28	AML	0
29	29	AML	0
30	30	AML	0
31	31	AML	0
32	32	AML	0
33	33	AML	0
34	34	AML	0

Fig. 8 Data for prediction

	patientid <int>	cancer <fctr>	out <dbl>
25	25	ALL	1
26	26	ALL	1
27	27	ALL	1
28	28	AML	0
29	29	AML	0
30	30	AML	0
31	31	ALL	1
32	32	AML	0
33	33	ALL	1
34	34	AML	0

Fig. 9 Experimental data for prediction

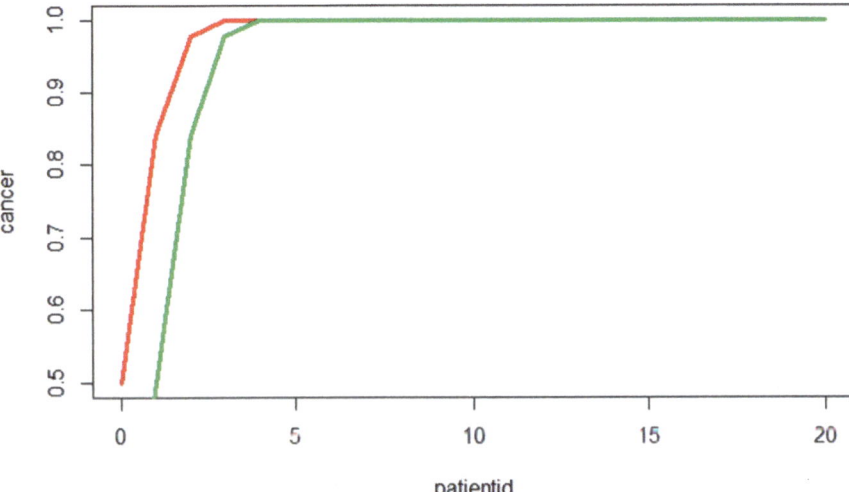

Fig. 10 A plot between actual and predicted data

5 Conclusion

We proposed a model using the Random Forest method which is trained with the gene expression data set. Although we have predicted the given cancer type is AML or ALL. The process tells the Leukemia classification problem to which class the input image belongs. The main concentration was on patient records which consist of gene accession number, gene descriptions, and experiments regarding particular genes. The feature extraction and classification both play a major role in a single frame. Feature scrutiny may include classification of the model that is: using patient medical history data AML regarding the information from a healthy individual and time to time results. Tissues should be recognized at the test during the Leukemia (ALL or AML). This model can be correlated with various architectures of random forest which may have a low error rate than the present model and with the models of

SVM, KNN for training the data. Then we have compared the model of measurement accuracy and each confidence model. The result clearly shows that the Random Forest algorithm can be implemented very well on prediction data when compared to other models.

References

1. Chu, F., Xie, W., Wang, L.: Gene selection and cancer classification using a fuzzy neural network, vol. 2, pp. 555–559 (2004)
2. Nahar, J., Chen, Y.-P.P., Shawkat Ali, A.B.M.: Micro-array classification and rule based cancer identification, pp. 43–46 (2007)
3. Wang, L., Chu, F., Xie, W.: Accurate cancer classification using expression of very few genes **4**(1), 40–53 (2007)
4. Xu, R., Anagnostopoulos, G.C., Wunsch, D.C.: Multiclass cancer classification using semisupervised ellipsoid ARTMAP and particle swarm optimization with gene expression data **4**(1), 65–77 (2007)
5. Yukinawa, N., Oba, S., Kato. K., Ishii, S.: Optimal aggregation of binary classifiers for multiclass cancer diagnosis using gene expression profile **6**(2), 333–343 (2009)
6. Luo, W., Wang, L., Sun, J.: Feature selection for cancer classification based on support vector machine **4**, 422–426 (2009)
7. Bilen, M., Işik, A.H., Yiğit, T.: A hybrid artificial neural network genetic algorithm approach for classification of micro array data, pp. 339–342 (2015)
8. Ganesan, T., Rajarajeswari, P.: Genetic algorithm based optimization to improve the cluster lifetime by optimal sensor placement in WSN's. Int. J. Innov. Technol. Explor. Eng. (IJITEE) **8**(8) (2019). ISSN: 2278-3075
9. Tasci, A., Ince, T., Guzelis, C.: A comparison of feature selection algorithms for cancer classification through gene expression data. In: 2017 10th International onference on Electrical and Electronics Engineering (ELECO), pp. 1352–1354 (2017)
10. Ganesan, T., Rajarajeswari, P.: Genetic algorithm approach improved by 2D lifting scheme for sensor node placement in optimal position. In: Second International Conference on Intelligent Sustainable Systems IEEE xplore, ISBN: 978-1-5386-7798-8978 (2019)
11. Harvey, B.S., Ji, S.-Y.: Cloud-scale genomic signals processing for robust large scale cancer genomic micro-array data analysis **21**(1), 238–245 (2017)
12. Kavitha, K.R., Nair Harishankar, U., Akhil, M.C.: PSO based feature selection of gene for cancer classification using SVM-RFE, pp. 1012–1016 (2018)
13. Guillen, P., Ebalunode, J.: Cancer classification based on microarray gene expression data using deep learning, pp. 1403–1405 (2016)
14. Zhu, Q.-X., Fan, Y., He, Y.-L., Xu, Y.: Effective cancer classification based on gene expression data using multidimensional mutual information ELM, pp. 954–958 (2018)
15. Ma, X., Tang, W., Wang, P., Guo, X., Gao, L.: Extracting stage specific and dynamic modules through analysing multiple networks associated with cancer progression **15**(2), 647–658 (2018)
16. Golub, et al.: Molecular classification of cancer: class discovery and class prediction by gene expression monitoring. Science **286**, 531–537
17. Supriyamenon, M., Rajarajeswari, P.: A review on association rule mining techniques with respect to their privacy preserving capabilities (KLEF). Int. J. Appl. Eng. Res. **12**(24), 15484–15488 (2017). ISSN 0973-4562
18. Amulya, P., Sai Meghana, S., Manisha, R.P.: A deep learning approach for brain tumor segmentation using convolution neural network. Int. J. Sci. Technol. Res. (2019)
19. Rajarajeswari, P., Supriya menon, M.: A contemporary way for enhancedmodeling of context aware privacy system in PPDM. J. Adv. Res. Dyn. Control Syst. **10**(01) (2018)

20. Krishna, N., Rajarajeswari, P., et al.: Recognition of fake currency note using convolutional neural networks. Int. J. Innov. Technol. Explor. Eng. (IJITEE) **8**(5) (2019). ISSN: 2278-3075
21. Jafarpisheh, N., Teshnehlab, M.: Cancer classification based on deep neural networks and emotional learning approach **12**(6), 258–263 (2018)

Estimation of Basic Reproduction Number and Herd Immunity for COVID-19 in India

Poulami Majumder and Partha Pratim Ray

Abstract In recent times, the rapid rise of the COVID-19 has imparted a devastating effect on human society. India has been perceiving the significant impacts of the COVID-19 in many ways. Estimation of basic reproduction number and herd immunity has become an important question which might support policy makers to take decisions for the improvement of the current scenario. In this chapter, the autoregressive integrated moving average (ARIMA) tool has been used to estimate confirm cases, discharge, deaths, and case fatality rate due to COVID-19 in India during March 1st–May 6th, 2020. The sequential bayesian (SB) method, Wallinga and Teunis approach (TD), exponential growth (EG), and maximum likelihood (ML) techniques are used to estimate the basic reproduction number and herd immunity due to COVID-19 in India. The findings are: basic reproduction number in earlier method as follows, 1.6998 (95% CI, 1.4595–1.9210), 1.8043 (95% CI, 1.6287–1.9894), 1.4685 (95% CI, 1.4672–1.4698) and 1.8931 (95% CI, 1.8655–1.9210) in SB, TD, EG, and ML, respectively. The estimations of herd immunity as follows for SB, TD, EG, and ML, such as, 0.4116 (95% CI, 0.3148–0.4794), 0.4457 (95% CI, 0.3860–0.4973), 0.3190 (95% CI, 0.3184 0.3196), and 0.4717 (95% CI, 0.4639 0.4794), respectively. Results demonstrate the significant impact of epidemic dynamics of COVID-19 in India.

Keywords COVID-19 · Basic reproduction number · Herd immunity · Forecasting · Data analysis

P. Majumder (✉)
Department of Biotechnology, Maulana Abul Kalam Azad University of Technology, Kolkata, West Bengal 700064, India
e-mail: plm89.majumder@gmail.com

P. P. Ray
Department of Computer Applications, Sikkim University, Gangtok, Sikkim 737102, India
e-mail: ppray@ieee.org

1 Introduction

COVID-19 has imparted a significant impact on human civilization in recent times [1–12]. Scientific community is busy solving the mystery behind vaccination of the COVID-19 [13–17]. It is not clear when the world will receive the vaccine and other drugs in near future. In such uncertainty, one should seek the possible alternative aspects related to the COVID-19, especially data science specific approaches [18–22]. Prior knowledge of the basic reproduction number and herd immunity could be very helpful to manage and control the COVID-19 scenario [23–29].

India is one of the most vulnerable and highly affected countries due to COVID-19 [30–36]. Such state of severity leads to huge loss of lives and socioeconomic breakdown in India [37–40]. Thus, it demands an estimation of basic reproduction number and herd immunity so that the policy makers of India could be served with the holistic data analytical results for decision-making. In this context, it can be referred that the basic reproduction number as the ratio of contagiousness or transmissibility of infectious agents [41–44]. Herd immunity refers to the proportion of the subjects with immunity in a given population [45, 46]. Thus, an approximation of such parameters could leverage significant amount of data insight for the dissemination of COVID-19 mitigation approaches.

Several studies have shown the effectiveness of ARIMA model to forecast COVID-19 in the recent past [47–59]. Thus, in this study, firstly we use the ARIMA models to forecast confirm daily cases, cure/discharge patients, deaths, and case fatality rates in India due to COVID-19. Secondly, we perform data analysis on the estimation of basic reproduction numbers in India. Lastly, the approximation of the herd immunity for Indian scenario has been done by using four different techniques namely the sequential bayesian method [60], Wallinga and Teunis approach [61], exponential growth [62, 63], and maximum likelihood [64].

The paper is organized as follows. Section 2 presents various methods and data related information used in this study. Section 3 shows important results and discusses their significance. Section 4 concludes this article.

2 Data and Method

2.1 Data Collection

The data was collected from the worldwide repository of the COVID-19 for India in the https://www.worldometers.info/coronavirus/country/india/ during March 1st–May 6th, 2020.

2.2 Data Design

We prepared the dataset against the four key factors such as confirm (cnf) cases, cure/discharge/migrated (cdm) cases, deaths (det), and case fatality rate (cfr) during the specific time period.

We calculated the basic reproduction number and corresponding herd immunity columns on the specific dataset for in-depth analysis.

2.3 Data Analysis

The following operations on the dataset have been performed, such as (i) forecasting for 90 days starting from May 7th, 2020, (ii) finding R_0, and (iii) finding herd immunity.

2.4 Tools Used

We used the RStudio 1.2.5033, R 3.6.3 on top of Windows 10 Professional, Intel Core i7 7th generation, 8 GB RAM to perform the data analysis. The packages like "*forecast*" and "*ggplot2*" are used in this study. Some built-in functions like "*read.csv*", "*seq*", "*ts*", "*auto.arima*", "*acf*", "*pacf*", "*hist*", "*dnorm*", "*lines*", "*forecast*", "*plot*", "*Box.test*", and "*accuracy*" are also included to analyze the dataset from various perspectives in this study.

2.5 Forecasting Model

In this work these functions such as, "*seq*", "*ts*", "*auto.arima*", "*forecast*", and "*plot*" are taken for forecasting R_0 and herd immunity data for 90 days. The forecasting method called "*auto.arima*" is used to set the lag values and diffing the time series values to the stationary state.

In this study, we used the ARIMA method to perform forecasting over four key parameters like confirm cases, cure/discharge/migrated cases, death cases, and case fatality ratio. This study implied drifting (D), zero, and non-zero mean (Z) while analyzing the forecast. This work also leveraged both the interception and non-interception schemes to model the parameters.

This can represent an $ARIMA(p', q)$ model based on a time series data $X_t - \alpha_1 X_{t-1} - \cdots - \alpha_i X_{t-p'} = \epsilon_t + \theta_1 \epsilon_1 + \cdots + \theta_q \epsilon_{t-q}$ as (1), where L is the lag operator, α, θ, and ϵ refer to the component of autoregressive segment, moving average segment, and error terms, respectively.

$$\left(1 - \sum_{i=1}^{p'} \alpha_i L^i\right) X_t = \left(1 + \sum_{i=1}^{q} \theta_i L^i\right) \epsilon_t \tag{1}$$

The (1) can be generalized as (2), i.e., $ARIMA(p, d, q)$ with drift $= \frac{\delta}{1-\sum \phi_i}$ and multiplicity d.

$$\left(1 - \sum_{i=1}^{p'} \phi_i L^i\right)(1 - L)^d X_t = \delta + \left(1 + \sum_{i=1}^{q} \theta_i L^i\right) \epsilon_t \tag{2}$$

Forecasting was done by using (3) and (4) for non-stationary and stationary data.

$$Y_t = (1 - L)^d X_t \tag{3}$$

$$\left(1 - \sum_{i=1}^{p} \phi_i L^i\right) Y_t = \left(1 + \sum_{i=1}^{q} \theta_i L^i\right) \epsilon_t \tag{4}$$

We used 95% confidence interval (CI) while following $\hat{y}_{T+h|T} \pm 1.96 \sqrt{v_{T+h|T}}$, where $v_{T+h|T}$ is assumed to be the variance over $y_{T+h|T}$.

2.6 R_0 Estimation Schemes

In this study, four schemes are used such as (i) Time Dependent Reproduction Number by Bayesian Approach (SB), (ii) Time Dependent Reproduction Number by Wallinga and Teunis Approach (TD), (iii) Exponential Growth (EG), and (iv) Maximum Likelihood (ML) to assess the R_0 and herd immunity on the dataset.

2.6.1 Sequential Bayesian (SB) Approach

While considering all the data on daily basis, i.e., sequential form such as, $X_1, X_2 \ldots, X_n$ with a requirement of unknown parameter θ. With a prior distribution of $\Pi(\theta)$ at the time n the density of COVID-19 data on conditional θ can be represented as (5)

$$f(x_1, \ldots, x_n|\theta) = f(x_1|\theta) f(x_2|x_1, \theta) \ldots f(x_n|x_{n-1}, \theta) \tag{5}$$

where $X_i = (x_1, \ldots, x_i)$. Here, we don't consider $X_1, X_2 \ldots, X_n$ to be independent on θ. We can update the distribution of θ to the posterior as follows (6):

$$\Pi_n(\theta) = f(\theta|x_n) \alpha \Pi(\theta) f(x_n|\theta) \tag{6}$$

If a new observation is $X_{n+1} = x_{n+1}$, then we can update like follows (7):

$$\Pi_{n+1}(\theta) = f\left(\theta | x_{n|1}\right) \alpha \Pi_n(\theta) f\left(x_{n+1}, \theta\right) \tag{7}$$

New prior distribution based on the prior data can be written on the $n+1$ time as follows (8):

$$\tilde{\Pi}_{n+1}(\theta) \alpha \Pi_n(\theta) f\left(x_{n+1} | x_n, \theta\right) \tag{8}$$

2.6.2 Wallinga and Teunis (TD) Approach

Wallinga and Teunis method provided the daily estimation of basic reproduction number with help of probability estimation of i, i.e., infected COVID-19 person with a gap between the onset days of two infected persons.

It is assumed that case i on the onset time t_i. For a single infected person, the probability of i person infected by j person can be described as follows (9):

$$p_{ij} = \frac{w\left(t_i - t_j\right)}{\sum_{l \neq i} w\left(t_i - T_j\right)} \tag{9}$$

The reproduction number can be estimated on the consideration of $\sum_{l \neq i} p_{ij}$ with (10)

$$R_j = \sum_i p_{ij} \tag{10}$$

2.6.3 Exponential Growth (EG)

It is assumed that the exponential growth of COVID-19 to be r that can be estimated by following the least square fitting method by using log-scale i.e. $\log(N_t)$. If $f_G(t)$ represents the probability density function, then R_0 can be obtained by using the Euler–Lotka equation as (11)

$$\widehat{R} = \frac{1}{\int_0^\infty e^{-rt} f_G(t)dt} \tag{11}$$

2.6.4 Maximum Likelihood (ML)

It is assumed that t, N_t represent the day and number of confirmed cases on the t day, respectively. With serial interval k days, the infection followed the Poisson distribution. If the serial interval of an individual COVID-19 infected person in j days remain to be w_j then priory discretized Gamma can produce likelihood function as follows (12):

$$L(R, w) = \prod_{t=1}^{T} \frac{e^{-\mu} \mu_t^{N_t}}{N_t!} \tag{12}$$

where

$$\mu_t = R \sum_{j=1}^{\min\{k,t\}} N_{t-j} w_j$$

The reproduction number can be estimated as $\widehat{R}$ by applying maximized likelihood against the given w_j as follows (13):

$$\widehat{R} = \frac{\sum_{t=1}^{T} N_t}{\sum_{t=1}^{T} \sum_{j=1}^{\min\{k,t\}} N_{t-j} w_j} \tag{13}$$

2.7 Herd Immunity Estimation

Herd immunity (HIT) estimation in this study is based on the prior computation of reproduction number in the following form (14)

$$HIT = 1 - \frac{1}{R_0} \tag{14}$$

Thus, if the HIT is close to 0, it is better for the COVID-19 epidemic and closer to 1 is worse for the epidemic scenario.

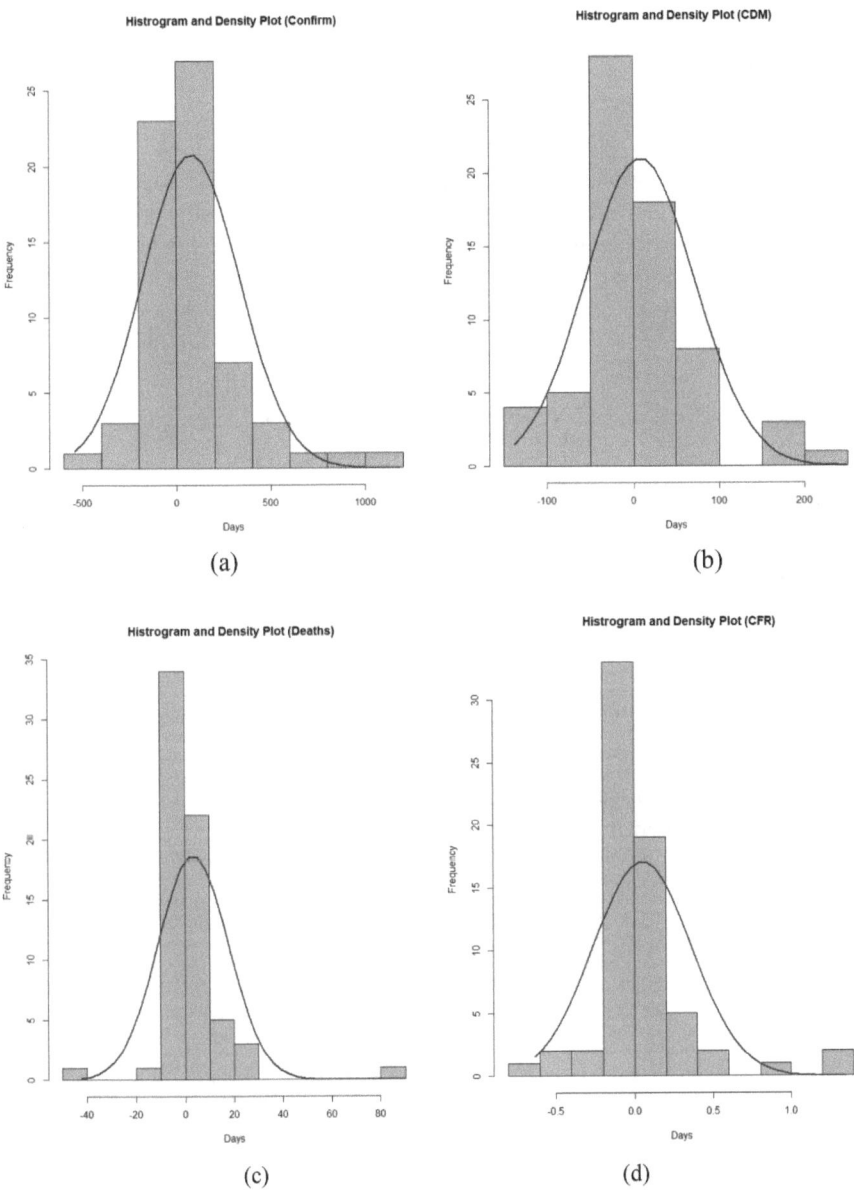

Fig. 1 Histogram and density plots of forecasting models, **a** cnf_forecast (90D), **b** cdm_forecast (90D), **c** det_forecast (90D), **d** cfr_forecast (90D)

3   Results and Discussion

3.1   Histogram and Density Plots

Various histogram and embedded density plots are presented in Fig. 1a–d for the cnf, cdm, det, and cfr variables, respectively. Kernel density estimation (KDE) has been done to estimate the density plot in this study. The KDE can be expressed as follows in Eq. (15) where K represents kernel over the density f which is based on a univariate sample set $(x_1, x_2, \ldots, x_n)$ with bandwidth $h > 0$ and a scaled kernel K_h.

$$\widehat{f}_h(x) = \frac{1}{n} \sum_{i=1}^{p} K_h(x - x_i) = \frac{1}{nh} \sum_{i=1}^{p} K\left(\frac{x - x_i}{h}\right) \tag{15}$$

Bandwidth selection was performed by asymptotic mean integrated squared error (AMISE) as (16).

$$h_{AMISE} = \frac{RK^{\frac{1}{5}}}{m_2(K)^{\frac{2}{5}} R(f'')^{\frac{1}{5}} n^{\frac{1}{5}}} \tag{16}$$

The bandwidth estimator is assumed to be Gaussian, that may formulate $h = \left(\frac{4\sigma^5}{3n}\right)^{\frac{1}{5}} \approx 1.06\sigma n^{\frac{-1}{5}}$, where n is the cardinality of the set.

The characteristic function (15) may be expressed with help of Fourier transform as (17), where the density estimator is $\widehat{f}(x)$ and ψ is the damping function.

$$\begin{aligned} \widehat{f}(x) &= \frac{1}{2\pi} \int_{-\infty}^{+\infty} \widehat{\varphi}(t)\psi_h(t)e^{-itx} dt \\ &= \frac{1}{2\pi} \int_{-\infty}^{+\infty} \frac{1}{n} \sum_{j=1}^{n} e^{it(x_j - x)} \psi(ht) dt = \frac{1}{nh} \sum_{j=1}^{n} K(\frac{x - x_j}{h}) \end{aligned} \tag{17}$$

3.2   Forecasting Model Parameters

Forecasting models are fitted and validated by utilizing the metrics like standard error (S.E.), log likelihood method, σ^2, Akaike information criterion (AIC), AIC correlation (AICC), Bayesian information criterion (BIC).

S.E. is the estimation of error in the standard deviation of the mean as expressed in (18), where σ and n are standard deviation and number of the population, respectively. We used (19) to find the S.E. of sample s of size n.

$$\sigma^- x = \frac{\sigma}{\sqrt{n}} \tag{18}$$

$$s^- x = \frac{s}{\sqrt{n}} \tag{19}$$

Log likelihood measures how good sample data are for fitting into a statistical model. Probability functions could be either discrete, continuous, or mixed. Discrete probability likelihood function is measured as $l(\theta|x) = p_\theta(x) = P_\theta(X = x)$, where θ, p, X represent a parameter, discrete random number, probability, respectively. Similarly, continuous likelihood function may be expressed as $l(\theta|x) = f_\theta(x) = p(X = x|\theta)$. The same could be written as $l(\theta|x) = f(x|\theta)$ for the parameterized model. Likelihood ratio refers to a ratio between two likelihood functions as $\lambda(\theta_1 : \theta_2|x) = \frac{l(\theta_1|x)}{l(\theta_2|x)}$ over a likelihood region $\{\theta : R(\theta) \geq \frac{p}{100}\}$. On the other hand, profile likelihood $\widehat{\beta_1} = \left(X_1^T\left(I - X_2(X_2^T X_2)^{-1}X_2^T\right)X_1\right)^{-1} X_1^T (I - X_2(X_2^T X_2)^{-1}X_2^T)y$. Finally, the log of likelihood could be expressed as $\log\frac{l(A)}{l(B)} = \log l(A) - \log l(B) = l(A) - l(B)$.

Variance is measured as $\sigma^2 = \frac{\sum(x_i - \mu)}{n}$, where μ is the mean of n sample data. AIC is computed as in (20)

$$AIC = -2\log(l) + 2(p + q + k) \tag{20}$$

AICC is computed as in (21)

$$AICC = AIC + 2\frac{(p + q + k)(p + q + k + 1)}{(T - p - q - k - 1)} \tag{21}$$

BIC is computed as in (22)

$$BIC = AIC + (\log(T) - 2)(p + q + k) \tag{22}$$

Here, l, p, q, k represent the likelihood of the sample data, order of autoregressive, moving average, and intercept of the underlying ARIMA model. Intercept depends on k, if it is 0 no intercept if 1 then intercept.

Figure 2a–d present the forecasting trends of four key parameters, (a) cnf_forecast (90D), (b) cdm_forecast (90D), (c) det_forecast (90D), (d) cfr_forecast (90D). Table 1 presents model forecasting parameters.

3.3 Model Accuracy

In this work, we performed the Ljung-Box test for finding the chi-squared (χ^2) distribution of the forecasting model and associated p value. If the p-value is less

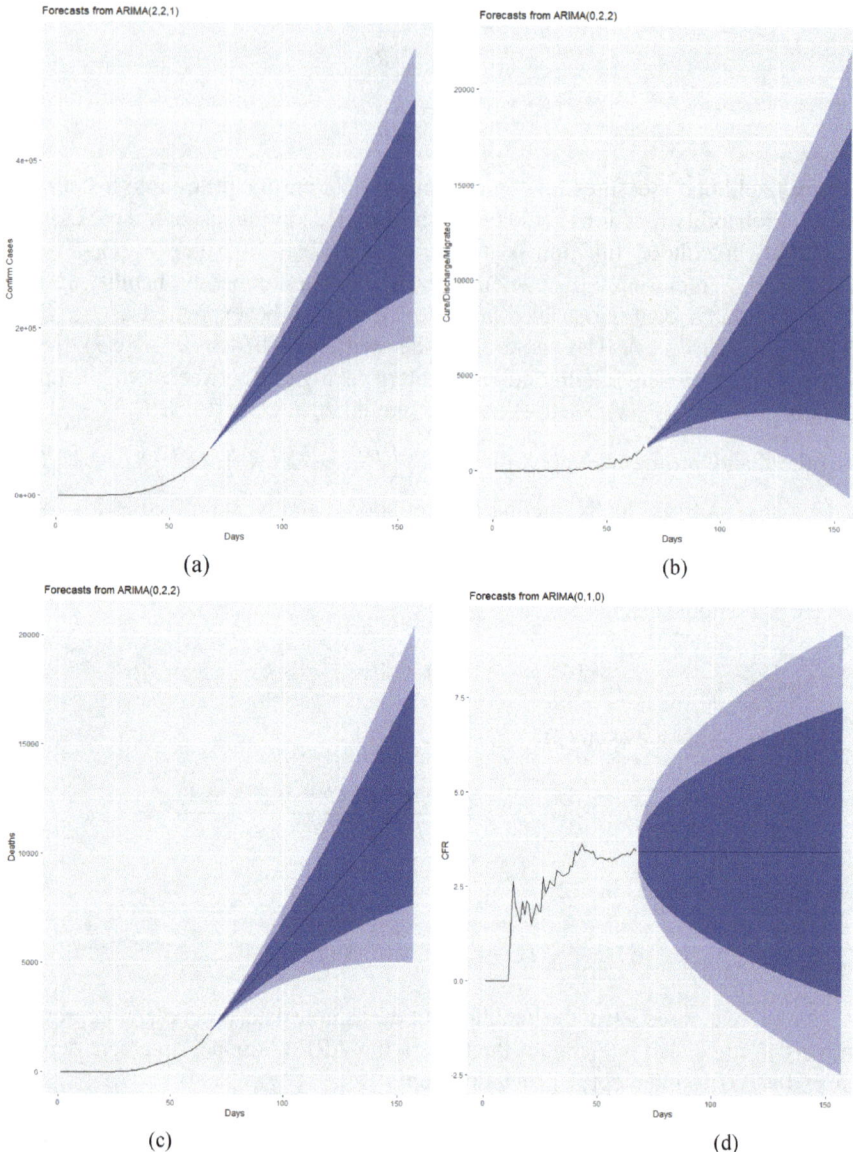

Fig. 2 Forecasting trends of key parameters, **a** cnf_forecast (90D), **b** cdm_forecast (90D), **c** det_forecast (90D), **d** cfr_forecast (90D)

Table 1 Comparison of forecasting model parameters

	Cnf	Cdm	det	cfr
ar1	−1.3367	0	0	0
ma1	0.8885	−1.4543	−0.8261	0
S.E	0.1228, 0.0919	0.0826	0.1653	0
σ^2	77,057	4327	227.2	227.2
Log(Likelihood)	−456.85	−364.61	−267.91	−17.79
AIC	921.7	735.21	541.83	37.65
AICC	922.36	735.6	542.22	37.65
BIC	390.36	741.73	548.35	39.78
Drift	0	0	0	0

than 0.05, then it is statistically significant. Otherwise, at 95% CI, it can be concluded that there is little evidence of non-zero autocorrelation in the in-sample forecast errors that lags 1 to df. Thus, further forecasting could be done. All the tests were conducted at 20 degree of freedom (df). The main aim of performing the Ljung–Box test was to check whether the autocorrelation of a group of time series data was different from 0, thus it carried total randomness on top of lag values.

The Ljung–Box test statistic could be expressed as (23)

$$Q = n(n+2) \sum_{k=1}^{h} \frac{\hat{\rho}_k^2}{n-k} \tag{23}$$

The randomness was measured by following $Q > \chi^2_{1-\alpha,h}$ with $n, k, h, \hat{\rho}$ refer to total number of sample data, lag, behind the lag, and autocorrelation, respectively.

We conducted error tests like mean error (ME), root mean square error ($RMSE$), mean absolute error (MAE), mean percentage error (MPE), mean absolute percentage error ($MAPE$), mean absolute scaled error ($MASE$), and autocorrelation of error at lag 1 ($ACF1$) for check proof the forecasting model. Table 2 presents the comparison of model accuracy in this study.

MAE is expressed as (24) to measure the average error in the forecasted value.

$$MAE = \frac{1}{n} \sum_{i=1}^{n} (|x_i - \hat{x}_i|) \tag{24}$$

$RMSE$ measures are quadratic of average error in the forecast.

$$RMSE = \sqrt{\frac{1}{n} \sum_{i=1}^{n} (|x_i - \hat{x}_i|)^2} \tag{25}$$

Table 2 Comparison of forecasting model accuracy

	Cnf	Cdm	Det	cfr
ME	78.685	8.352	3.466	0.0514
RMSE	267.032	63.766	14.616	0.314
MAE	150.94	34.893	6.711	0.1644
MPE	1562	−Inf	3.495	2.545
MAPE	6.59	Inf	9.547	9.050
MASE	0.188	0.8556	0.248	0.985
ACF1	−0.072	−0.1432	−0.039	−0.0342
χ^2	14.652	17.25	6.818	19.639
P	$p\,(0.796) > 0.05$	$p\,(0.6367) > 0.05$	$p\,(0.9972) > 0.05$	$p\,(0.4807) > 0.05$

Table 3 Comparison of point forecasting parameters for 90 days

Cnf	cdm	det	cfr
ARIMA(2, 2, 1)	ARIMA(0, 2, 2)	ARIMA(0, 2, 2)	ARIMA(0, 1, 0)

MPE is expressed as (26) to measure an average percentage error in the forecasted value that differs from the actual value.

$$MPE = \frac{100\%}{n} \sum_{i=1}^{n} \frac{a_t - f_t}{a_t} \tag{26}$$

$MAPE$ is expressed as (27) to measure an average absolute percentage error in the forecasted value that differs from the actual value.

$$MAPE = \frac{1}{n} \sum_{i=1}^{n} \frac{a_t - f_t}{a_t} \tag{27}$$

$MASE$ is expressed as (28) to measure non-seasonal scaled error $|e_i|$ for a time series forecasting.

$$MASE = mean\left(\frac{|e_i|}{\frac{1}{T-1} \sum_{t=2}^{T} |Y_t - Y_{t-1}|}\right) = \frac{\frac{1}{J} \sum_i |e_i|}{\frac{1}{T-1} \sum_{t=2}^{T} |Y_t - Y_{t-1}|} \tag{28}$$

Table 4 Comparison of point forecasting and maximum possible range for 90 days

	Average	Max (80% CI)	Max (95% CI)
cnf	362,432	478,386	539,769
cdm	10,383	2665	18,101
det	12,795	17,866	20,551
cfr	3.446%	7.298%	9.337%

3.4 Point Forecasting

Table 3 shows comparisons of pointwise forecasting for 90 days duration of COVID-19 parameters of India. The comparisons against cnf, cdm, det, and cfr parameters have been conducted. This work also estimated the futuristic achievable values. The various $ARIMA(p, d, q, X)$ schemes are included to ensure the quality of the forecasting models.

Notations of following $ARIMA(p, d, q, X)$ could be assumed as (i) $ARIMA(0, 1, 0)$ represents a random walk in the dataset and (ii) $ARIMA(0, 2, 2)$ represents the Holts' linear model with error in the dataset.

Table 4 shows the comparison of point forecast, maximum of 80% CI, and maximum of 95% CI for 90 days forecasting in India.

3.5 R_0 Estimation

Table 5 presents a comparison among four types of resultants of basic reproduction number (R_0) for example, SB: time dependent reproduction number by Bayesian approach, TD: time dependent reproduction number by Wallinga and Teunis approach, EG: exponential growth, and ML: maximum likelihood. In all cases, R_0 values exceed 1, i.e., epidemic persistence. Figure 3 represents the dynamics of R_0 during the computational period.

Table 5 Comparison of basic reproduction numbers

	SB	TD	EG	ML
R_0	1.6998	1.8043	1.4685	1.8931
95% CI Lo	1.4595	1.6287	1.4672	1.85655
95% CI Hi	1.9210	1.9894	1.4698	1.9210

$R_0 > 1$: Epidemic

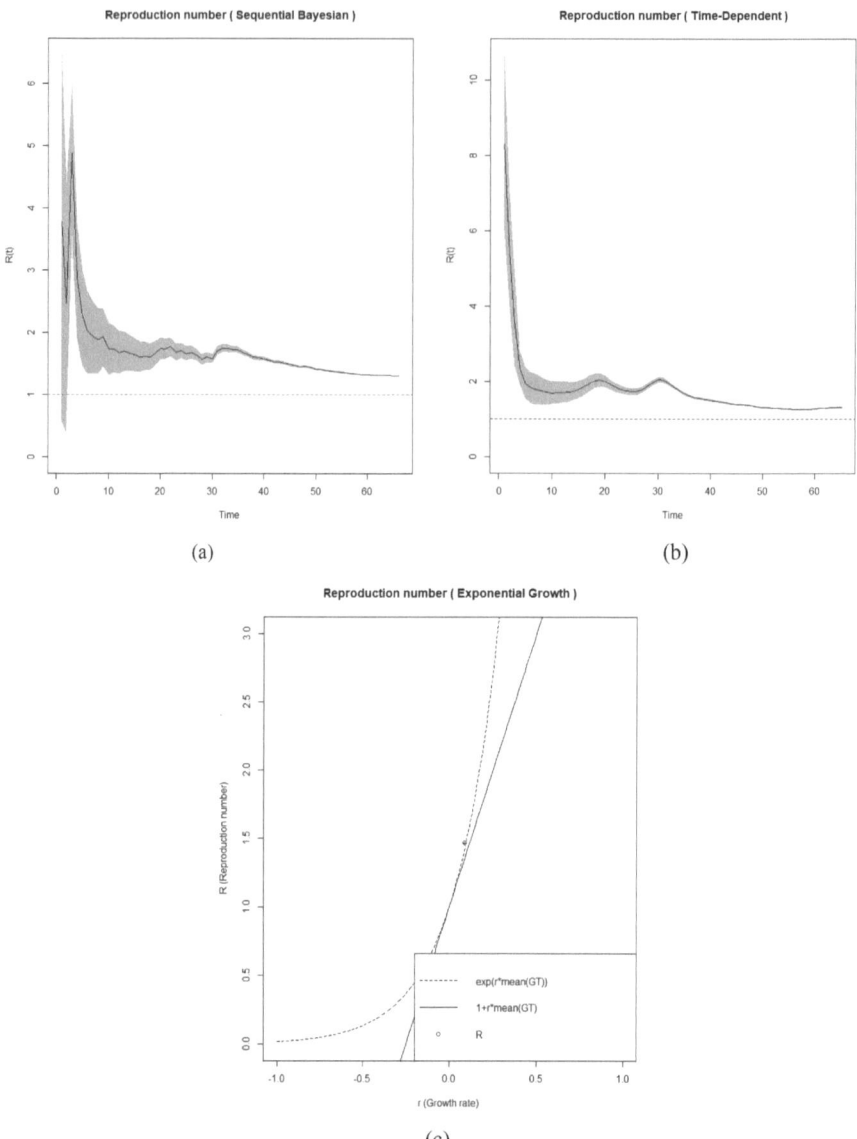

Fig. 3 Comparison of basic reproduction number charts, **a** SB, **b** TD, **c** EG

3.6 HIT Estimation

Table 6 presents the comparison between HIT estimation against the R_0 obtained in the earlier section. It is assumed that it is better if HIT goes towards 0, worse if moves towards 1. In the present scenario, HIT seems to be in worse dynamics.

Table 6 Comparison of herd immunity (HIT)

	SB	TD	EG	ML
R_0	0.411	0.4557	0.319	0.4717
95% CI Lo	0.3148	0.3860	0.3184	0.4639
95% CI Hi	0.4794	0.4970	0.3196	0.4794

$0 \leq HIT \leq 1$: Epidemic. Better if towards 0, worse if towards 1

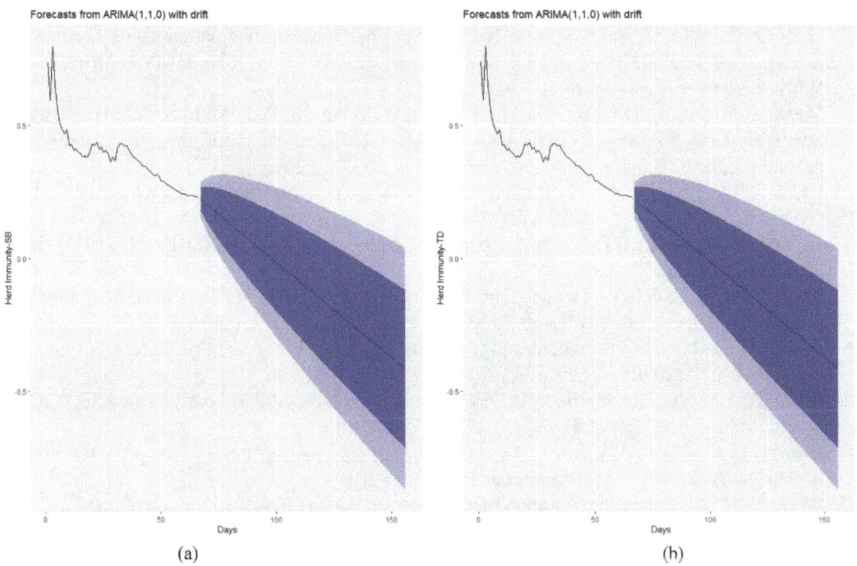

(a)   (h)

Fig. 4 Comparison of 90 days forecasting of herd immunity, **a** SB, **b** TD

Figure 4 compares values of 90 days forecasting of the herd immunity following SB and TD methods.

4 Conclusion

In this study, we estimated approximated values of basic reproduction number and corresponding herd immunity due to COVID 19 in India. We also performed forecasting of cnf, cdm, det, and cfr points estimation for 90 days using ARIMA. This study reveals the impactful effect of data analytics on the existing COVID-19 situation in India. Though herd immunity has not been achieved at the time of this study, however, it is expected to gain herd immunity during January–April, 2021. As the R_0 is linearly related to the herd immunity, thus the epidemic level of current COVID-19 spread-dynamics may be nullified during the aforementioned time. The key parameters such as daily confirmed cases, cure rate, deaths, and death rate are expected to get stabilize during early to mid, 2021, upon fulfilling all the preventive and curative measures as directed by the WHO and local administrative bodies.

References

1. COVID, Team CDC, and Response Team: Severe outcomes among patients with coronavirus disease 2019 (COVID-19)-United States, February 12–March 16, 2020. MMWR Morb. Mortal Wkly. Rep. **69**(12), 343–346 (2020)
2. Mehta, P., McAuley, D.F., Brown, M., Sanchez, E., Tattersall, R.S., Manson, J.J., HLH Across Speciality Collaboration: COVID-19: consider cytokine storm syndromes and immunosuppression. Lancet (London, England) **395**(10229), 1033 (2020)
3. Fauci, A.S., Clifford Lane, H., Redfield, R.R.: Covid-19: navigating the uncharted 1268–1269 (2020)
4. Hollander, J.E., Carr, B.G.: Virtually perfect? Telemedicine for COVID-19. N. Engl. J. Med. **382**(18), 1679–1681 (2020)
5. Bai, Y., Yao, L., Wei, T., Tian, F., Jin, D.-Y., Chen, L., Wang, M.: Presumed asymptomatic carrier transmission of COVID-19. JAMA **323**(14), 1406–1407 (2020)
6. Cao, X.: COVID-19: immunopathology and its implications for therapy. Nat. Rev. Immunol. **20**(5), 269–270 (2020)
7. Dong, E., Hongru, Du., Gardner, L.: An interactive web-based dashboard to track COVID-19 in real time. Lancet. Infect. Dis **20**(5), 533–534 (2020)
8. Rothan, H.A., Byrareddy, S.N.: The epidemiology and pathogenesis of coronavirus disease (COVID-19) outbreak. J. Autoimmun. 102433 (2020)
9. World Health Organization: Coronavirus disease 2019 (COVID-19): situation report **72** (2020)
10. Velavan, T.P., Meyer, C.G.: The COVID-19 epidemic. Tropical Med. Int. Health **25**(3), 278 (2020)
11. Lipsitch, M., Swerdlow, D.L., Finelli, L.: Defining the epidemiology of Covid-19—studies needed. N. Engl. J. Med. **382**(13), 1194–1196 (2020)
12. Liu, W., Zhang, Q., Chen, J., Xiang, R., Song, H., Shu, S., Chen, L., et al.: Detection of Covid-19 in children in early January 2020 in Wuhan, China. N. Engl. J. Med. **382**(14), 1370–1371 (2020)
13. Le, T.T., Andreadakis, Z., Kumar, A., Gomez Roman, R., Tollefsen, S., Saville, M., Mayhew, S.: The COVID-19 vaccine development landscape. Nat. Rev. Drug. Discov. **19**(5), 305–306 (2020)
14. Hotez, P.J., Corry, D.B., Bottazzi, M.E.: COVID-19 vaccine design: the Janus face of immune enhancement. Nat. Rev. Immunol. **20**(6), 347–348 (2020)
15. Peeples, L.: News feature: avoiding pitfalls in the pursuit of a COVID-19 vaccine. Proc. Natl. Acad. Sci. **117**(15), 8218–8221 (2020)
16. Graham, B.S.: Rapid COVID-19 vaccine development. Science **368**(6494), 945–946 (2020)
17. Corey, L., Mascola, J.R., Fauci, A.S., Collins, F.S.: A strategic approach to COVID-19 vaccine R&D. Science **368**(6494), 948–950 (2020)
18. Ray, D., Salvatore, M., Bhattacharyya, R., Wang, L., Du, J., Mohammed, S., Purkayastha, S., et al.: Predictions, role of interventions and effects of a historic national lockdown in India's response to the COVID-19 pandemic: data science call to arms. Harvard Data Sci. Rev. **2020**(Suppl 1) (2020)
19. Latif, S., Usman, M., Manzoor, S., Iqbal, W., Qadir, J., Tyson, G., Castro, I., et al.: Leveraging data science to combat COVID-19: a comprehensive review (2020)
20. Wang, C.J., Ng, C.Y., Brook, R.H.: Response to COVID-19 in Taiwan: big data analytics, new technology, and proactive testing. JAMA **323**(14), 1341–1342 (2020)

21. Ting, D.S., Wei, L.C., Dzau, V., Wong, T.Y.: Digital technology and COVID-19. Nat. Med. **26**(4), 459–461 (2020)
22. Ienca, M., Vayena, E.: On the responsible use of digital data to tackle the COVID-19 pandemic. Nat. Med. **26**(4), 463–464 (2020)
23. Randolph, H.E., Barreiro, L.B.: Herd immunity: understanding COVID-19. Immunity **52**(5), 737–741 (2020)
24. Kwok, K.O., Lai, F., Wei, W.I., Wong, S.Y.S., Tang, J.W.T.: Herd immunity–estimating the level required to halt the COVID-19 epidemics in affected countries. J. Infect. **80**(6), e32–e33 (2020)
25. Syal, K.: COVID-19: herd immunity and convalescent plasma transfer therapy. J. Med. Virol. (2020)
26. Park, H., Kim, S.H.: A study on herd immunity of COVID-19 in South Korea: using a stochastic economic-epidemiological model. Environ. Resour. Econ. 1–6 (2020)
27. Britton, T., Ball, F., Trapman, P.: A mathematical model reveals the influence of population heterogeneity on herd immunity to SARS-CoV-2. Science **369**(6505), 846–849 (2020)
28. Chaves, L.F., Hurtado, L.A., Rojas, M.R., Friberg, M.D., Rodríguez, R.M., Avila-Aguero, M.L.: COVID-19 basic reproduction number and assessment of initial suppression policies in Costa Rica. Math. Modell. Natl. Phenom. **15**, 32 (2020)
29. Patrikar, S.R., Kotwal, A., Bhatti, V.K., Banerjee, A., Chatterjee, K., Kunte, R., Tambe, M.: Incubation period and reproduction number for novel coronavirus 2019 (COVID-19) infections in India. Asia Pacif. J. Publ. Health (2020). 1010539520956427
30. Singhal, T.: A review of coronavirus disease-2019 (COVID-19). Indian J. Pediatr. 1–6 (2020)
31. Roy, D., Tripathy, S., Kar, S.K., Sharma, N., Verma, S.K., Kaushal, V.: Study of knowledge, attitude, anxiety and perceived mental healthcare need in Indian population during COVID-19 pandemic. Asian J. Psychiatry 102083 (2020)
32. Pramesh, C.S., Badwe, R.A.: Cancer management in India during Covid-19. N. Engl. J. Med. **382**(20), e61 (2020)
33. Sarkar, K., Khajanchi, S., Nieto, J.J.: Modeling and forecasting the COVID-19 pandemic in India. Chaos, Solitons Fractals **139**, 110049 (2020)
34. Sharma, S., Zhang, M., Gao, J., Zhang, H., Kota, S.H.: Effect of restricted emissions during COVID-19 on air quality in India. Sci. Total Environ. **728**, 138878 (2020)
35. Chatterjee, K., Chatterjee, K., Kumar, A., Shankar, S.: Healthcare impact of COVID-19 epidemic in India: a stochastic mathematical model. Med. J. Armed Forces India (2020)
36. Dsouza, D.D., Quadros, S., Hyderabadwala, Z.J., Mamun, M.A.: Aggregated COVID-19 suicide incidences in India: fear of COVID-19 infection is the prominent causative factor. Psychiatry Res. 113145 (2020)
37. Ozili, P.K., Arun, T.: Spillover of COVID-19: impact on the global economy. Available at SSRN 3562570 (2020)
38. Paital, B., Das, K., Parida, S.K.: Inter nation social lockdown versus medical care against COVID-19, a mild environmental insight with special reference to India. Sci. Total Environ. 138914 (2020)
39. Chakraborty, I., Maity, P.: COVID-19 outbreak: migration, effects on society, global environment and prevention. Sci. Total Environ. 138882 (2020)
40. Wasdani, K.P., Prasad, A.: The impossibility of social distancing among the urban poor: the case of an Indian slum in the times of COVID-19. Local Environ. **25**(5), 414–418 (2020)
41. Delamater, P.L., Street, E.J., Leslie, T.F., Tony Yang, Y., Jacobsen, K.H.: Complexity of the basic reproduction number (R_0). Emerg. Infect. Dis. **25**(1), 1 (2019)
42. Zhao, S., Lin, Q., Ran, J., Musa, S.S., Yang, G., Wang, W., Lou, Y., et al.: Preliminary estimation of the basic reproduction number of novel coronavirus (2019-nCoV) in China, from 2019 to 2020: a data-driven analysis in the early phase of the outbreak. Int. J. Infect. Dis. **92**, 214–217 (2020)
43. Zhou, T., Liu, Q., Yang, Z., Liao, J., Yang, K., Bai, W., Xin, Lu., Zhang, W.: Preliminary prediction of the basic reproduction number of the Wuhan novel coronavirus 2019-nCoV. J. Evid. Based Med. **13**(1), 3–7 (2020)

44. Van den Driessche, P., Watmough, J.: Further notes on the basic reproduction number. In: Mathematical Epidemiology, pp. 159–178. Springer, Berlin, Heidelberg (2008)
45. John, T.J., Samuel, R.: Herd immunity and herd effect: new insights and definitions. Eur. J. Epidemiol. **16**(7), 601–606 (2000)
46. Brisson, M., Edmunds, W.J.: Economic evaluation of vaccination programs: the impact of herd-immunity. Med. Decis. Making **23**(1), 76–82 (2003)
47. Ceylan, Z.: Estimation of COVID-19 prevalence in Italy, Spain, and France. Sci. Total Environ. 138817 (2020)
48. Singh, R.K., Rani, M., Bhagavathula, A.S., Sah, R., Rodriguez-Morales, A.J., Kalita, H., Nanda, C., et al.: Prediction of the COVID-19 pandemic for the top 15 affected countries: advanced autoregressive integrated moving average (ARIMA) model. JMIR Publ. Health Surveill. **6**(2), e19115 (2020)
49. Benvenuto, D., Giovanetti, M., Vassallo, L., Angeletti, S., Ciccozzi, M.: Application of the ARIMA model on the COVID-2019 epidemic dataset. Data in Brief 105340 (2020)
50. Yang, Q., Wang, J., Ma, H., Wang, X.: Research on COVID-19 based on ARIMA Model∆— Taking Hubei, China as an example to see the epidemic in Italy. J. Infect. Publ. Health (2020)
51. Ribeiro, M.H.D.M., da Silva, R.G., Mariani, V.C., dos Santos Coelho, L.: Short-term forecasting COVID-19 cumulative confirmed cases: perspectives for Brazil. Chaos, Solitons Fractals 109853 (2020)
52. Chintalapudi, N., Battineni, G., Amenta, F.: COVID-19 disease outbreak forecasting of registered and recovered cases after sixty day lockdown in Italy: a data driven model approach. J. Microbiol. Immunol. Infect. (2020)
53. Pourghasemi, H.R., Pouyan, S., Farajzadeh, Z., Sadhasivam, N., Heidari, B., Babaei, S., Tiefenbacher, J.P.: Assessment of the outbreak risk, mapping and infection behavior of COVID-19: application of the autoregressive integrated-moving average (ARIMA) and polynomial models. Plos one **15**(7), e0236238 (2020)
54. Payne, J., Morgan, A.: COVID-19 and violent crime: a comparison of recorded offence rates and dynamic forecasts (ARIMA) for March 2020 in Queensland, Australia (2020)
55. Kufel, T.: ARIMA-based forecasting of the dynamics of confirmed Covid-19 cases for selected European countries. Equilib. Quart. J. Econ. Econ. Policy **15**(2), 181–204 (2020)
56. Moftakhar, L., Mozhgan, S.E.I.F., Safe, M.S.: Exponentially increasing trend of infected patients with COVID-19 in Iran: a comparison of neural network and ARIMA forecasting models. Iran. J. Publ. Health **49**, 92–100 (2020)
57. Chakraborty, T., Ghosh, I.: Real-time forecasts and risk assessment of novel coronavirus (COVID-19) cases: a data-driven analysis. Chaos, Solitons Fractals 109850 (2020)
58. Fadly, F., Sari, E.: An approach to measure the death impact of Covid-19 in Jakarta using autoregressive integrated moving average (ARIMA). Unnes J. Publ. Health **9**(2) (2020)
59. Ilie, O.-D., Cojocariu, R.-O., Ciobica, A., Timofte, S.-I., Mavroudis, I., Doroftei, B.: Forecasting the spreading of COVID-19 across nine countries from Europe, Asia, and the American Continents using the ARIMA models. Microorganisms **8**(8), 1158 (2020)
60. Kadi, A.S., Avaradi, S.R.: A bayesian inferential approach to quantify the transmission intensity of disease outbreak. Comput. Math. Methods Med. (2015)
61. Wallinga, J., Teunis, P.: Different epidemic curves for severe acute respiratory syndrome reveal similar impacts of control measures. Am. J. Epidemiol. **160**(6), 509–516 (2004)
62. Obadia, T., Haneef, R., Boëlle, P.-Y.: The R_0 package: a toolbox to estimate reproduction numbers for epidemic outbreaks. BMC Med. Inform. Decis. Mak. **12**(1), 1–9 (2012)
63. Glass, K., Mercer, G.N., Nishiura, H., McBryde, E.S., Becker, N.G.: Estimating reproduction numbers for adults and children from case data. J. R. Soc. Interface **8**(62), 1248–1259 (2011)
64. You, C., Deng, Y., Hu, W., Sun, J., Lin, Q., Zhou, F., Pang, C.H., Zhang, Y., Chen, Z., Zhou, X.-H.: Estimation of the time-varying reproduction number of COVID-19 outbreak in China. Int. J. Hyg. Environ. Health 113555 (2020)

Artificial Intelligence in Medicine: Diabetes as a Model

Gumpeny R. Sridhar⊙ and Gumpeny Lakshmi⊙

Abstract Despite making a late entry into clinical medicine, artificial intelligence (AI) is finding a role in diverse fields: in imaging (radiology, pathological images, skin conditions, retinal conditions of the eye), in the diagnosis of disease, predicting disease onset, treatment outcomes, and recently unraveling previously hidden associations. AI-based applications are available for identifying diabetic eye changes. As AI comes into mainstream medicine, issues of privacy, security, and ethics must be addressed. AI systems promise to improve medical care by supplementing rather than supplanting human interventions.

Keywords Deep learning · Diagnosis · Imaging · Neural networks · Ethics · Security · Clinical · Health economics · Holistic

1 Introduction

Artificial intelligence refers to 'machines performing human-like cognitive functions (e.g., learning, understanding, reasoning, and interacting)' [1]. This can at best be considered a starting point, because one must first define what is meant by 'intelligence' and by 'artificial'. The origin of artificial intelligence can be traced back to the late 1940s and early 1950s, with progressive approximation of abilities between machines and humans [2]. The operative word is 'artificial' in AI, where the intention is not to imitate the intelligence of humans, but to 'explore the ability to build intelligent artefacts' [2]. Such form of AI is called 'General Artificial Intelligence'. Therefore, AI doesn't aim at imitating humans, but seeks to be inspired by them. It may be considered a discipline that 'uses the computer-processing capabilities of

G. R. Sridhar (✉)
Endocrine and Diabetes Centre, 15-12-15 Krishnanagar, Visakhapatnam, India
e-mail: sridharvizag@gmail.com

G. Lakshmi
Assistant Professor, Department of General Medicine, Gayatri Vidya Parishad Institute of Healthcare & Medical Technology, Visakhapatnam, India
e-mail: laukhhi.gumpeny@gmail.com

© The Author(s), under exclusive license to Springer Nature Singapore Pte Ltd. 2021   283
K. G. Srinivasa et al. (eds.), *Artificial Intelligence for Information Management: A Healthcare Perspective*, Studies in Big Data 88,
https://doi.org/10.1007/978-981-16-0415-7_14

symbols to find generic methods for automating perceptual, cognitive and manipulative activities via algorithms' [2]. The functional areas relate to problem-solving, knowledge representation and reasoning, planning of actions, learning, communication, perception and action, and finally philosophical and cognitive foundation [2]. When applied to clinical medicine, it straddles the fields of natural science, social science, and technical science [3]. Broadly speaking, it can be utilized in the hospital setting before identification, in the identification, and after identification of disease.

The definition of AI is not merely teleological. Different choices can lead to different directions of research. Defining the definition is not unique to the field of AI; while discussing the concept of 'probability', Carnap identified four aspects to be considered: similarity to the explicandum, exactness, fruitfulness, and simplicity. Wang elaborated on how these could be applied to arrive at a working definition of AI [4].

The presentation is divided into the following sections: Availability of data for analysis, broad scope and need for AI in clinical care, their potential applications and concerns, particular applications to diabetes and related metabolic disorders, use in diabetic retinopathy from India and from around the world, guidelines for the use in telehealth, the current status, and outlook for the future.

1.1 Availability of Data

The foundation of data mining and artificial intelligence lies in the availability of sufficient data. Until advances in information technology were widely available, capture and analysis of data formed the bottleneck in biological and clinical sciences [5]. The widespread use of electronic medical record system [6], omics data from nucleotides, proteomics, and metabolomics [7], images and data captured in electronic format from sensors in the hospitals, as well as outside (e.g. smartwatches, continuous glucose monitoring, blood pressure monitoring) [8] changed the equation: the constraint lay not in the availability of data, but in the ability to analyze and put it to appropriate use for improving clinical care [9, 10].

Once data became available, there were 'unprecedented opportunities—and daunting challenges' [11]. A wide variety of clinical sciences appear to embrace AI: some are logical and incremental such as identifying eye conditions using digital images, others are game-changing such as identifying the risk of heart disease from images of the eye. Other areas include diagnosing skin diseases, some forms of cancer using histopathological images, interpreting x-rays, computerized tomographic scans, and predictive methods to calculate patients who are at risk of developing complications in the intensive care units. On a broader scale, the 'flattened earth' enables expertise to reach remote communities where experts cannot be physically present. However, there are issues yet to be resolved: how can one translate these advances into routine clinical practice? How much can one depend merely on AI for clinical decisions? Do they offer a logical and understandable explanation for the advice that is provided, rather than as a 'black box' as in non-human related decision-making. How and when does one prefer the AI system's decision to be based on providing an understandable explanation, rather than appearing to come out of a 'black box'. Can insisting on the former compromise the efficiency of the latter? A gaze into the crystal ball suggested that in a little over 40 years hence, there is a 50% chance that machines can outperform tasks done by humans [12]. As things stand, the challenges are in integrating AI tools and platforms, rather than their replacing humans in expertise.

1.2 Scope and Need for AI in Clinical Care

While some of the developed nations spend nearly 18% of GDP on health, the outcomes are not proportionate to the money spent. Simultaneously, there is a burgeoning amount of data that is being generated as alluded to earlier: from medical images, biosensor information, genome sequences, and electronic medical records. Some of the poor outcomes of health spending result from an inability to synthesize and use the large amount of data to make proper decisions [13]. AI has the potential to bypass some of the deficiencies such as errors in diagnosis, treatment mistakes, inefficient workflow, and limited availability of time to interact with patients. One can expect pattern recognition using deep neural networks to be incorporated in routine clinical care.

Technically it should be feasible for a medical decision to be reviewed by a team of appropriate experts who would then give guidance, but that time is not yet arrived [14]. Before one moves ahead, it is necessary to realize that there is no clear distinction between machine learning methods and traditional statistical models. The machine learning model is able to learn from examples and does not need any pre-specified rules. Humans can analyze and make associations using a limited amount of data. Currently, machine learning requires a lot more data, although this limitation is being addressed. The greater the amount of data that is available, the better the output from machine learning methods; besides, machines do not have attention lapses unlike human beings [14].

1.3 Potential Applications of AI in Medical Care

Before one can integrate AI into routine clinical care, there are barriers, the chief of which is data stored in electronic medical records. Often the records exist in silos, limited to a single institution or a group of institutions. They exist in different forms: numeric, free text, images, and sometimes as digitized handwritten notes. It is necessary to first homogenize data from their disparate forms and make them suitable for analysis; this is in addition to ensuring that a valid diagnosis is agreed upon by the medical experts themselves [15].

Broadly AI can be useful in various areas such as (a) **Radiology**: for suspecting pneumonia in chest x-ray, fractures of wrist, of the vertebrae in the spine, nodules in the lung, liver masses. (b) **Pathological images**: Digitizing pathological images from slides has been slower compared to radiological imaging. However, deep learning algorithms were developed to classify different classes of cancer in the lung and in the breast. When validated by a trained pathologist, the use of AI speeded up the review of slides. Another advantage with deep learning is the ability to sharpen out of focus images. (c) **Skin diseases**: Deep learning network diagnosis of skin cancer by using images was compared with that of domain experts (dermatologists). When a large training set of more than 125,000 photographs was employed, the diagnostic ability was at least as good as that of US board certified dermatologists. Similar results were obtained in diagnosing a variety of other skin conditions. One must realize that comparison was made by using only images. They were not studied in clinical conditions, where the doctor performs physical inspection and acquires other relevant information. (d) **Diseases of the eye**: It i s i ndentifying eye diseases that the performance of algorithms has been the most widely studied. Specifically, validation has been reported for the identification of different forms of diabetic eye disease (diabetic retinopathy) using AI. Other eye conditions such as glaucoma (increased intraocular pressure) and papilledema (swelling of the optic disc) can also be detected by AI. A more detailed account will be provided in later sections dealing with the application of AI to eye diseases. (e) **Others**: AI has been applied to other conditions such as heart disease (interpreting electrocardiograms), gastrointestinal disorders (polyps of the intestine), and to psychiatry [13].

AI can be profitably employed as an initial screening tool before referral to a specialist. This would lower the workload on the specialist, who can then carefully deal with those who have suspected disease requiring specific attention and treatment.

1.4   Potential Concerns in Implementing AI in Medical Care

Although the potential for AI use in clinical medicine is vast, one must consider the current limitations. In their present form, most AI models are classifiers, rather than being able to provide precise prediction in an *individual* subject; secondly being able to extract (incomplete) data in many forms from the records is a significant problem in itself. Lastly, other variables that are not traditionally recorded may play a significant role in risk assessment. These include socioeconomic, psychological, behavioral and of late, sensor data [13]. In addition, it is difficult to apportion blame when an error occurs as a result of using AI in decision-making: who is to blame when there are so many sources of variability—the provider of training data, the developer of the algorithm or the clinician who employed the system? This brings to the fore an ability to clarify the logic behind decisions arrived at by the AI system, and the limitation in the efficiency of the system if clarity is sought for each decision that is made. In the interest of patients, AI platforms must adhere to the same standards of outcome as any other medical platform, because the health outcome of an individual is at stake [13].

Not only is data needed for initial training, but it must be continually fed for ongoing training, validation, and improvement. This entails availability in a usable form that is deidentified from various sources, bringing forth issues of cybersecurity. Concerns may arise on the sharing of data. The original model must be fine-tuned for local conditions by being trained with local data. Similarly, transparency in the development of algorithms may not be provided by commercial organizations, leading to concerns of safety and culpability [16].

Finally, usability issues could be the weakest part of the link: the AI should be integrated into the clinical workflow to be useful in real-life settings. This requires financial commitments including training of healthcare workers, which may not produce immediate returns.

2 Application of Deep Neural Network Models in Non-communicable Diseases

Diabetes forms a substantial part of non-communicable diseases that include cardiovascular disease, cancers, and chronic diseases of the lung. As their causation is complex, it is difficult to foresee their development before they are clinically manifest. Because the clinician must deal with many variables in a limited time, it is difficult to assimilate all the data and come to an accurate decision. Neural network models can aid in the prediction of chronic diseases by considering them as a multi-label classification problem [17].

2.1 Chronic Disease Prediction

Multi-label classification belongs to a supervised learning problem where an event may have multiple simultaneous labels. These methods are employed in a variety of conditions—not only in disease prediction but also in image classification and semantic analysis. Problem transformation methods, which employ multi-label algorithms first 'convert multi-label classification problem into several binary classification problems or a multi-class classification problem'. Secondly, they are handled by applying original machine learning algorithms [17]. Zhang et al. used a convolutional neural network method for classifying chronic diseases based on records of physical examination. By employing a group block, the number of convolution parameters was reduced to improve the performance in classification. They also introduced a novel architecture 'GroupNet to classify multiple chronic diseases, which improved the classification by devising 'correlated loss' [17]. Efforts are being made to enhance its learning ability.

2.2 Employing Machine Learning for Clustering of Cardiometabolic Risk Factors

Diabetes can manifest with differences in the risk of complications. Unlike nonmodifiable factors which by definition cannot be modified, if modifiable risk factors can be identified, there is a potential for correcting them to reduce complications. Liao X et al. employed machine learning method to assess the contribution of different risk factors [18]. Using data from a large sample of adults from a wellness improvement program (n: 2,17,254), a logistic regression method was employed to study the relation between distinct risk factors and cardiometabolic risk. A ranking of variables was then identified by supervised machine learning methods, followed by clustering method to identify subpopulations of interests. Predictions were divided as being nonmodifiable and modifiable. In addition to the modifiable risk factors identified by the logistic regression model, machine learning recognized other risk factors (lipids, intake of fruits and vegetables, sleep, and physical exercise). More variables will be available with the deployment of new digital ecosystems, which can be incorporated in future machine learning algorithms. However missing data in such large pools is an ever-present limitation that must be addressed. It can be developed into an integrated system with continuous analysis of data and provision of feedback to correct modifiable risk factors [18].

2.3 Prediction of Different Aspects of Diabetes Using Machine Learning

Diabetes mellitus is diagnosed by the measurement of blood glucose. Zou et al. employed machine learning to predict diabetes mellitus [19]. Training set, comprising of 14 attributes obtained from a hospital physical examination database (n: 68,994), comprised 14 attributes of data from 68,994 healthy persons and those with diabetes. Diabetes was predicted by the use of different methods such as decision tree, neural network, and random forest. Earlier, other methods were used: support vector machine, decision tree and logistic regression, principal component analysis and neuro fuzzy inference, quantum particle swarm optimization algorithm, and weighted least squares support vector machine [19]. In the current study, the authors used decision tree, random forest, and neural network. The physical examination variables were age, pulse and respiratory rate, diastolic pressure of left arm and of right arm, height of the individual, body weight, fasting plasma glucose, waist circumference, LDL cholesterol and HDL cholesterol.

Classification was determined by using decision tree, random forest, and neural network. The hidden layer number was set to 10 for improved performance. Standard validation methods were used for the model; five-fold cross validation method was used to train and test whole samples of the dataset.

Feature selection was carried out by principal component analysis and other measures for ensuring max Euclidean distances. To measure the effectiveness of classification, sensitivity, specificity, accuracy, and Matthews correlation coefficient were used [19]. When glucose was excluded as a variable from the dataset, the random forest decision showed the best performance.

In this proof of principle study, machine learning was found to be potentially useful in predicting diabetes. It is necessary to find suitable attributes, classifier, and data mining methods.

Psychological stress is being increasingly recognized to have a role in the causation and course of diabetes [20]. Employing clinical and biochemical inputs, we devised neural network predictive models for the outcome of various psychological states. From a cohort of 241 subjects with diabetes, we developed a multi layer perceptron neural network model. A back-propagation algorithm was used for training.. Predicted measures were well-being (depression, anxiety, energy, and positive well-being) [21]. We further used the same method to predict the quality of life in diabetes [22]. Both studies led to clinically relevant results. The method has the potential to provide greater time for the clinician to be involved in with patient management rather than spend time in identifying the set of problems [21, 22].

Later we developed two prototype models to predict well-being in diabetes: the first was a multi level perceptron neural network with back-propagation algorithm; the second was a support vector regression model [23]. Both methods gave similar results in terms of error values, although the support vector regression model provided lower error values. The performance is expected to improve by the provision of greater inputs to the system.

Later, a multi layer perceptron neural network-based diagnostic method was developed, with the addition of another input variable, viz brain derived neurotrophic factor (BDNF) level. BDNF, a member of the neurotrophic factor family has a principal role in neuronal growth, differentiation, connections, and repair. It has a role in causing diabetes and insulin resistance [24]. We demonstrated a relationship between BDNF, type 2 diabetes mellitus and psychological variables [25], strengthening the results of our earlier studies [21, 22].

A proof of concept study on six healthy volunteers (age 22 ± 3 years; 3 men, 3 women) employed a personal health system that wirelessly collected bio-monitoring sensor data (electrocardiography recordings and three-axial accelerometer to monitor activity). It was possible to assess real-time stress levels, with the potential to add other sensor inputs over longer periods of time. The individual would be able to make suitable proactive changes to avoid stress [26]. This model has been expanded for use in monitoring and dealing with stress among students [27].

3 Application of Machine Learning Techniques in Diabetes

Treatment of diabetes consists not just of medication, but a combination of lifestyle changes including regulated diet, physical exercise, and personal habits. Different kinds of medicines are available, which must be taken on time. Efficacy of treatment must be monitored to ensure that blood glucose and other parameters stay in the normal range. In addition, periodic tests are done to identify and treat any complications. The availability of biosensors (that monitor glucose levels in the body, blood pressure variations, physical activity by step counter, as well as patterns of sleep) increases the volume of analyzable data.

A surge in the number of patients with diabetes, and inadequate healthcare workforce in addition to the complexity of managing the various modifiable factors leads to sub-optimal care. Artificial intelligence can improve care by automating and aiding in decision-making, so that physicians are not overwhelmed by having to examine all patients; pre-screening by AI can allow only those requiring a specialist evaluation to be referred.

3.1 Use of Deep Neural Network for Image Processing

The most evolved area where neural network is applied in clinical medicine is, image processing: identification of diseased cells and tissues and recognizing abnormalities in the interior of the eye from digital images. In fact, the first FDA approved application of using AI in patient care is for 'automated' identification of eye changes in diabetes [13].

3.2 Methods to Identify Diabetic Retinopathy

Considering the mismatch between the burden of identifying diabetic retinopathy and the availability of experts to interpret the changes, screening by retinal photography was introduced in the 1980s. Initially, pictures were obtained on films, which were then interpreted by an eye specialist [28]. With the advent of digital photography, films were replaced by pixels. Photographs could be taken through the pupil which was either undilated or dilated; the area of the fundus that was photographed traditionally covered 30°–50°, including the macula, which is the area of greatest color identifying region, and the optic disc, where the optic nerve leaves the eye on its way to the brain. To include a greater area, photographs taken from a wider area were 'stitched' together as a montage. Ultra-wide field camera can image the periphery of the retina to more than 80% of the total retinal area.

Initially, the eye specialist had to be physically present to identify abnormal images that would need treatment. With digital technology, the images could be transmitted to a remote location for interpretation. It was associated with an asymmetry in communication, besides a heavy workload. AI was introduced to address both these issues [29].

Machine learning, a subfield of AI can analyze data without being given specific instructions. Fed with large data, it can identify patterns based on past experience. In medical imaging, deep convolutional neural network methods (CNN) are commonly employed because they are more accurate.

3.3   Concepts and Methods of AI in Diabetic Retinopathy (DR)

Classification and performance level depends on the model architecture. In DR, because of the limited availability of training images, hybrid approach may be used for low-level detection. A second and important factor to be considered is the need for computing resources. One has to make a trade-off between performance and speed [29].

Different approaches to DR include [29]: (a) **Ensembling**, where different independent machine learning models are combined for arriving at a classifier model; the performance of the combined model is better than that of its constituent models (b) **Transfer learning** adopts a model trained on identifying images from a different domain. In DR, common features consist of corners and edges, which may be similar to the original learning model. The merging of the two may involve using pretrained weights to initialize and to proceed with training, while allowing weight values to be updated. In contrast, pretrained weights may be fixed, using the pretrained model to extract features by replacing the output layer. Ultimately optimal selection depends on the purpose for which it is employed which is then determined empirically (c) **Weakly supervised and active learning** is necessary, as annotated image data is often unavailable. The initial model, trained on labeled trained data classifies unlabelled training data, which in turn, becomes labeled data. This continual refinement by active learning occurs from a 'gold standard', often a human expert (d) **Joint learning**: DR often coexists with other conditions such as hypertension and glaucoma. Joint learning trains the model to identify multiple conditions simultaneously.

3.4   Study of Retinal Vessels Segmentation by Deep Learning Models

Identifying diabetic retinal vessel changes by high performance segmenting of retinal images helps in diagnosis. Islam et al. performed a meta-analysis of deep learning algorithms to evaluate retinal vessel segmentation [29]. The **Convolutional Neural**

Network (CNN) has the advantage of not needing feature extraction. They are automatically extracted in a hierarchical manner and are further classified; the next layer uses a convolutional function of digital images as the input variable. A filter is moved over the images. The output is employed as the input of the next layer. In general, deeper network performs better with large datasets. The convolutional layers are subject to activation functions such as ReLu, tanh, or sigmoid. The former is commonly used because it can reduce the exploding/vanishing gradient problem. For reducing the feature size, max pooling allows the output to be smaller than the previous layer, which is then connected to every neuron present in the fully connected layer [29].

Features of vessels must be differentiated from unrelated noise by machine learning methods to identify vessels by generating low-level feature vectors. The problem of retinal vessel segmentation is taken as a pixel-wise binary classification issue [29].

A meta-analysis of 31 studies published between 2015 and 2019, evaluated the performance of DL algorithm in retinal vessel segmentation. The principal conclusions were that DL algorithms performed well in terms of specificity and sensitivity, comparable to that of professional medical experts [30].

3.5   Critical Aspects in Application to Clinical Care

Despite the apparent advantages of AI methods, one must consider their limitations in translation to clinical care. These must be validated to document that they are robust and applicable among clinicians, eye care providers, and scientists. Secondly, insufficient availability of data sets is a limitation: large annotated data sets as the gold standard are often lacking. Finally, the 'black box' nature of the algorithms is a stumbling block in translation to routine care, because incorrect decisions must be accountable, which hinders physicians from trusting the system [29].

Ultimately, AI/DL can be employed in a screening setup where professional resources are scarce. It improves the speed of screening, reduces cost, and provides better care for patients [31]. One should not overlook that the value of this technology is achieved only when downstream interventions, namely prevention and treatment are provided [32].

4   Studies in the Application of AI to Identify Diabetic Retinopathy

Diabetes mellitus is caused by an absolute or relative deficiency of the hormone insulin, secreted by the beta cells of the pancreas. Even though it is associated with many other changes in metabolism, the principal complications leading to disability result from vascular dysfunction, i.e., involvement of blood vessels supplying the eyes, nerves, kidneys, heart, brain, and other organs.

Involvement of the eye vessels (retinopathy) can be detected by examining the retina through the pupil of the eye. A doctor can physically look, using an ophthalmoscope. Limitations of ophthalmoscopy include lack of trained specialists and the subjective nature of assessment. Diabetic retinopathy (DR) must be identified early [33]. Often it does not cause problems until a late stage when vision is threatened; by then treatment options are both limited and expensive. When identified at an early stage, prevention and treatment can be initiated to prevent or delay its progression.

To ensure that widespread screening is available, fundus photography was established. A trained technician or non-specialist doctor can take a picture and transmit it to an eye specialist for interpretation and further action. Even though digital images made it possible for remote transmission, it was still limited by the need for physical assessment by a specialist. To work around this, deep learning methods were devised to enable the identification of normal and abnormal images, and to refer only those subjects with significant DR to an eye specialist.

There have been large-scale studies demonstrating the feasibility of using artificial intelligence and deep learning methods in identifying DR, and they are at the threshold of being widely employed [34].

4.1 Employment of Retinal Fundus Camera to Identify Diabetic Retinopathy Using AI

Automated methods to identify DR from retinal images were reported for over 15 years from different geographic areas of the developed and developing world. While early reports came from the UK and USA, results of large-scale studies were published from Singapore, the Indian subcontinent, and African countries. Starting with proof-of-concept studies, recent publications employed deep learning methods to identify normal from abnormal images, as well as to flag those subjects who need intervention. Others showed that automated methods were comparable in terms of performance to qualified image readers, suggesting that they could be used to screen for DR. Recent economic analysis studies showed that they had a beneficial cost–benefit ratio. Retinal images were captured using fundus cameras, as well as portable devices such as smartphones.

4.2 Early Studies

Philip et al. demonstrated that it was possible to automatically identify 'disease/no disease' grading in DR. Using 14,406 images from 6722 patients obtained from nonmydriatic 45° fixed Canon fundus cameras attached to digital bodies, disease/no disease classification was done manually (by retinal screeners) and by automated grading system. The automatic system consisted of software to assess the quality of image and to detect whether or not fundus abnormalities were present. Automated grading was shown to be capable of reducing the burden of manual grading. The automated method software was less specific but more sensitive than manual grading [35]. The authors concluded that this method could reduce the burden of screening on manual readers.

Abramoff et al. performed a retrospective multi-centric study to detect diabetic retinopathy using automatic method built from published algorithms. The analysis was conducted on fundus pictures of 5,692 patients [36]. The algorithms were devised to automatically determine the image quality and perform segmentation of vessels. The optic disc was detected and masked, allowing the detection of abnormalities in the vessels (presence of bleeding and of microaneurysms) and detection of bright lesions (exudates, cotton-wool spots, drusen). The authors considered it as a first-step to being used in routine clinical practice.

In 2013, the Iowa Detection Program (IDP) was employed on 874 subjects to identify diabetic retinopathy that needed a referral to an ophthalmologist. The sensitivity of IDP for referable diabetic retinopathy was 96.8% and specificity 59.4%. The area under the receiver operating characteristic curve was 0.937. With high sensitivity and specificity to identify referable diabetic retinopathy, the IDP was deemed to be safe for use in DR screening [37].

4.3 Studies from Asia

Roy et al. from southern India evaluated the ability of retinal grading system to screen for DR. The images were processed using the 'Retmarker' automated DR screening software. 'Retmarker', is a patented software developed by Critical Health SA, certified as a CE mark Class II a medical device; classifier training was performed to ensure the reproducibility and objectivity of the algorithm. From 1445 subjects with diabetes, 5780 images of ocular fundus were screened into two categories: 'DR' (Diabetic retinopathy present), 'no DR' (no Diabetic retinopathy). In the group with high and medium image quality (n: 1,188), specificity and sensitivity for identifying DR ranged from (0.59, 0.91) to (0.11, 0.95) [38].

Patchiyappan et al. described an automatic screening method to identify DR and glaucoma using fundus photographs and cortical coherence tomography. They applied morphological operations, filters, and thresholds to identify DR, and active contours based deformable snake algorithm to estimate the thickness of the retinal nerve fiber layer. A pilot study on 89 images showed that the system was accurate and robust from South India [39].

A recent study reported the prospective validation of the performance of an automated system to recognize DR compared with manual grading. The subjects comprised of 3049 subjects with diabetes who presented to two major specialist eye centers. The performance of the algorithm equaled or exceeded that of retinal specialists and trained graders [40]. Of particular clinical relevance, the images were obtained from real-world settings using nonmydriatic retinal cameras that are more likely to be used in developing countries.

Recently, Shah et al. published a study validating a deep convolutional neural network-based algorithm for detecting DR. An internal dataset of fundus images centering on the macula were used; the external validation set was obtained from MESSIDOR [41]. The internal validation set showed a sensitivity of 99.7% and specificity of 98.5% for the detection of any DR detection; for prompt referral, it was 98.9 and 94.84%. The corresponding area under the curve was 0.991 and 0.969. The external validation set gave a sensitivity and specificity of 90.4%. There was good agreement between the neural network and clinician in both datasets [41].

An international study by Keel et al. reported that patient acceptability with AI detection of DR was good. It took an average of 6.9 min for automated screening of DR. More than 95% were satisfied with the automated method. Over 75% preferred the automated model over manual screening [42].

4.4 Studies from Africa

The Iowa Detection Program was carried out in Kenya (Kenyan Nakuru Study; KNS). Automated identification of diabetic eye diseases was compared with grading by trained eye specialists at Moorfields Reading Centre [43]. The NW6 Topcon Digital Retinal camera was employed to take retinal images of 4,381 participants. Human graders first classified the images into those having DR and those without DR. Those with DR were further sub-divided into DR that required referral to an expert and those that did not. The software was employed for those who had retinopathy to categorize the stage of disease [43]. The Study, which was begun in 2007/08, comprised a complete eye examination (n: 4,382), and fundus imaging through dilated pupils (n: 3460). DR was graded later. Images consisted of two fields: one centered on the optic disc; the other on the fovea. The software [37], analyses each pixel in the image for abnormalities indicative of DR. With a combination of image quality and lesion detection, a dr-index is provided, which is a numerical output ranging between 0 and 1. If the number is close to 1, it is more likely that either the eye disease is present or the possibility that the image is ungradable [43]. The main interest was on comparing how well the software performed in comparison with trained specialists.

Of 3,460 images that could be graded, the software detected eye changes with a sensitivity of 91.0%; area under the curve (AUC) was 0.878. The negative predictive value was 98% [43].

The accuracy of deep learning to identify DR was studied in Zambia [44]. An ensemble AI model was employed: two convolutional neural networks and a residual neural network classified fundus images. Training set consisted of 76,370 retinal images from 13,099 diabetes subjects from SIDRP (Singapore Integrated Diabetic Retinopathy Program). Clinical validation was performed on 1574 subjects with diabetes from Zambia at a mobile screening camp. The AUC for the AI system for

DR that needed referral was 0.973 (95% CI 0.969–0.978); sensitivity was 92.25% (90.10–90.12), specificity 89.04% (87.85–90.28). Performance of both AI and of human graders was comparable [44].

The validation of the predictive model in a different ethnic population ensured that there was no inbuilt bias in the model [45]. There are, however, practical issues that have to be addressed such as price of fundus cameras, software, and access to the internet.

4.5   Smart Phone Images to Identify Diabetic Retinopathy Using AI

Considering the widespread availability of smartphones and the drawbacks in using expensive fundus cameras, smartphones were used to screen for DR using AI [46].

Rajalakshmi et al. used AI to assess smartphone-based retinal images, which were validated against the grading of an eye specialist. Remidio 'Fundus on phone' was used to take fundus pictures from 301 subjects with type 2 diabetes; they were graded by a validated AI DR software (EyeArt™), which can identify the severity of the disease, as well as give recommendations for further action. It was possible to grade retinal images of 296 patients. With AI, there was a 95.8% sensitivity (95% CI 92.8–98.7) and specificity of 80.2% (95% CI 72.6–87.8) to detect any DR; for detecting sight-threatening DR, it had a sensitivity of 99.1% and a specificity of 80.4% [46].

Natarajan et al. analyzed retinal images using a smartphone employing offline automated analysis [Medios AI (Remidio)] [47] through a dilated pupil. This was performed on subjects with diabetes who attended government dispensaries in Mumbai. Photographs were taken of the posterior pole, nasal and temporal fields. Assessment was done by the AI system and by an ophthalmologist. Among 213 subjects whose eye images were available, the sensitivity and specificity of the offline AI system to diagnose referable DR was made with a sensitivity of 100.0% and specificity of 88.4%. For diagnosing any DR, the sensitivity was 85.2% and the specificity 92.0%. All these were in comparison with a trained eye specialist who graded the same images [47].

4.6   AI to Predict Progression of DR

As a step forward from merely identifying DR, using 7-field color fundus photographs at baseline, Arcadu et al. used deep learning to predict the progression of DR [48]. This is an exciting application that can show the trajectory of the possible future course of DR. They reported that by including peripheral parts of the retina in the image, the predictive ability of DL algorithm was enhanced.

Ting et al. identified other risk factors in the prevalence of DR by AI screening. In a cross-sectional multi-ethnic multi-site study (n: 18,912 subjects; 93,292 images), risk factors by using forest plot meta-analysis and by human assessors were, ie, longer duration of diabetes elevated levels of HbA1c and higher readings of systolic blood pressure [49]. The potential time taken to assess the 93,293 retinal images is dramatically shortened by DLS (it would have taken >2 years for a human assessor to complete reading all the images. In contrast, it took about 10 h for the DLS [49]. It is thus possible to combine clinical information and DLS assessment of retinal images to provide a more nuanced risk stratification. A similar risk factor assessment with DR was performed by Bellemo et al. in the Zambian population [44].

4.7 Health Economic and Safety Issues in AI Applications for DR Screening

AI technology to screen for DR requires substantial manpower and financial commitments. Therefore, health economic assessment of patient safety must be assessed to allocate resources [50]. Methods for health economic assessment include cost-utility/cost-effectiveness analysis, cost-minimization analysis, and cost–benefit analysis. One must also consider false negatives and false positives in screening, besides locally available trained manpower and resources.

Xie et al. carried out an economic analysis modeling study for use of AI in teleophthalmology-based DR screening national programme [51]. The potential simulated savings to DL methods were assessed by a cost-minimization analysis. A comparison of the actual cost for screening by AI method and of trained specialists was determined by the decision tree model. From a health system view, the model costing the least was a semi-automated screening method [51].

4.8 Guidelines for Ocular Telehealth–Diabetic Retinopathy

The DRTPG (Diabetic Retinopathy Telehealth Practice Guidelines Working Group) published their guidelines in 2020, based on the evidence-based best practices to design, implement and operate a telehealth diabetic retinopathy programme [52]. Emphasis was made on the use to which it can be put clinically and on the degree of security and of data integrity. At the outset, the importance of communication among the clients and care givers was emphasized. Guidelines were provided about the qualifications of the medical supervisors, patient care coordinator, personnel who review images, and operate information systems.

Equipment ratified by the national regulatory body (FDA in USA) must be used. Factors to be considered included sufficient resolution; accuracy of diagnosis depends on the field of view and whether the photograph is taken with a dilated pupil or without dilation.

Features of image analysis refer to computer algorithms to improve the digital quality of retinal images or to provide an automated identification of retinal abnormalities. Stress has been laid that algorithmic DR assessment undergoes rigorous clinical validation.

On data management, interoperability is desirable. Attention must be paid to compression ratio, data communication and transmission, archival, and retrieval. One must also ensure reliability and redundancy. Finally, documentation must be done in an appropriate format.

Administrative guidelines are also provided for health insurance portability (where applicable), privileging and credentialing, as well as the risk of fraud and abuse of data. Quality of care with corrective actions and financial issues must also be factored in.

5 Application of AI to Identify Conditions Other Than DR from Retinal Images

There have been exciting possibilities of using AI in retinal images to predict and diagnose conditions other than DR.

Visual loss in DR results mainly from *macular edema* where extracellular fluid accumulates within the retina, disturbing its architecture. Sahisten et al. described a deep learning method to identify two eye conditions that are common in diabetes: retinopathy and macular edema [53]. They showed that the performance is affected by training with fewer images. Their DL method was equal to or better than other methods [40] accomplished by the use of nearly a fourth the number of training images compared to others.

Glaucoma, which occurs commonly in diabetes results from increased pressure in the eye, leading to the death of retinal ganglion cells [54]. Li et al. described a DL system to detect glaucomatous optic neuropathy needing referral, with good sensitivity and specificity [55]. Employing fundus images downloaded from an online dataset LabelMe, they used Inception-v^3 architecture, a convolutional neural network. On a sample of 48,116 fundus photographs, the DL method showed a sensitivity of 95.6%, and specificity of 92.0%, with an AUC of 0.986 [55].

An interesting application of DL of retinal images consisted of *differentiating individuals with and without type 2 diabetes.* Heslinga et al. used deep neural networks viz, multi-target learning approach to simultaneously identify retinal changes and diabetes mellitus [56]. Even though retinopathy may be present when diabetes is first diagnosed clinically, retinal vascular geometry is not studied in the early stages. DL model was employed to distinguish individuals with diabetes from those without diabetes using retinal photographs. Images of both eyes were captured and subjected to Channel-wise global contrast normalization. Among the different model set ups, the best performance was observed with the MTL approach with random initialized weights [56]. It offered a unique screening method using smartphone fundus photography; however further studies must validate the findings before it can be recommended for general screening.

DL algorithms were employed to *predict cardiovascular risk factors* from retinal images. Data from 284,335 patients were used for training and validated on two independent datasets. It could predict the risk of cardiovascular disease from retinal images while considering other variables such as the age and gender of the individual, history of smoking, level of glycosylated hemoglobin, and systolic blood pressure [57].

Papilledema refers to a swelling of the optic disc. Recently, Milea et al. studied whether AI could identify papilledema and other abnormalities of the optic disk using fundus photographs [58]. In a collection of digital color ocular fundus images, training, validation, and external-testing were carried by a DL system. Training set comprised 14,341 images from 11 countries; external testing was performed on 1505 pictures in five other countries. The images were classified as normal optic disc, papilledema due to intracranial hypertension, and disc with other abnormalities. The DL consisted of U-Net, a segmentation network to identify the optic disc, and DenseNet a classification network to classify the images into one of the three categories. The strength of the study lay in employing diverse sample images. They were obtained from different ethnic backgrounds having variations in pigmentation, ages and were taken with different kinds of fundus cameras. In the validation set, DL could discriminate normal disc with those having papilledema with an area under the curve of 0.99); and normal from abnormal discs with an AUC of 0.99% (95% CI 0.99–0.99) [58].

6   Current Status of AI in Ophthalmology

There is broad scope for AI in the field of ophthalmology, from the detection of DR to glaucoma, metabolic diseases, to providing referral guidelines. In future, integration with electronic medical records can enhance its usefulness in clinical care [59]. As of now, AI and DL can supplement, not supplant human intervention. Medico-legal, ethical and cybersecurity issues need to be addressed [60, 61]. FDA approved iDx-DR to be used in adults with diabetes who are aged 22 years or older for automatic detection of more than mild DR, in subjects not known to have DR; it can be used in primary care, with referral to an eye specialist if indicated [16].

A confluence of DL with human intervention has the ability to provide the best possible care: DL is not limited by fatigue, but humans can recognize 'out of-set' variations more easily [62]. Ultimately a holistic approach is needed where, apart from technology, one must 'gather all the key components of clinical care' if the potential of AI is to be fully met [63].

7 Outlook for the Future

Because AI is so complex to define, Panch et al. attempted to make it *simple*, but in deference to Einstein *not any simpler* [64]: *Artificial intelligence* is the broad field that 'aims to understand and develop systems that display properties of intelligence'. It has roots in a wide range of fields including philosophy, mathematics, and computer science. *Machine learning* refers to a sub discipline of AI where algorithms (computer programs) 'learn associations of predictive power from examples in data'. *Deep Learning* methods 'allow a machine to be fed with large quantities of raw data and to discover the representations necessary for detection or classification'. *Supervised learning* involves 'training computer programs to learn associations between inputs and outputs in data through analysis'; outputs of interest are generally defined by a human supervisor. *Unsupervised Learning* refers to 'computer programs that learn associations in data without an external definition of associations of interest'. Often they are employed to discern previously unknown predictors. *Reinforcement Learning* are 'computer programs that learn actions based on their ability to maximize a defined reward.' This is influenced by the field of behavioral psychology.

We are poised at the cusp of a fascinating era, where AI is applied in previously inconceivable areas: a recent study showed that *anemia* can be detected from *electrocardiograms* by DL algorithms [65]. Integration of data from many related areas by AI (clinical, radiological, and genomic) helps in accurate diagnosis of disease and in predicting outcomes [66]. Despite the excitement, the World Health Organization had the following words of caution about digital health, of which AI is a component: 'The enthusiasm for digital health has also driven a proliferation of short-lived implementations and an overwhelming diversity in digital tools, with a limited understanding of their impact on health systems and people's well-being' [67].

With the availability of cloud-based services, application of artificial intelligence to data mining has been democratized; it is no longer esoteric. While this is laudable in being made more accessible, one must be careful in using them properly. One must not repeat the previous mistake of using powerful easily available off-shelf statistical software inappropriately.

Along with technical and humanitarian concerns, ethical aspects must be considered [68]. It is essential to align the capacity of algorithms with the insights that can be provided by humans. One must be aware of the risk of excluding marginal groups who pass under the radar of providing data for DL algorithms: Kalluri, in a recent opinion piece called it 'AI by and for the people' [69].

Just as AI can provide contact tracing abilities in situations such as the present Covid-19 pandemic, application of digital contact tracing raises issues of consent and confidentiality [70].

8 Conclusion

The growth and development of AI in health sciences, as in many other areas have profound implications. One must guard against 'the danger of leaving determinations around these issues in the hands of a small number of individuals ..., whose incentives and worldviews are often at odds with the interests of those who bear the consequences of such decisions' [71].

The development of AI, particularly in clinical medicine is unprecedented: one cannot look at the past to foresee the future. There is tremendous scope for its applications, which comes with responsibilities. Issues of trust, ability to explain, use in practical situations, and transparency must all be addressed. It needs coordination among those who provide data, the developers of AI systems along with the end-users—both from the health care team and the patients [72]. The availability of representative data often forms the bottleneck in developing AI system. Skewing by ethnicity, gender or phenotypes tends to introduce bias in the output, which is amplified. Trust and comprehensibility are new issues that must be addressed. More effective AI platforms tend to use a black-box approach in which the logic behind an outcome may not always be apparent to the users of the system. Unless the physicians and the patients can understand the way i n which a decision has been obtained, trust cannot be built, which is reflected in the reluctance to use AI technology. One must balance the different requirements to allow the power of AI to be harnessed in patient care.

Yet these must not hinder the potential applications of AI in future global health. Near universal availability of infrastructure for IT and mobile telephony, geographies permit the adoption of AI to improve health and health care across the world. It can be used for both communicable and non-communicable diseases, which are equally prevalent in low and middle income countries. A combination of machine learning and signal processing technologies can aid in identifying diseases, assessing disease burden and death rates, predicting the outbreak of infections, and guiding in health planning. Simultaneous broad-based attention must be paid to ethics, regulation, and practical applicability [73]. While it took more than 20 years for electronic medical records to evolve from an aspiration [74] to a robust clinical platform [75], AI applications are expected to have a shorter gestation.

References

1. Baruffaldi, S., van Beuzekom, B., Dernis, H., Harhoff, D., Rao, N., Rosenfeld D., Squicciarini, M.: Identifying and Measuring Developments in Artificial Intelligence: Making the Impossible Possible. OECD Science, Technology and Industry Working Papers 2020/05 (2020). https://doi.org/10.1787/5f65ff7e-en
2. Pereira, L.M., Lopes, A.B.: Machine Ethics. Studies in Applied Philosophy, Epistemology and Rational Ethics, vol. 53. Springer Nature Switzerland AG (2020)
3. Bao, T., Cheng, C.: Application research of artificial intelligence in medical information system. In: Cheng, C., et al. (eds.) Data Processing Techniques and Applications for Cyber-Physical

Systems (DPTA 2019). Advances in Intelligent Systems and Computing, vol. 1088, pp. 1935–1943. Springer Nature Singapore (2020)

4. Wang, P.: On defining artificial intelligence. J. Artif. Gen. Intell. **10**, 1–37 (2019)
5. Sridhar, G.R.: Diabetes and data in many forms. Int. J. Diabetes Dev. Ctries. **36**, 381–384 (2016)
6. Sridhar, G.R., Murali, G.: Computerization of data in diabetes centers. Int. J. Diabetes Dev. Ctries. **31**, 48–50 (2016)
7. Sridhar, G.R., Duggirala, R., Padmanabhan, S.: Emerging face of genetics, genomics and diabetes. Int. J. Diabetes Dev. Ctries. **33**, 183–185 (2013)
8. Chang, H.Y., Jung, C.K., Woo, J.I., Lee, S., Cho, J., Kim, S.W., Kwak, T.Y.: Artificial intelligence in pathology. J. Pathol. Transl. Med. **53**, 1–12 (2019)
9. Ayanian, J.Z., Markel, H.: Donabedian's lasting framework for health care quality. N. Engl. J. Med. **375**, 205–207 (2016)
10. Sevakula, R.K., Yeung, W.T.M.A., Singh, J.P., Heist, E.K., Isselbacher, E.M., Armoundas, A.A.: State-of-the-art machine learning techniques aiming to improve patient outcomes pertaining to the cardiovascular system. J. Am. Heart Assoc. **9**, e013924 (2020). https://doi.org/10.1161/JAHA.119.013924
11. Koch, M.: Artificial intelligence is becoming natural. Cell **173**, 531–533 (2018)
12. Grace, K., Salvatier, J., Dafoe, A., Zhang, B., Evans, O.: When Will AI Exceed Human Performance? Evidence from AI Experts. arXiv:1705.08807 [cs.AI] (2017)
13. Topol, E.J.: High-performance medicine: the convergence of human and artificial intelligence. Nat. Med. **25**, 44–56 (2019)
14. Rajkomar, A., Dean, J., Kohane, I.: Machine learning in medicine. N. Engl. J. Med. **380**, 1347–1358 (2019)
15. Greene, J.A., Lea, A.S.: Digital futures past—the long arc of big data in medicine. N. Engl. J. Med. **381**, 480–485 (2019)
16. He, J., Baxter, S.L., Xu, J., Xu, J., Zhou, X., Zhang, K.: The practical implementation of artificial intelligence technologies in medicine. Nat. Med. **25**, 30–36 (2019)
17. Zhang, X., Shao, H., Zhang, S., Li, R.: A novel deep neural network model for multi-label chronic disease prediction. Front. Genet. **10**, 352 (2019). https://doi.org/10.3389/fgene2019.00351
18. Liao, X., Kerr, D., Morales, J., Duncan, I.: Application of machine learning to identify clustering of cardiometabolic risk factors in US adults. Diabetes Technol. Ther. **21**, 1–9 (2019)
19. Zou, Q., Qu, K., Luo, Y., Yin, D., Ju, Y., Tang, H.: Predicting diabetes mellitus with machine learning techniques. Front. Genet. **9**, 515 (2018). https://doi.org/10.3389/fgene.2018.00515
20. On psychology and psychiatry in diabetes. Indian J. Endocr. Metab. **24**, 387–395 (2020)
21. Narasingarao, M.R., Manda, R., Sridhar, G.R., Madhu, K., Rao, A.A.: A clinical decision support system using multilayer perceptron neural network to assess well being in diabetes. J. Assoc. Physicians India **57**, 127–133 (2009)
22. Narasinga Rao, M.R., Sridhar, G.R., Madhu, K., Appa, R.A.: A clinical decision support system using multi-layer perceptron neural network to predict quality of life in diabetes. Diabetes Metab. Syndr.: Clin. Res. Rev. **4**, 57–59 (2010)
23. Narasinga Rao, M.R., Padmaja, T.M., Sridhar, G.R., Lind, M., Madhu, K., Ramakrishna, V.: Assessment of well being in diabetes—a comparison of MLP with back-propagation and support vector regression. J. Life Sci. **1**, 55–60 (2013)
24. Rozanska, O., Uruska, A., Ziolkiewicz, D.Z.: Brain-derived neurotrophic factor and diabetes. Int. J. Mol. Sci. **21**, 841 (2020). https://doi.org/10.3390/ijms21030841
25. Devarapalli, D., Apparao, A., Narasinga Rao, M.R., Kumar, A., Sridhar, G.R.: A multi layer perceptron (MLP) neural network based diagnosis of diabetes using brain derived neurotrophic factor (BDNF) levels. Int. J. Adv. Comput. **35**, 422–427 (2012)
26. Tartarisco, G., Baldus, G., Corda, D., Raso, R., Arnao, A., Ferro, M., Gaggioli, A., Pioggia, G.: Personal Health System architecture for stress monitoring and support to clinical decisions. Comput. Commun. **35**, 1296–1305 (2012)

27. Verma, P., Sood, S.K.: A comprehensive framework for student stress monitoring in fog-cloud IoT environment: m-health perspective. Med. Biol. Eng. Comput. **57**, 231–244 (2019)
28. Sridhar, G.R., Satish, K., Ahuja, M.M.: Nonmydriatic retinal color photography in young Indian diabetic patients. Ann. Ophthalmol. **25**, 187–190 (1993)
29. Lim, G., Bellemo, V., Xie, Y., Lee, X.Q., Yip, M.Y.T., Ting, D.S.W.: Different fundus imaging modalities and technical factors in AI screening for diabetic retinopathy: a review. Eye Vis. **7**, 21 (2020). https://doi.org/10.1186/s40662-020-00182-7
30. Islam, M.M., Poly, T.N., Walther, B.A., Yang, H.C., Li, Y.C.J.: Artificial intelligence in ophthalmology: a meta-analysis of deep learning models for retinal vessels segmentation. J. Clin. Med. **9**, 1018 (2020). https://doi.org/10.3390/jcm9041018
31. Islam, M.M., Yang, H.C., Poly, T.N., Jian, W.S., Li, Y.C.J.: Deep learning algorithms for detection of diabetic retinopathy in retinal fundus photographs: a systematic review and meta-analysis. Comput. Methods Programs Biomed. **191**, 105320 (2020). https://doi.org/10.1016/j.cmpb.2020.105320
32. Wong, T.Y., Sabanayagam, C.: Strategies to tackle the global burden of diabetic retinopathy: from epidemiology to artificial intelligence. Ophthalmologica **243**, 9–20 (2020)
33. Sabanayagam, C., Banu, R., Chee, M.L., Lee, R., Wang, Y.X., Tan, G., Jonas, J.B., Lamoureux, E.L., Cheng, C.Y., Klein, B.E., Mitchell, P., Klein, R., Cheung, C.M.G., Wong, T.Y.: Incidence and progression of diabetic retinopathy: a systematic review. Lancet Diabetes Endocrinol. **7**, 140–149 (2019)
34. Sosale, A.R.: Screening for diabetic retinopathy—is the use of artificial intelligence and cost-effective fundus imaging the answer? Int. J. Diabetes Dev. Ctries. **39**, 1–3 (2019)
35. Philip, S., Fleming, A.D., Goatman, K.A., Fonesca, S., Mcnamee, P., Scotland, G.S., Prescott, G.J., Sharp, P.F., Olson, J.A.: The efficacy of automated "disease/no disease" grading for diabetic retinopathy in a systematic screening programme. Br. J. Ophthalmol. **91**, 1512–1517 (2007)
36. Abramoff, M.D., Viergever, M.A., Niemeijer, M., Russell, S.R., Schulten, M.S.A.S., Ginneken, B.V.: Evaluation of a system for automatic detection of diabetic retinopathy from color fundus photographs in a large population of patients with diabetes. Diabetes Care **31**, 193–198 (2008)
37. Abramoff, M.D., Folk, J.C., Han, D.P., Walker, J.D., Williams, D.F., Russell, S.R., Massin, P., Cochener, B., Gain, P., Tang, L., Lamard, M., Moga, D.C., Quellec, G., Niemeijer, M.: Automated analysis of retinal images for detection of referable diabetic retinopathy. JAMA Ophthalmol. **131**, 351–357 (2013)
38. Roy, R., Lob, A., Pal, B.P., Oliveira, C.M., Raman, R., Sharma, T.: Automated diabetic retinopathy imaging in Indian eyes: a pilot study. India J. Ophthalmol. **62**, 1121–1124 (2014)
39. Pachiyappan, A., Das, U.N., Murthy, T.V.S.P., Tatavarti, R.: Automated diagnosis of diabetic retinopathy and glaucoma using fundus and OCT images. Lipids Health Dis. **11**, 73 (2012). https://www.liidworld.com/content/11/1/73
40. Gulshan, V., Rajan, R.P., Widner, K., Wu, D., Wubbels, P., Rhodes, T., Whitehouse, K., Coram, M., Corrado, G., Ramasamy, K., Raman, R., Peng, L., Webster, D.R.: Performance of a deep-learning algorithm vs manual grading in detecting diabetic retinopathy in India. JAMA Ophthalmol. **137**, 987–993 (2019)
41. Shah, P., Mishra, D., Shanmugam, M.P., Doshi, B., Jayaraj, H., Ramanjulu, R.: Validation of deep convolutional neural network-based algorithm for detection of diabetic retinopathy—artificial intelligence versus clinician for screening. Indian J. Ophthalmol. **68**, 398–405 (2020)
42. Keel, S., Lee, P.Y., Scheetz, J., Li, Z., Kotowicz, M.A., MacIsaac, R.J., He, M.: Feasibility and patient acceptability of a novel artificial intelligence-based screening model for diabetic retinopathy at endocrinology outpatient services: a pilot study. Sci. Rep. **8**, 4330 (2018). https://doi.org/10.1038/s41598-018-22612-2
43. Hansen, M.B., Abramoff, M.D., Folk, J.C., Mathenge, W., Bastawrous, A., Peto, T.: Results of automated retinal image analysis for detection of diabetic retinopathy from the Nakuru Study, Kenya. PLoS One **10**, e0139148 (2015). https://doi.org/10.1371/journal.pone.0139148
44. Bellemo, V., Lim, Z.W., Lim, G., Nguyen, Q.D., Xie, Y., Yip, M.Y.T., Hamzah, H., Ho, J., Lee, X.Q., Hsu, W., Lee, M.L., Musonda, L., Chandran, M., Mutati, G.C., Muma, M., Tan,

G.S.W., Sivaprasad, S., Menon, G., Wong, T.Y., Ting, D.S.W.: Artificial intelligence using deep learning to screen for referable and vision-threatening diabetic retinopathy in Africa: a clinical validation study. Lancet Digit. Health **1**, e35–e44 (2019)

45. Mathenge, W.C.: Artificial intelligence for diabetic retinopathy screening in Africa. Lancet Digit. Health **1**, e6–e7 (2019)

46. Rajalaksmi, R., Subashini, R., Anjana, R.M., Mohan, V.: Automated diabetic retinopathy detection in smartphone-based fundus photography using artificial intelligence. Eye **32**, 1138–1144 (2018)

47. Natarajan, S., Jain, A., Krishnan, R., Rogye, A., Sivaprasad, S.: Diagnostic accuracy of community-based diabetic retinopathy screening with an offline artificial intelligence system on a smartphone. JAMA Ophthalmol. **137**, 1182–1188 (2019)

48. Arcadu, F., Benmansour, F., Maunz, A., Willis, J., Haskova, Z., Prunotto, M.: Deep learning algorithm predicts diabetic retinopathy progression in individual patients. NPJ Digit. Med. **2**, 92 (2019). https://doi.org/10.1038/s41746-019-0172-3

49. Ting, D.S.W., Cheung, C.Y., Nguyen, Q., et al.: Deep learning in estimating prevalence and systemic risk factors for diabetic retinopathy: a multi-ethnic study. NPJ Digit. Med. **2**, 24 (2019). https://doi.org/10.1038/s41746-019-0097-x

50. Xie, Y., Gunasekeran, D.V., Balaskas, K., Keane, O.A., Sim, D.A., Bachmann, L.M., Macrae, C., Ting, D.S.W.: Health economic and safety considerations for artificial intelligence applications in diabetic retinopathy screening. Transl. Vis. Sci. Technol. **9**, 22 (2020). https://doi.org/10.1167/tvst.9.2.22

51. Xie, Y., Nguyen, Q.D., Hamzah, H., Lim, G., Bellemo, V., Gunasekeran, D.V., Yip, M.Y.T., Lee, X.Q., Hsu, W., Lee, M.L., Tan, C.S., Wong, H.T., Lamoureux, E.L., Tan, G.S.W., Wong, T.Y., Finkelstein, E.A., Ting, D.S.W.: Artificial intelligence for teleophthalmology-based diabetic retinopathy screening in a national programme: an economic analysis modelling study. Lancet Digit. Health **2**, E240–E249 (2020)

52. Horton, M.B., Cavallerano, J., Barker, G., Crockett, C.H., Karth, P., Newman, C.D., et al.: Practice guidelines for ocular telehealth—diabetic retinopathy. Third Edition. Telemed. e-Health **26**, 495–543 (2020)

53. Sahisten, J., Jaskari, J., Kivinen, J., Turunen, L., Jaanio, E., Hietala, K., Kaski, K.: Deep learning fundus image analysis for diabetic retinopathy and macular edema grading. Sci. Rep. **9**, 10750 (2019). https://doi.org/10.1038/s41598-019-47181-w

54. Zhao, Y.X., Chen, X.W.: Diabetes and risk of glaucoma: systematic review and a meta-analysis of prospective cohort studies. Int. J. Ophthalmol. **10**, 1430–1435 (2017)

55. Li, Z., He, Y., Keel, S., Meng, W., Chang, R.T., He, M.: Efficacy of a deep learning system for detecting glaucomatous optic neuropathy based on color fundus photographs. Ophthalmology **125**, 1199–1206 (2018)

56. Heslinga, F.G., Pluim, J.P.W., Houben, A.J.M.H., Schram, M.T., Henry, R.M.A., Stehouwer, D.A., van Greevenbroek, M.J., Berendschot, T.T.J.M., Veta, M.: Direct classification of type 2 diabetes from retinal fundus images in a population-based sample from the Maastricht Study. arXiv:1911.10022 [eess.IV]. To be published in the proceeding of SPIE—Medical Imaging (2020)

57. Poplin, R., Varadarajan, A.V., Blumer, K., Liu, Y., McConnell, M.V., Corrado, G.S., Peng, L., Webster, D.R.: Predicting cardiovascular risk factors from retinal fundus photographs using deep learning. Nat. Biomed. Eng. **2**, 158–164 (2018)

58. Milea, D., Najjar, R.P., Zhubo, J., Ting, D., Vasseneix, C., Xu, X., et al.: Artificial intelligence to detect papilledema from ocular fundus photographs. N. Engl. J. Med. **382**, 1687–1695 (2020)

59. Mcneil, R.: Coming to terms with AI. Eye News **26**(2) (2019)

60. Ting, D.S., Gunasekeran, D.V., Wickham, L., Wong, T.Y.: Next generation telemedicine platforms to screen and triage. Br. J. Ophthalmol. **104**, 299–300 (2020)

61. Finlayson, S.G., Bowers, J.D., Ito, J., Zittrain, J.L., Beam, A.L., Kohane, I.S.: Adversarial attacks on medical machine learning. Science **363**, 1287–1289 (2019)

62. Ballemo, V., Lim, G., Rim, T.H., Tan, G.S.W., Cheung, C.Y., Sadda, S., et al.: Artificial intelligence screening for diabetic retinopathy: the real-world emerging application. Curr. Diabetes Rep. **19**, 72 (2019). https://doi.org/10.1007/s11892-019-1189-3

63. Ting, D.S.W., Lin, H., Ruamviboonsuk, P., Wong, T.Y., Sim, D.A.: Artificial intelligence, the internet of things, and virtual clinics: ophthalmology at the digital translation forefront. Lancet Digit. Health **2**, e8-9 (2020)

64. Panch, T., Szolovits, P., Atun, R.: Artificial intelligence, machine learning and health systems. J. Glob. Health **8**, 020303 (2018). https://doi.org/10.7189/jogh.08.020303

65. Kwon, J.M., Cho, Y.H., Cho, S.H., et al.: A deep learning algorithm to detect anaemia with ECGs: a retrospective, multicentre study. Lancet Digit. Health **2**, e358–e367 (2020)

66. Chang, H.Y., Jung, C.K., Woo, J.I., Lee, S., Cho, J., Kim, S.W., Kwak, T.Y.: Artificial intelligence in pathology. J. Pathol. Transl. Med. **53**, 1–12 (2018)

67. WHO Guideline: Recommendations on digital interventions for health system strengthening. World Health Organization. License: CC BY-NC-SA 3.0 IGO (2019)

68. Coyle, D., Weller, A.: "Explaining" machine learning reveals policy challenges. Science **368**, 1433–1434 (2020)

69. Kalluri, P.: Don't ask if AI is good or fair, ask how it shifts power. Nature **583**, 169 (2020)

70. Darbysire, T.: Do we need a Coronavirus (Safeguards) Act 2020? Proposed legal safeguards for digital contact tracing and other apps in the COVID-19 crisis. Patterns **1**, 1–2 (2020). https://doi.org/10.1016/j.patter.2020.100072

71. Crawford, K., Dobbe, R., Dryer, T., Fried, G., Green, B., Kazinuas, E., et al.: AI Now 2019 Report. New York. AI Now Institute. https://ainowinstitute.org/AI_Now_2019_Report.html (2019)

72. Cutillo, C.M., Sharma, K.R., Foschini, L., Kundu, S., Mackintosh, M., Mandl, K.D., and MI in Healthcare Workshop Working Group: Machine intelligence in health—perspectives on trustworthiness, explainability, usability and transparency. NPJ Digit. Med. **3**, 47 (2020). https://doi.org/10.1038/s41746-020-0254-2

73. Schwalbe, N., Wahl, B.: Artificial intelligence and the future of global health. Lancet **395**, 1579–1586 (2020)

74. Sridhar, G.R., Venkat, Y.: Information technology and endocrine sciences in the new millennium. Indian J. Endocrinol. Metab. **4**, 70–80 (2000)

75. Sridhar, G.R.: Expanding scope of information technology in clinical care. In: Khosrow, M. (ed.) Encyclopedia of Information Science and Technology, pp. 1888–1900. IGI Global, Hershey, PA (2021). https://doi.org/10.4018/978-1-7998-3479-3.ch131

Smart Healthcare: Using IoT and Machine Learning-Based Analytics

Pramod Sunagar, R. Hanumantharaju, D. Pradeep Kumar, B. J. Sowmya, S. Seema, and Anita Kanavalli

Abstract Smart medicinal services is an inventive procedure of synergizing the advantages of sensors, Internet of things (IoT), and large information Analytics to convey improved patient consideration while lessening the human services costs. The Medical Services industry faces tremendous difficulties to spare the information produced and to process it to separate information out of it. The expanding volume of human services information created through IoT gadgets, electronic health, mobile health, and telemedicine screening requires the advancement of new strategies and approaches for their taking care of. In this chapter, we discuss a portion of the healthcare challenges and information analysis development. To screen the health status of an individual, support from sensors and IoT gadgets is fundamental. The goal of this examination is to give healthcare services administrations to the sick just as sound populace through remote observation utilizing keen calculations, instruments, and methods with quicker investigation and master intervention for better treatment suggestions. The analysis is done on the Blood Pressure data and Heart Disease dataset by collecting the data from the IoT sensors and the framework is able to

P. Sunagar (✉) · R. Hanumantharaju · D. Pradeep Kumar · B. J. Sowmya · S. Seema · A. Kanavalli
Department of Computer Science and Engineering, M S Ramaiah Institute of Technology (Affiliated to VTU), Bangalore, India
e-mail: pramods@msrit.edu

R. Hanumantharaju
e-mail: hmrcs@msrit.edu

D. Pradeep Kumar
e-mail: pradeepkumard@msrit.edu

B. J. Sowmya
e-mail: sowmyabj@msrit.edu

S. Seema
e-mail: seemas@msrit.edu

A. Kanavalli
e-mail: anithak@msrit.edu

© The Author(s), under exclusive license to Springer Nature Singapore Pte Ltd. 2021
K. G. Srinivasa et al. (eds.), *Artificial Intelligence for Information Management: A Healthcare Perspective*, Studies in Big Data 88,
https://doi.org/10.1007/978-981-16-0415-7_15

307

predict the disease. It can likewise be gainful for distantly checking chronic diseases, which require essential physical data, biological, and hereditary information.

Keywords Smart healthcare · Internet o f Things (IoT) · Machine learning · K-Nearest Neighbor (KNN)

1 Introduction

One of the conspicuous ailments that influence numerous individuals during middle or mature age is coronary illness, and much of the time it inevitably prompts lethal entanglements. Heart infections are more common in men than in ladies. According to statistics, it was estimated from the WHO that 24% of the passage in India due to non-transferable diseases is caused by heart disease. The risks of having coronary heart disease based on danger factors are difficult to determine objectively. Be that as it may, AI strategies are valuable to anticipate the yield from existing information. Subsequently, we should submit one of those AI procedures called the grouping of risk factors for predicting cardiovascular disease. It likewise attempts to improve the precision of foreseeing coronary illness chance utilizing a methodology named troupe. IoT (Internet of Things) is often a system which makes use of advances including sensors; arrange correspondence, man-made brainpower, and big data to give genuine arrangements. These arrangements and frameworks are intended for ideal control and execution. Internet of Things (IoT) is also an event technology due to the developments in interconnected technologies such as sensor, connectivity, and computing.

The main focus is prediction using the techniques of machine learning. Machine learning was already commonly used in certain business applications, including e-commerce, and many more. Prediction has been one of the fields where such machine learning is used, our focus is to predict heart disease by analyzing the patient's dataset and patient data to which we will predict the risk of a heart attack.

Combine cloud and machine learning paradigms into a web-based IoT-oriented platform targeting to derive useful details between produced data. Guidance to achieve this is provided at the backend IoT server by using implementations based on Machine Learning to learn data signatures of interest immediately, based on the data already obtained.

The IoT and Cloud Computing technologies merged together to solve problems in many domains but not suitable for applications where high network latency requires real time responses. This can be overcome by using MatLab computing that pushes the computation, thereby reducing network latencies but results in concerns related to real time responses, battery power use, bandwidth costs, data protection, and privacy.

Following objectives are achieved in this work

1. Collection of a relevant dataset of heart sensors (ECG, EKG, and other).
2. The framework sends the client's detected information to the web for investigation and representation.

3. Clinical specialists can screen and control the patient remotely at any area.

Expected to structure and execute an easy to use and brilliant system for a human heartbeat rate observing and control framework. This methodology utilized the utilization of sensors and web of things (IoT) innovation to deliver an incorporated model to ease checking and control of heart related issues.

Heart diseases are one of the common diseases that have become a part of our lives. Any disorder related to the heart can be termed a heart disease. One of the major causes of the deaths is due to heart related diseases. Due to unhealthy lifestyles and food habits, heart diseases have been the reason for the many deaths in India, in the past few decades. According to a survey, one in 4 deaths in India is due to heart diseases. Identifying heart related problems at an early stage and preventing it has become the need of the hour to save the lives of the people. Machine learning algorithms can play a major role in addressing these challenges. Classification algorithms can help in predicting if a person will have health related diseases or not. Training the models on a proper dataset and then testing to accurately predict if a person will have heart disease or not.

Integrating cloud computing and Machine Learning paradigms into a Distributed computing-based IoT Framework targeting to extract relevant information among huge data generated. Guidance to achieve this is provided at the backend IOT server by using implementations based on Machine Learning to be able to automatically learn data signatures of interest based on the data it has already received. Providing an intelligent model which analyzes the medical data precisely and transmits it with very low latency for Computation, we build a Dataset generation system that generates data as real as patients suffer health conditions. All these data are analyzed and passed to computing servers which further applies the machine learning algorithms. We consider various machine algorithms for the best and quick predictions.

2 Literature Survey

Kusiak et al. [1] utilized mechanisms of preprocessing, transformation and a data mining strategy to pick up information on the connection between huge numbers of the parameters estimated related to the patient's survival. Two separate mining algorithms were used, specified in the form of decision rules for extricating data. A Decision-making algorithm utilized certain principles which foresee the endurance of new unseen patients. For their clinical aspects, significant boundaries were found by data mining. In their exploration work, they built up a standard which was applied and tried utilizing information acquired at four dialysis locations. The technique set out in their paper brings down expenses and profitability.

Abhishek et al. [2] have utilized a pair of neural system techniques, Back Propagation Algorithm (BPA), Radial Basis Function (RBF), and a non-straight Support Vector Machine (SVM) classifier, were utilized and estimated by their effectiveness and accuracy. For usage, they utilized WEKA 3.6.5 instrument to locate the best method among the three Kidney Stone Diagnosis calculations referenced previously. The fundamental motivation behind their postulation work was to propose the best apparatus for clinical finding, for example, ID of the kidney stone, to lessen the hour of determination, and improve adequacy and exactness. BPA altogether improved the classification technique which was used in the trial results.

Ashfaq Ahmed et al. [3] introduced methods of AI, in particular supporting vector machines [SVM] and Random Forest [RF]. These were utilized to test, distinguish, and contrast informational indexes and distinctive portion and piece boundaries for malignant growth, liver, and coronary illness. Aftereffects of Random Forest and Support Vector Machines were thought about for various informational collections, for example, dataset for bosom malignant growth malady, dataset for liver ailment, and dataset for coronary illness. The discoveries were custom fitted to the right arrangement of boundaries for explicit parts. Results were better investigated to build up better prescient learning strategies. It is reasoned that various results have been seen with various SVM grouping strategies with various piece capacities.

Kara et al. [4] analyzing design electroretinography signals with the guide of a neural network, on the conclusion of optic nerve illness. Executed multilayer feed forward ANN furnished with back proliferation calculation Levenberg Marquart (LM). The final product was set safe and wiped out. The outcomes announced recommended that the proposed PERG approach could permit a compelling interpretation.

Sweety Bakyarani et al. [5] describes Data as Knowledge, with the age of information overload, Data Analytics approaches have effectively given solutions for many problems encountered by industries. Healthcare is an area which also requires the approaches or techniques of data analytics in solving many problems. Authors have proposed the schema where Medicinal services investigation benefits patients, as well as all the central members engaged with the social insurance division. The expected utilization of examination being to prevent outbreak of diseases, early identification of diseases, reduced cost in operation, and administrative cost of hospitals, provisioning the betterment of government health care policies, which in turn, improves the quality of life. Authors have reviewed key machine learning algorithms grouped into Supervised learning, Unsupervised learning, and Reinforcement learning. Also, the paper has showcased the steps involved in Machine learning for processing the data collected by the Healthcare sector. The conclusive evidence gives the inference that the chosen algorithm has a direct dependence on the type of data collected. Also, authors interpret that Big data is very much suited for machine learning by making use of distributed computing platforms like Apache Spark and Apache Hadoop.

Shinde et al. [6] have introduced machine learning algorithms and methods utilized in infection and its related treatment warnings acquired from different distributed clinical papers. The goal was to show Natural Language handling (NLP) and AI methods utilized for the portrayal of data removed from crude information and arranging the calculations that are most appropriate for distinguishing and grouping pertinent clinical data. The proposed framework in Fig. 1, its design features integrates with any clinical administration framework to settle on better choices in checking patients which runs on biomedical data and diagnostics. Likewise, the

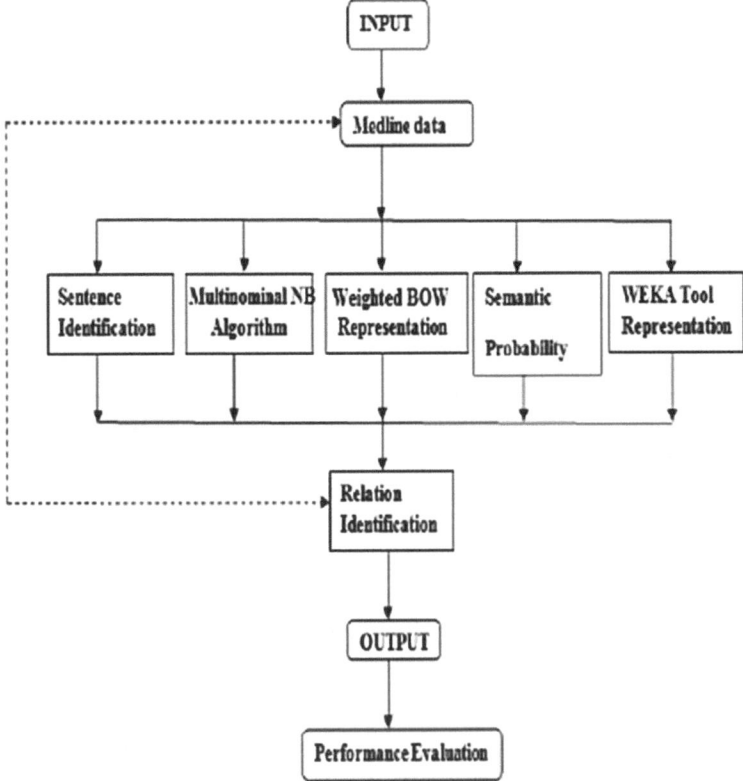

Fig. 1 System architecture [6]

proposed framework expels undesirable information from the MEDLINE and results in a book record containing just specific illness and its important manifestations, its causes and the finding required for it. The consequences of the work are deciphered by limiting the time and the heap of specialists in dissecting the patient's data and their checking and medicines. The model is valuable for all the stakeholders like a patients, doctors, and medical team.

Sarwar et al. [7] delineates the need for analytics and the convenience of it in industry and the scholarly world for the information, data that are devised from big data. Additionally, big data and distributed computing give new rising diagnostic approaches for the various segments which incorporate traffic checking, climate anticipating, extortion location, training strengthening, and human services. Authors have addressed the disadvantages of existing machine learning approaches for healthcare. Because of quick upgrades in enormous analytics and prediction, the medicinal services area has gotten important consideration in ongoing hardly in the years to come. Existing conventional machine learning approaches take a lot of time proportional to the collected data. Thus, in the medicinal services area, immense information is gathered from various sources and analysts consistently attempt to make issues less complex to patients. In large information, we can discover astounding and concealed data that can help in understanding the idea of an issue all the more profoundly. Since the algorithms face disadvantages, there is a need of combining various techniques. Authors additionally propose the best methodology for the connection among information and its affiliation. Since there is a consistent requirement for discovering better connections between maladies for the need of comparable treatment. Apriori calculation is applied in relationship to discover the connection among things and furthermore to perform partition between comparable just as various things. PSO enhancement approach is for the most part joined. Creators likewise look at covering approach and channel approaches dependent on computational expense for taking care of enormous information issues.

Padmashree et al. [8] have proposed a framework that targets improving human services on the board by dissecting wellbeing boundaries like pulse, internal heat level, pulse, and anticipating heart issues. The favorable position is being made when a patient is versatile. The framework examinations different wellbeing boundaries and alarms for any variations from the norm. The checking is done through representation where the patient can see his wellbeing information on his telephone, with the specialist seeing all the patients he treats. A large portion of the Healthcare frameworks is intended for heart maladies. The created framework is to foresee heart related issues by thinking about boundaries of pulse, internal heat level, pulse. The data is depicted carefully to all the partners. These boundaries are given as a contribution to the Weka library that is coordinated to the android application. Multilayer perceptron calculation in Weka is utilized to discover the likeness in design between the prepared informational collection which comprises wellbeing boundaries of patients with heart issues and test information which contains the wellbeing information of the application clients.

Healthcare is a framework producing heterogeneous information, which requires insightful frameworks for the intelligent examination of wellbeing information which is picking up ubiquity in wellbeing the board in overseeing asset advancements and the quality in wellbeing results. authors have conveyed the significance of health analytics from the astute strategies from computerized reasoning and the enormous information. In this paper Abidi et al. [9] have analyzed wellbeing information on its size, clarified the working of man-made consciousness-based logical techniques, additionally definitive proof of what bits of knowledge inferred range of wellbeing information investigation strategies will improve framework the board, information disclosure, and medicinal services development.

The growing healthcare industry has colossal measures of information identified with patients, treatment experienced, installments made, and protection inclusions included pulling in logical examination. Writers have considered many peer reviewed journals/articles which have tended to assortments of information in an alternate measurement from Healthcare, however, they need incomprehensive builds. Anyway, writers in this paper have introduced a survey of Healthcare examination utilizing information mining and enormous information utilizing a PRISMA rule, for the database search somewhere in the range of 2015 and 2016. The characterization for the viable great writing review initiated is as appeared in Fig. 3. Additionally, Islam et al. [10] has led a methodological overview on chose articles with the chose watchwords to manufacture a system chart. The system chart gives a perception of high recurrence words with white and blue circles as portrayals which speak to the recurrence of the event of catchphrases in articles. Anyway, basic components of the examinations in human services were extricated to give an efficient view being developed of information mining methods, kinds of investigation, and the information sources to be utilized. The current techniques incorporate the utilization of health related informations generated via various sensors to help in improving the field of medicinal services (Fig. 2).

Pentek et al. [11] has introduced one of a kind e-Health information distribution center usage dependent on Med-I-Hub engineering. The executed model gathers and investigates information from sources like wellness gears, shrewd gadgets, and so on. The prime focal point of the paper is on the design stage and its qualities. This framework gives an answer for incorporating sensor information into a medicinal services framework by means of APIs. The proposed is tried for versatility and it is adaptable and extensible. The executed framework captures, assesses, and totals the

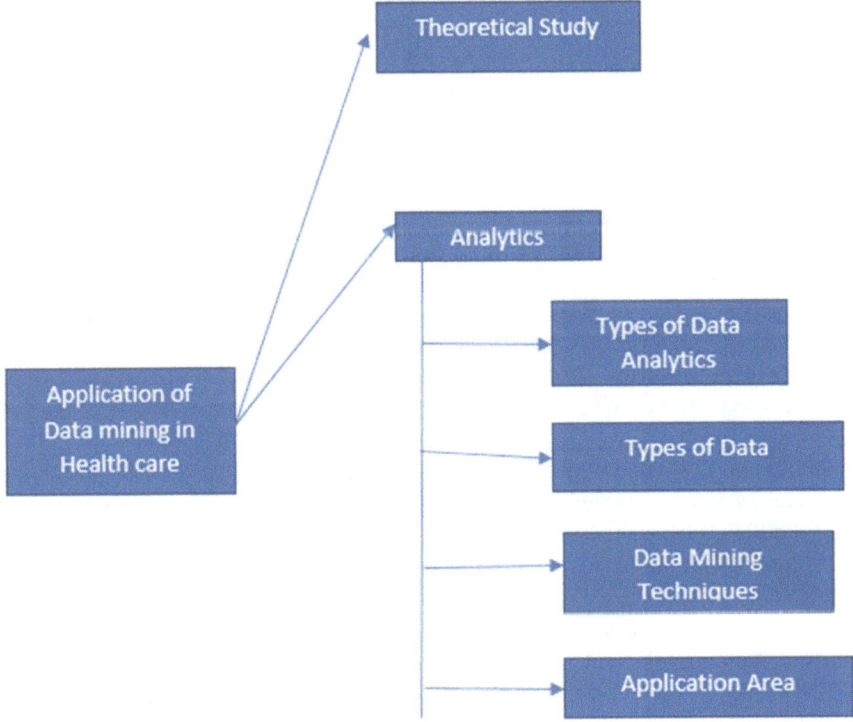

Fig. 2 Classification of literature

bio tactile human data streams. The Med-I-Hub arrangement is equipped for empowering interoperability among various human services frameworks. The current form works with open source innovations with worldwide guidelines. The advancement will prompt the intellectual social insurance benefits that can be incorporated with the Medihub framework. The futurist of the proposed work needs to improve individual help, screen complex investigation utilizing executed information stockroom arrangements.

Isravel et al. [12] have considered Heart ailment as a basic sickness which influences individuals of various age gatherings. The proposed procedure is a preprocessing strategy to improve the exactness of the ECG signals, since the crude information contains clamor which diminishes the precision of grouping. The misshaped ECG signals are done through preprocessing procedure. The proposed framework assesses the exhibition of arrangement is tried utilizing different order calculations, for example, KNN, Naïve Bayes, and Decision tree to recognize ordinary and strange heartbeat rhythms. The proving ground demonstrates that pre- preparing improves the precision of the general framework. The exploratory examination demonstrated that the choice tree beats KNN and Naive Bayes with exactness, affectability, and accuracy. Creators infer that the paper gives a significant forward leap for the medicinal services industry to analyze heart related issues utilizing IoT stages and AI calculations. From this time forward inferring that pre-handling demonstrates as a successful methodology to analyze heart related ailments.

Rastogi et al. [13] delineates according to the insights there are 30 million heart patients, and being a medicinal services industry immense volumes of information is being created, which isn't regularly utilized adequately. The information produced will consistently have some shrouded designs which are utilized to remove the connections. There are less instruments to get information from clinical conclusions. The proposed approach utilizes input highlights, for example, sexual orientation, cholesterol, circulatory strain, TTH, and worry to foresee the patient's danger of coronary illness. The proposed approach utilizes Data Mining procedures, for example, gullible bayes, Decision trees, Support vector machines to investigate the coronary illness database. The precision of the calculations is estimated and looked at; the consequence of the examination is 0 or 1, which represents no risk or peril to the person.

Dinh et al. [14] have proposed a gadget which utilizes electrocardiogram signal produced from incorporated sensors and the photoplethysmogram signal from the fingers which gives out systolic and diastolic blood pressures for each heartbeat. The proposed framework contains the sensors expected to drive in ECG highlights. Creators infer this is a minimal effort, little size, and low force utilization gadget which can be utilized to screen significantly other heart related highlights, for example, untimely ventricular compression and venous throbs.

Kirtana et al. [15] has proposed a pulse fluctuation (HRV) which is a proportion of variety between back to back heart thumps. HRV being exceptionally touchy connected with cardiovascular ailment. Observing HRV boundaries is required for clinical consideration at most occasions. In this paper, creators have proposed an easy Remote HRV checking framework with the utilization of IoT. The information is gotten from Zigbee based remote sensors, sent to a worker utilizing MQTT convention associated with an Arduino board. The worker gathers and investigates the information, in case of any variations from the norm, the taker and specialists are told through short message administration (SMS) for sufficient clinical assistance. The proposed framework joins the double advantages of Zigbee and Wi-Fi innovation. Thusly, it effectively satisfies all the perfect attributes of a far-off wellbeing observing framework as far as ease, long range, security, speediness, and simple-to-utilize that serves in sparing lives.

3 Design

The overall engineering of IoT applications can be isolated into three layers: The Sensing layer, the transport layer, and what's more, the application layer. This sort of design is clear and adaptable enough for our checking framework, in this way we plan the framework design dependent on that broad model.

The compact IoT framework is intended to work with sensors and microcontrollers. The segments that are utilized for setting up the compact framework are:

- LM35 Temperature Sensor
- Heartbeat Sensor
- AD8232 ECG Sensor
- Raspberry Pi.

These 3 sensors are associated with the Raspberry Pi microcontroller to gather the internal heat level, heartbeat rate, and what's more, ECG signals. The diverse perusing of the patient's essential signs is assembled and sent for testing by the classifier model which is utilizing the dataset for distinguishing the anomalies.

Figure 3 shows the steps involved in collecting the data from sensors and storing it in the cloud for further processing. To include more amounts of data even the data is collected from several online sources. The recorded wellbeing information of the patient was taken from the heart disease dataset for preparing the classifier. The dataset utilized for preparing the classifier for testing the exactness, affectability, and accuracy of order is the heart disease dataset.

Determination of detecting gadgets ought to be founded on two issues: which boundaries to be observed, and what is the examining recurrence for every boundary. As the point of our monitoring framework is to help far-off specialists to know about patients' wellbeing status and to analyze or gauge hazardous conditions, fulfilling the necessity of clinical analysis of heart ailments and obeying rules in clinical practice are fundamental for parameters selection and sampling frequencies. Figure 4 represents the sensors that are carried by the patients.

Fig. 3 Collection of data

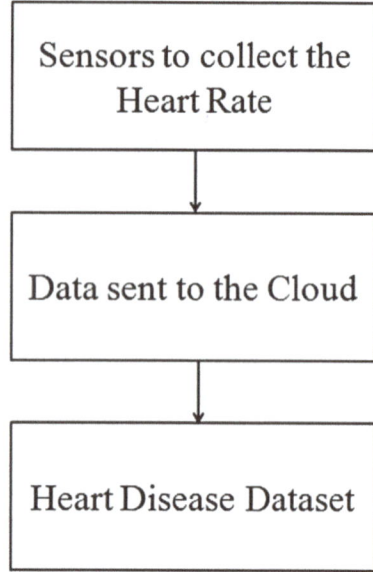

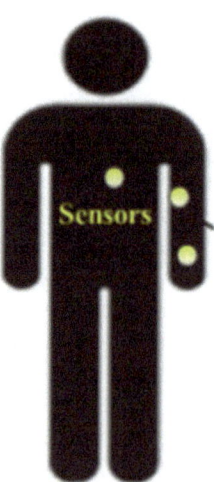

Fig. 4 Sensors carried by patients

Figure 5 represents the system architecture for the work. It consists of several modules such as data collection phase, Building classification model, and finally the evaluation of the performance module.

a. **IoT Module**

IoT based patient observing framework has three sensors. Initial one is a temperature sensor, second is a Heartbeat sensor and the others are Blood Pressure and ECG

Fig. 5 Workflow of all the modules in the architecture

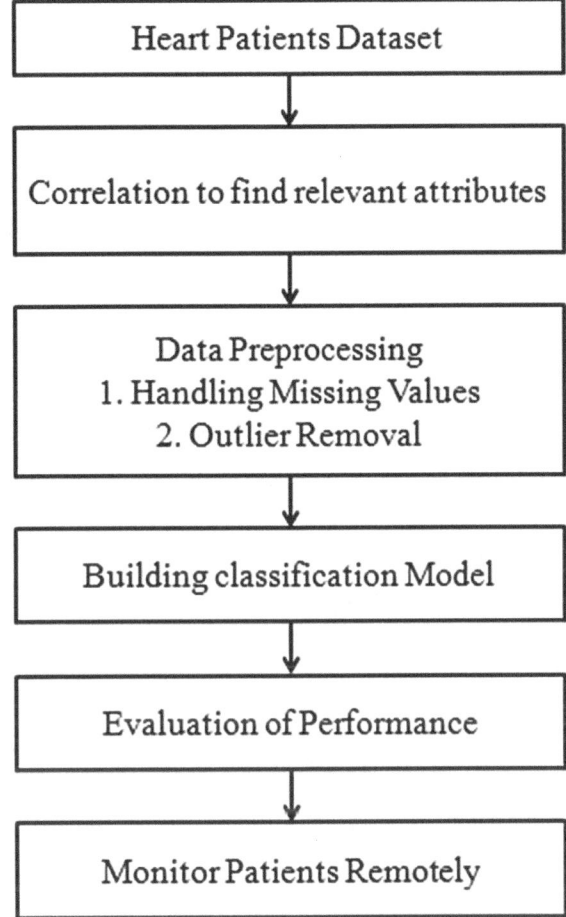

Heart Patients Dataset

Correlation to find relevant attributes

Data Preprocessing
1. Handling Missing Values
2. Outlier Removal

Building classification Model

Evaluation of Performance

Monitor Patients Remotely

sensors. All these boundaries are then taken care of to the Raspberry pi pack, where the different tasks are performed like examination of various parameters of healthcare and afterward at long last sent to Server. The Raspberry pi ceaselessly inspects duty from these sensors. By then it sends this information to the cloud by sending aggregated information to a specific URL/IP address. This activity of sending information to IP is rehashed after a specific timeframe. For example, in this assignment, we will develop the module which will send the patients information at normal stretches related to the Wi-Fi association using a Wi-Fi module. After getting the crucial data from distant patients, the master specialist will send a treatment plan to the patient promptly and henceforth sparing the valuable life.

b. **Data Pre-processing and Correlation to find relevant attributes**

Information preprocessing is a data mining method which is used to change the rough data in an important and beneficial manner.

The various steps in data preprocessing

Data Cleaning

The information can have various unimportant and missing parts. To remove and to work exactly with data for analyzing this part, data cleaning is finished. The data cleaning incorporates the activities related to the handling of missing data, loud data

Unavailability of data:

> Data set consists of information in terms of rows and columns, some attribute values can be missing. During that time several activities are carried out, the following are the activities
> Eliminate the tuples

This philosophy is fitting exactly when the dataset we have is tremendous and different characteristics are missing inside a tuple.

Fill the Missing characteristics:

There are different approaches to manage this obligation. You can decide to fill the missing attributes genuinely, by property mean or the most possible worth.

Noisy Data:

Noisy information is aimless information that can't be deciphered by machines. It can be produced because of broken information assortment, information passage blunders, and so forth. This task can be handheld effectively by using Regression, Clustering, and Binning techniques.

Data Transformation

This movement is taken in order to change the data in fitting structures sensible for the mining cycle.

> *Normalization:*
> It is done so as to scale the information esteems in a predefined go (-1.0 to 1.0 or 0.0 to 1.0)
> *Selection of Attributes:*
> In this procedure, new traits are built from the given arrangement of credits to enable the mining to process.
> *Discretization:*
> This is done to supplant the crude estimations of numeric characteristics by span levels or reasonable levels.
> *Generation of Hierarchy based on Conceptual criteria:*
> Here characteristics are changed from level to more elevated level in progressive systems. For Example—The trait "city" can be changed over to "nation".

Data Reduction

Since data mining is a methodology that is used to manage a colossal proportion of data. While working with an enormous volume of data, examining that volume of data is more important. But all the data is not important to examine. In order to discard this, we use the data decline method. It hopes to extend the limit capability and decline data storing and assessment costs.

There are various sequence of procedures involved in this reduction process, they are as follows.

Data Cube Aggregation, Attribute Subset Selection, Numerosity Reduction, Dimensionality Reduction.

Correlation to find relevant attributes

Is an approach to comprehend the connection between numerous factors and traits in your dataset. Utilizing Correlation, you can get a few experiences, for example,

- One or numerous traits rely upon another quality or a reason for another property.
- One or various qualities are related to different traits.

Connection can help in predicting one quality from another (Great way to deal with credit missing characteristics).

Connection can (now and again) exhibit the closeness of a causal relationship.

Connection is used as a basic sum for some showing systems.

c.   Building Classification Model

Classification is a data mining task that gives out things in a collection to target orders or classes. The path toward finding a model that delineates and perceives data classes and thoughts. Request is the issue of recognizing which of a great deal of classes (subpopulations), another discernment has a spot with, in view of a planning set of data containing observations and whose groupings enrollment is known.

It is a two-advance system, for instance

- Learning Step (Training Phase): This progression is intended to develop the Classification Models. Different Algorithms are used to gather a classifier by making the model get the hang of using the arrangement set available. The model must be ready for the desire for precise results.
- Classification Step: Model used to foresee class names and testing the created model on test data and consequently check the precision of the portrayal rules.

The preparation set is given to a learning calculation, which determines a classifier. At that point, the classifier is tried with the test set, where all class items are covered up.

On the off chance that the classifier groups most cases in the test set effectively, it very well may be expected that it works precisely likewise on the future information else it might be an off-base model picked.

For implementing a heart disease prediction model, our approach implements six machine algorithms such as Logistic Regression, Naive Bayesian, Support Vector

Machines, K-Nearest Neighbors, Decision Trees, and Random Forest. These algorithms are trained on heart disease dataset and utilized to analyze and predict if a person is having any heart related diseases or not. Once the models are trained and deployed, the application will test if a person has any heart disease or not by analyzing the data received from the sensors and are stored on the cloud.

Logistic Regression: The Logistic regression algorithm is applied to illustrate the classification of patients into having heart related issues and not having heart related issues. Here using this approach, the Heart disease will be predicted based on various factors

Support Vector Machines: The Support Vector Machine (SVM) is a managed AI calculation which can be applied for both order or relapse difficulties. Nevertheless, it is for the most part used in characterization disputes. In the SVM calculation, we plot every information as a point in n-dimensional space with the approximation of each element being the assessment of a specific arrangement. Here n represents the number of highlights. Now perform organization by finding the best hyperplane that divides the two classes clearly. Here in our data set the Algorithm characterizes the data into Heart disease person and non-diseased person by drawing the linear hyperplane to classify the same.

KNN: K-nearest neighbors (KNN) calculation is a kind of regulated ML evaluation which can be applied for both arrangements just as relapse prescient issues. Be that as it may, it is mostly utilized for grouping prescient issues.

Decision Trees: A decision tree has a flowchart-like structure in which every inner node is a test criterion and each branch is the result of the test. The final tree will have the structure for predicting heart disease and the different parameters considered to predict the heart diseases.

Random Forest: The Random Forest algorithms build multiple decision trees for the dataset. The time taken to train and test using random forest will be always on the higher side compared to other algorithms. The one tree with the highest accuracy will be selected when random forest algorithms are implemented. The accuracy of the random forests will always be higher compared to decision trees.

d.   **Monitor the patients remotely**

In advancement to engage seeing of patients outside of standard clinical settings (for instance in the home), which may construct admittance to mind and decreasing social protection movement costs. Merging RPM in perpetual infirmity the chiefs can essentially improve an individual's very own fulfillment.

We characterize far off patient checking as the arrangement of exercises that meet four key rules: (1) information on patients is gathered distantly and analyzed over the cloud (2) the information gathered is sent to a human services supplier in an alternate area; (3) the information is assessed and care suppliers are told, varying; and (4) care suppliers impart significant information driven bits of knowledge and intercessions to patients.

4 Implementation and Results

The heart disease dataset [16] is created by considering the information related to 303 individuals. The task is to predict whether an individual will have heart disease or not based on the given information. The machine learning algorithms will help us to detect and as the system can take necessary steps for treatment of the individuals.

Dataset

The dataset consists of the details of 303 individuals. There are 14 columns in the dataset. The details of the dataset are given below.

1. Age: Candidate's Age
2. Sex: Candidate's Gender

    - Male $= 1$
    - Female $= 0$

3. Chest pain type: Different types of chest-pains.

    - Angina Typical represents the 1st type
    - Angina Atypical represents the 2nd type
    - Non-Anginal Pain represents the 3rd type
    - Asymptotic is represented by 4th type

4. Blood Pressure(Resting): Candidate's blood pressure reading in mm Hg
5. Serum Cholesterol: low and high density lipoprotein in person's blood mg/dl
6. Blood Sugar (fasting): blood glucose value of a candidate is compared with 120 mg/dl. If glucose level in fasted state is more than 120 mg/dl then: true $=$ 1 else: false $= 0$
7. ECG(resting):

    - Normalcy is indicated by 0Normalcy is indicated by 0
    - abnormalities in ST-T wave is indicated by 1
    - hypertrophy in the left ventricle is indicated by 2

8. heart rate (Max): Maximum rate of heart attained by a candidate.
9. Angina (by means of exercise):

    - Yes is indicated by 1Yes is indicated by 1
    - No is indicated by 0

10. ST depression caused by exercise in relation with rest: Value is either in integer or floating point.
11. Peak exercise ST segment:

    - Upsloping is indicated by 1
    - Flat is indicated by 2
    - Downsloping is indicated by 3

12. Count of major vessels (0–3) colored by fluoroscopy: Value is either a floating point or an integer.
13. Thal: Displays the thalassemia:

   - Normal represented by 3Normal represented by 3
   - Fixed Defect represented by 6
   - Reversable Defect represented by 7

14. Examination of heart's condition: Indication if the candidate is having heart condition (risk).

   - No Heart Disease is indicated by 0
   - Suffering from Heart Disease indicated by 4,3,2,1

Model Training and Prediction

The six machine learning models will be trained on this dataset as we know whether an individual is having heart disease or not. This process is identified as a supervised Technique. Model that is trained will be able to forecast if a user is suffering from a heart condition or not. The process of training the model and predicting is illustrated as follows:

Splitting

The entire dataset is partitioned as training and testing dataset. In this work, the dataset is divided in the ratio of 80:20 to train and test the model. Classifier makes use of the training dataset to train and testing dataset is used for predicting whether an individual has heart disease or not.

Understanding the dataset

The heart disease dataset [16] consists of 303 entries. Every row consists of data for various attributes like age, sex, chest pain, resting blood pressure, etc. The final attribute target indicates if the person has a heart condition or he does not. The value 1 indicates the heart condition that needs immediate attention and 0 means no heart condition and the details are referred to as in Fig. 6.

Figure 7 displays the heart disease frequency for the female and male population in the dataset. The female population has more heart related diseases than the male

	age	sex	cp	trestbps	chol	fbs	restecg	thalach	exang	oldpeak	slope	ca	thal	target
0	63	1	3	145	233	1	0	150	0	2.3	0	0	1	1
1	37	1	2	130	250	0	1	187	0	3.5	0	0	2	1
2	41	0	1	130	204	0	0	172	0	1.4	2	0	2	1
3	56	1	1	120	236	0	1	178	0	0.8	2	0	2	1
4	57	0	0	120	354	0	1	163	1	0.6	2	0	2	1

Fig. 6 Details of the heart disease dataset

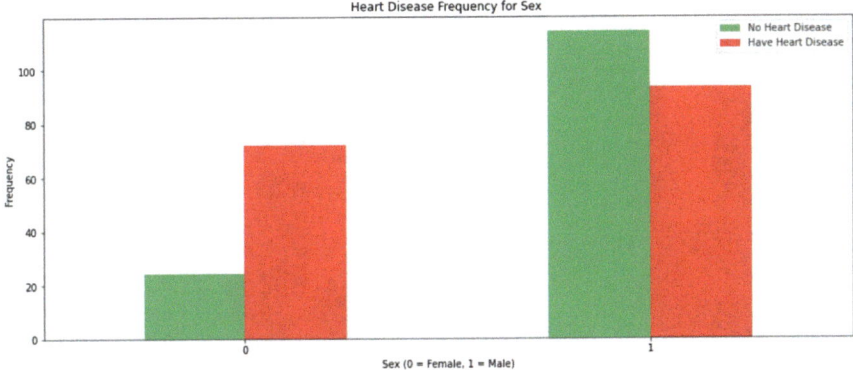

Fig. 7 Details of the heart disease frequency for Male and Female population

population. The green bar plots and red bar plots show the people with no heart disease and with heart disease, respectively.

Figure 8 displays the heart disease frequency for different ages. The blue bar plots are for those patients who do not have any heart related issues. The orange bar plots show that the patients in that age have heart related diseases. The data shows that the cases of heart related disease are more in the age range of 40–60 (Fig. 9).

The chest pain types assessed for this dataset are 0 for Typical Angina, 1 for Atypical Angina, 2 for Non-Anginal Pain, and 3 for Asymptotic. In Fig. 10, it is evident that people with chest pain type 2 are more prone to heart related diseases. People with typical angina have low probabilities of getting heart related disease.

The heart rates also play a vital role in deciding about heart disease. People with more heart rates are prone to heart related diseases. In Fig. 10, it is clearly visible that the individuals with more heart rates are more prone to heart related diseases. Age factor also drives the heart related diseases but the plot shows more heart rates and more heart related issues.

To predict heart disease, totally 6 algorithms in machine learning are considered namely logistic regression, support vector machines, naïve bayes, random forest,

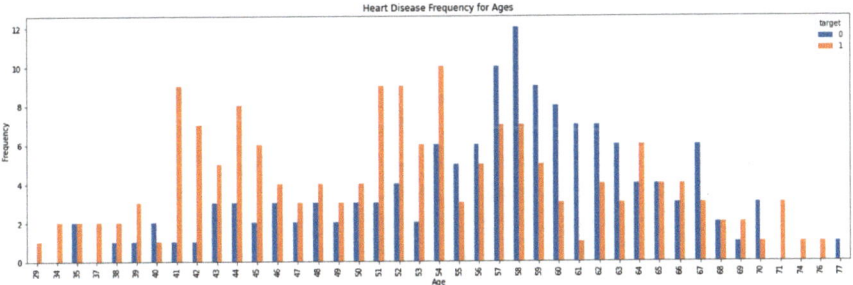

Fig. 8 Details of the heart disease frequency for Ages

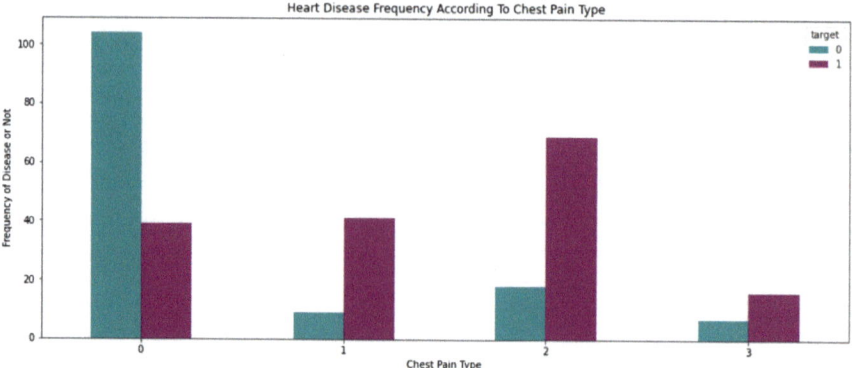

Fig. 9 Heart disease frequency for chest pain types

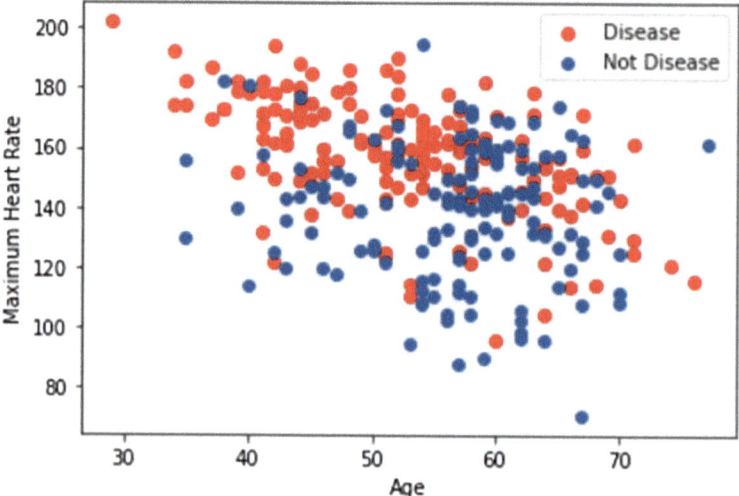

Fig. 10 Heart disease prediction from heart rate

k-nearest neighbors, and decision trees. The dataset used was Heart Disease UCI dataset which has 303 entries. The training to test split is 80:20. Figure 11 shows the time taken by the different algorithms to output the results. Except for the random forest, all the other algorithms needed less than a second to test the accuracy of the models. Random forest generates multiple decision trees and selects the one with the best accuracy. Hence, the time needed by the random forest is 296.81 s.

The selection of machine learning classifiers for a job is based on multiple parameters like accuracy of the algorithm, time taken to train the model, time taken to test the model, etc. Among these, the main factor is the accuracy of the algorithm considered. Figure 12 shows accuracy comparison between different classifiers considered.

	machine learning algorithms	time in seconds
0	logistic_regression	0.120973
1	naive_bayes	0.009753
2	support_vector_machine	0.831958
3	knearest_neighbors	0.085096
4	decision_tree	0.560878
5	random_forest	296.813749

Fig. 11 Prediction time in seconds for different machine learning classifiers

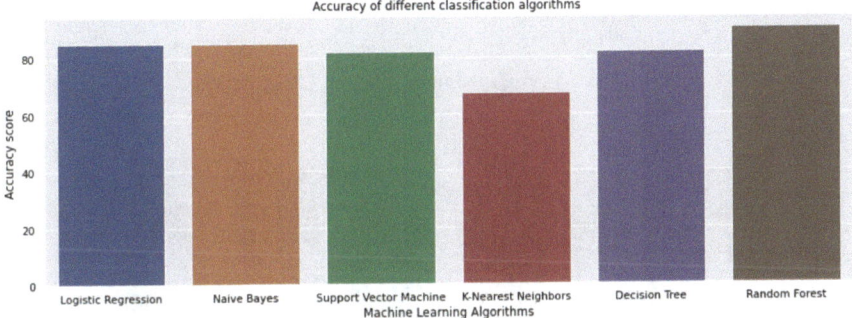

Fig. 12 Accuracy comparisons of different machine learning classifiers

Random forest algorithm has demonstrated the highest accuracy with 90% and above. K-Nearest neighbor has displayed low accuracy of around 67.21%. Other classifiers have demonstrated an accuracy of above 80% (Table 1).

Evaluation Metrics

In order to assess the effectiveness of these classifiers, we need some metrics to perform the comparison of the algorithms. We have used Accuracy, Recall, Precision, and F1 Score to compare the effectiveness of the algorithms (Fig. 13 and Table 2).

Accuracy: It is one of the simplest metrics and is deliberated as the number of aptly predicted classes divided by the total count of predictions made.

$$Accuracy = \frac{Number\ of\ Correct\ Prediction}{Total\ Number\ of\ Predictions\ Made} \tag{1}$$

Recall: It is one more key metric and is calculated as the count of True Positives over the sum of False Negative and True Positive.

Table 1 Comparison of training and testing accuracy of the classifiers

Algorithms	Training accuracy (%)	Testing accuracy (%)	Prediction time (s)
Logistic Regression	84.71	85.25	0.120973
Naïve Bayes	83.47	85.25	0.009753
Support Vector Machine	84.71	81.97	0.831958
K-Nearest Neighbor	72.31	67.21	0.085096
Decision Tree	100	81.97	0.560878
Random Forest	100	90.16	296.813749

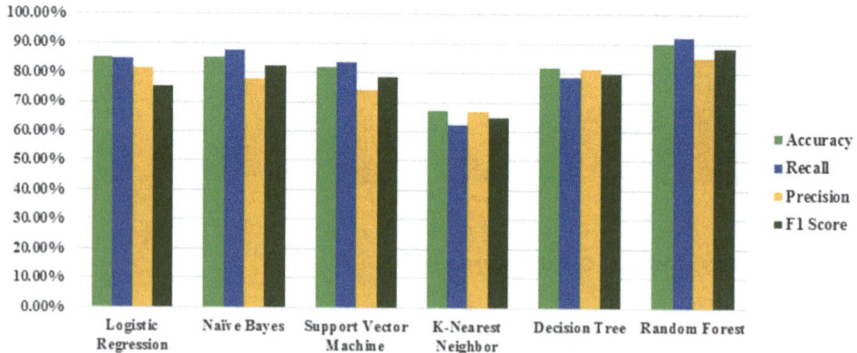

Fig. 13 Comparison of machine learning algorithms on Accuracy, Recall, Precision, and F1 Score

Table 2 Comparison of Machine Learning Algorithms on different evaluation metrics

	Logistic Regression (%)	Naïve Bayes (%)	Support Vector Machine (%)	K-Nearest Neighbor (%)	Decision Tree (%)	Random Forest (%)
Accuracy	85.25	85.25	81.97	67.21	81.97	90.16
Recall	84.61	87.5	83.34	62.06	78.57	92
Precision	81.48	77.78	74.07	66.67	81.48	85.18
F1 Score	75.16	82.35	78.43	64.53	79.99	88.45

$$Recall = \frac{TruePositive}{(TruePositives + FalseNegatives)} \tag{2}$$

Precision: It is deliberated as the count of True Positives over the summation of false Positive and true Positive.

$$Precision = \frac{TruePositives}{(TruePositives + FalsePositives)} \tag{3}$$

F1 Score: This metric unites the Recall and Precision into one metric. It is the harmonic mean of precision and recall and is calculated as follows:

$$F1\ Score = 2 * \frac{1}{\frac{1}{Precision} + \frac{1}{Recall}} \tag{4}$$

Confusion Matrix:

The performance of machine learning classifiers can be analyzed by a confusion matrix using the test data whose true values are known. A confusion matrix is simple to understand. Following are the terminologies associated with the confusion matrix.

- **True Positives (TP)**: Count of individuals correctly guessed as having heart related diseases.
- **True Negatives (TN)**: Count of individuals correctly guessed as not having heart related diseases.
- **False Positives (FP)**: The number of individuals who do not have heart related disease but the classifier has detected them as having heart disease.
- **False Negatives (FN)**: The number of individuals who have heart related disease but the classifier has detected them as not having any heart related disease.

Confusion matrix for the Logistic Regression, Naive Bayes, Support Vector Machine, K-Nearest Neighbors, Decision Tree, and Random Forest is shown in Fig. 14. The random forest has the maximum number of predictions that are true compared to other algorithms. K-Nearest neighbors have the highest number of false predictions for the dataset considered.

5 Conclusion

IoT has been changing the way computing was performed traditionally in all application areas especially healthcare. This paper presents a major improvement that can be brought about in healthcare in the way patients are remotely monitored for various health conditions by using the IoT platform. Wearable sensors can be put to use in healthcare, especially in the treatment of chronic heart ailments. The systems can

Confusion Matrixes

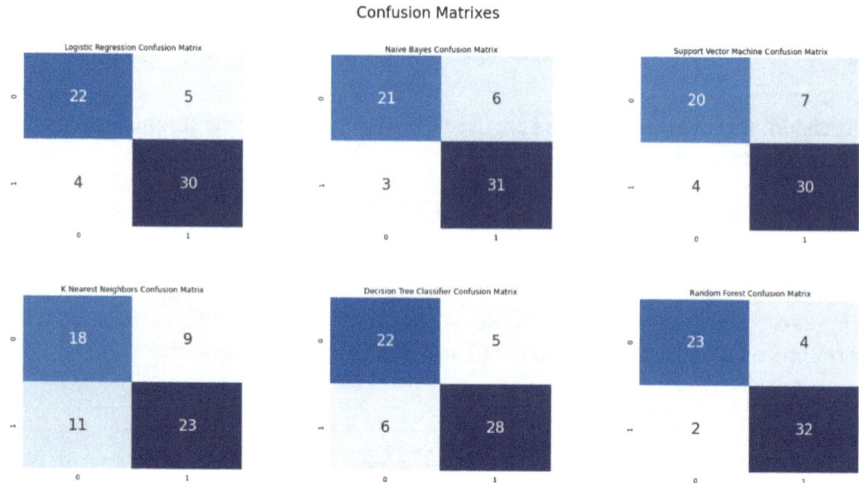

Fig. 14 Confusion matrix for the machine learning algorithms

monitor and predict risk and help in saving the lives of patient, particularly when they are residing in remote locations where health care centers are not available. The patient monitoring system is designed as low cost, user friendly, and reliable solution with Sensory hardware implementation consisting of the raspberry pi kit with ECG, Heart Beat, Blood Pressure, and Temperature Sensors by combining the benefits of cloud computing and internet technologies to solve many limitations concerning consumption of power, security in the network, and efficiency in the interchange of data. Techniques to preprocess and correlate have been implemented to enhance the efficiency to classify data algorithmically using machine learning by selection of the optimal features. To classify the algorithm used to train the system are logistic regression, Naïve bayes, KNN, random forest, decision trees, and support vector machines. The preprocessing technique has enhanced the performance of random forest as it performs better than other algorithms to classify with better precision, sensitivity, and accuracy. The predicted accuracy of various algorithms is evaluated. This system can be utilized to identify abnormalities in the heart data collected and aides in diagnosis in the earlier stages of the heart conditions of the patient. The healthcare system proposed here functions to help monitor user's heart health and also derive insights from the pool of data collected from various conditions to address it as early as possible. The results prove that the methodology achieves a greater level of accuracy in comparison with the other existing approaches. In future, we can work to conduct more experiments to improve the performance of the predictive classifier for heart disease diagnosis by employing other feature selection and optimization techniques.

References

1. Kusiak, A., Dixonb, B., Shaha, S.: Predicting survival time for kidney dialysis patients: a data mining approach. Comput. Biol. Med. **35**, 311–327 (2005). Elsevier Publication
2. Abhishek, G.S.M.T., Gupta, D.: Proposing efficient neural network training model for kidney stone diagnosis. Int. J. Comput. Sci. Inf. Technol. **3**(3), 3900–3904 (2012)
3. Ashfaq Ahmed, K., Aljahdali, S., Hussain, S.N.: Comparative Prediction performance with support vector machine and random forest classification techniques. Int. J. Comput. Appl. **69**(11), 12–16 (2013)
4. Kara, S., Guvenb, A., Urk Onerc, A.O.: Utilization of artificial neural networks in the diagnosis of optic nerve diseases. Comput. Biol. Med. **36**, 428–437 (2006). Elsevier Publication
5. Sweety Bakyarani, E., Srimathi. H., Bagavandas, M.: A survey of machine learning algorithms in health care. Int. J. Sci. Technol. Res. **8**(11). ISSN 2277-8616
6. Shinde, P., Jadhav, S.: Int. J. Comput. Sci. Inf. Technol. **5**(3), 3928–3933 (2014)
7. Sarwar, M.U., Hanif, M.K., Talib, R., Mobeen, A., Aslam, M.: A survey of Big Data analytics in healthcare. Int. J. Adv. Comput. Sci. Appl. **8**(6) (2017)
8. Padmashree, T., Cauvery, N.K., Anirudh, V.C, Kumar, P.: Int. J. Innov. Eng. Technol. (IJIET) **8**(1) (2017). ISSN 2319-1058
9. Abidi, S.S.R., Abidi, S.R.: Intelligent health data analytics: a convergence of artificial intelligence and big data Healthcare Management Forum 1-5 ª2019. The Canadian College of Health Leaders (2019)
10. Islam, M.S., Hasan, M.M., Wang, X., Germack, H.D., Noor-E-Alam: A systematic review on healthcare analytics: application and theoretical perspective of data mining. Healthcare, **6**, 54 (2018). 10.3390/healthcare6020054
11. Pentek, I., Adamko, A.: Hungary bio-sensory data warehouse with analytics for e-health solutions. In: 10th IEEE International Conference on Cognitive Infocommunications—CogInfoCom 2019 October 23–25, 2019 Naples, Italy (2019)
12. Isravel, D.P., Vidya Priya Darcini, S., Silas, S.: Improved heart disease diagnostic IoT model using machine learning techniques. Int. J. Sci. Technol. Res. **9**(02) (2020). ISSN 2277-8616
13. Rastogi, R., Chaturvedi, D.K., Satya, S., Arora, N.: Intelligent heart disease prediction on physical and mental parameters: a ML based IoT and big data application and analysis. In. Machine Learning with Health Care Perspective: Machine Learning and Healthcare, pp. 199–236. Springer International Publishing (2020)
14. Dinh, A., Luu, L., Cao, T.: Blood pressure measurement using finger ECG and photoplethysmogram for IoT. In: 6th International Conference on the Development of Biomedical Engineering in Vietnam (BME6) 2018, pp. 83–89. Springer, Singapore (2018)
15. Kirtana, R.N., Lokeswari, Y.V.: IEEE International Conference on Computer, Communication, and Signal Processing (ICCCSP-2017) 978-1-5090-3716-2/17/$31.00 ©2017 IEEE (2017)
16. Blake, C.L., Merz, C.J.: Repository of machine learning databases, University of California, Irvine. http://www.ics.uci.edu/~mlearn/mlrepository.html,1998 (1998)